Clinical implications of laboratory tests

Clinical implications of laboratory tests

SARKO M. TILKIAN, M.D.

Director of Medical Education, Northridge Hospital;
Staff Physician, Northridge Hospital Foundation, Northridge, California;
Valley Presbyterian Hospital, Van Nuys, California; and
Tarzana Medical Center, Tarzana, California

MARY BOUDREAU CONOVER, R.N., B.S.N.Ed.

Instructor in basic and advanced electrocardiography and
arrhythmia courses, West Hills and West Park Hospitals, Canoga
Park, California; faculty, National Critical Care Institute,
Orange, California

ARA G. TILKIAN, M.D., F.A.C.C.

Assistant Clinical Professor of Medicine, University of
California, Los Angeles; Associate Director of Cardiology,
Holy Cross Hospital and Valley Presbyterian Hospital,
San Fernando Valley, California

SECOND EDITION
with 45 illustrations

The C. V. Mosby Company

ST. LOUIS • TORONTO • LONDON 1979

SECOND EDITION

Printed in the United States of America

The C. V. Mosby Company
11830 Westline Industrial Drive, St. Louis, Missouri 63141

Library of Congress Cataloging in Publication Data

Tilkian, Sarko M 1936-
Clinical implications of laboratory tests.

Bibliography: p.
Includes index.
1. Diagnosis, Laboratory. I. Conover, Mary B., joint author. II. Tilkian, Ara G., 1944- joint author. III. Title. [DNLM: 1. Diagnosis, Laboratory. QY4.3 T573c]
RB37.T54 1979 616.07'5 78-16221
ISBN 0-8016-4962-5

CB/VH/VH 9 8 7 6 5 4 3 2 1 3/D/310

Lovingly dedicated to

our parents

Garabed and Nevart Tilkian

Essel and Eleanor Boudreau

PREFACE

This book is designed for persons in the nursing and allied health professions who need a concise reference and comprehensive guide to the clinical significance of laboratory tests. It is our intention to bridge the gap between the voluminous clinical pathology textbooks and the handbooks that merely list the conditions associated with abnormal laboratory results.

This second edition includes the following additions:

1. A special section on patient preparation and care has been added whenever special preparation or patient instruction must accompany the laboratory procedure or when particular aftercare is required to avoid complications.
2. The chapter on serodiagnostic tests has been replaced by two new ones on collagen vascular diseases and infectious diseases.
3. The chapter on gastrointestinal tests has been brought up to date by Dr. H. Steven Aharonian, a gastroenterologist. We are grateful to him for his expert contribution.
4. We have expanded the text to include new tests in current use, and the table of normal values in Appendix A has been corrected in the light of recent research. An appendix listing the effect of drugs on clinical laboratory tests has been added.

The discussions of tests in the routine laboratory screening panel (Unit One) suggest one or several possible disease entities that could be suspected when a particular laboratory test or combination of laboratory tests is abnormal. The table provided at the end of Unit One will guide the reader to the page in Unit Two where further discussion of the suspected disease entity and additional laboratory tests can be found that will help confirm the diagnosis.

In Unit Two the anatomy and physiology of the system involved are discussed briefly before the specific laboratory tests so that the rationale behind the test and the nomenclature and limitations of the specific tests may be better understood. Pathophysiology is presented when it is necessary for the understanding of terminology. The laboratory tests related to the organ system are then described, and, in most chapters, their use in the clinical setting is given. Finally, specific disease entities are discussed, with emphasis on laboratory tests and the differential diagnosis. The purpose of this approach is to avoid "tunnel vision" in the interpretation of laboratory tests. It is common to find that a test, although reported to be within "normal" range, is significantly aberrant when evaluated in relation to the other parameters.

Except in particular situations where some knowledge of the procedure is vital for intelligent interpretation, we have not described the technical process involved in performing the laboratory tests, assuming that quality control is duly exercised by responsible institutions and laboratories.

We would like to express our appreciation to Catherine Parker Anthony and Dr. and Mrs. Byron Schottelius, for their kind permission to use the anatomical illustrations from their books, and to Rene Fontan, for his work on the remainder of the drawings.

We are grateful to the W. B. Saunders Company and to the editors of Todd-Sanford *Clinical Diagnosis by Laboratory Methods*, and to the Lea & Febiger Company and Dr. H. Feigenbaum, author of the book *Echocardiography*, for their kind permission to reproduce the tables of normal values from their books.

Dr. Ara Tilkian devoted his special attention to the chapters on the cardiovascular, renal, and pulmonary systems, and Dr. Sarko Tilkian to the remainder of the book.

Sarko M. Tilkian
Mary Boudreau Conover
Ara G. Tilkian

CONTENTS

UNIT ONE

Routine multisystem screening tests

UNIT ONE

ROUTINE MULTISYSTEM SCREENING TESTS

An increase in the number, availability, and sophistication of laboratory tests has made them valuable tools in the study of clinical problems. In recent years multiphasic screening tests have been adopted widely to supplement the conventional history and physical examination. They are based on the fact that a group of laboratory determinations can now be carried out on a single specimen at a relatively low cost.

These helpful diagnostic procedures, however, do not release one from the careful study and observation of the patient, nor should they be ordered without an understanding and appreciation of their merits and limitations as well as their hazards and expense. When performed as part of the total physical examination they have the following advantages:

1. Biochemical aberrations that are usually undetectable by routine history and physical can be discovered more easily.
2. When the patient has a known disease, the screening panels serve as a gauge of the overall biochemical state relative to the existing malady.
3. When there is a diagnostic problem, the findings of the screening panels may help with the differential diagnosis.
4. They supply data concerning the biochemical parameters necessary for the safe administration of medications.

The most commonly used biochemical screening panels are routine blood chemistry, hematology, and urinalysis.

Blood chemistry usually includes calcium, phosphorus, glucose, uric acid, cholesterol, total protein, albumin, alkaline phosphatase, bilirubin, lactic dehydrogenase (LDH), serum glutamic oxaloacetic transaminase (SGOT), blood urea nitrogen (BUN), creatinine, and electrolytes.

Hematology consists of a white blood count and differential, red blood count, hematocrit, hemoglobin, mean corpuscular volume, mean corpuscular hemoglobin concentration, and sedimentation rate.

The urinalysis consists of determining the pH, specific gravity, glucose, blood, protein, and a microscopic examination.

1

BLOOD CHEMISTRY AND ELECTROLYTES

If an automated analyzer is used, a single specimen of blood may be used to determine levels of electrolytes and chemical constituents. The tests are listed in the order in which they usually appear on the automated report.

CALCIUM (Ca)

Over 98% of the calcium in the body is in the skeleton and teeth. Although the calcium in the extracellular fluid is only a small fraction of the total, its level and the level of phosphorus are regulated precisely by the parathyroid gland and the total serum protein, rarely varying more than 5% above or below normal.

Of the total plasma calcium, 50% is ionized, while most of the rest is protein bound. The ionized calcium is important in blood coagulation, in the function of the heart, muscles, and nerves, and in membrane permeability.

The parathyroid hormone raises the plasma ionized calcium concentration by acting directly on osteoclasts to release bone salts into the extracellular fluid, thus affecting both calcium and phosphate levels in the plasma. The parathyroid hormone also increases the rate of absorption of calcium from the intestines and acts on the renal tubular cells, causing calcium to be saved and phosphorus to be lost.

Two other factors important in calcium metabolism are vitamin D and the potent hypocalcemic hormone, calcitonin. Vitamin D increases the efficiency of intestinal calcium absorption; calcitonin has opposite effects of the parathyroid hormone in that it increases renal calcium clearance.

NORMAL SERUM CALCIUM

Ionized:	4.2-5.2 mg/dl
	2.1-2.6 mEq/L or 50% to 58% of total
Total:	9.0-10.6 mg/dl
	4.5-5.3 mEq/L
Infants:	11-13 mg/dl

Most frequently, a normal serum calcium value along with a normal overall biochemical screening panel rules out any significant disease entity involving calcium metabolism. However, a normal calcium value may reflect significant disease in the presence of an abnormal level of phosphorus. In serum, the product of Ca × P (mg/100 ml) is normally about 50 in children. This product may be below 30 in rickets.

A normal blood calcium level in association with an elevated blood urea nitrogen (BUN) would be very suggestive of one of two things: (1) secondary hyperparathyroidism, in which case the uremia and acidosis have initially lowered the serum calcium, which in turn will stimulate the parathyroid, resulting in a normal serum calcium or (2) primary hyperparathyroidism, which would initially elevate the serum calcium. The development of secondary kidney disease and uremia would then lower the elevated calcium to normal by phosphate retention.

A normal serum calcium associated with a marked decrease in serum albumin should be considered abnormal hypercalcemia. Since about 50% of the total serum calcium is protein bound, the blood level of calcium should be depressed in the presence of hypoproteinemia. Since free calcium ions are not measured directly, the concentration of serum proteins is an important factor in estimating the level of ionized calcium in the blood.

Hypercalcemia

If all other biochemical values are normal an elevation of calcium should raise the possibility of laboratory error, and a second determination of calcium and phosphorus should then be made.

Hypercalcemia associated with hypophosphatemia is characteristic of hyperparathyroidism.

Hypercalcemia associated with hypergammaglobulinemia indicates three main possibilities: (1) sarcoidosis, (2) multiple myeloma, or (3) malignancies.

Hypercalcemia associated with metabolic alkalosis should raise the possibility of milk-alkali syndrome, particularly if there is a history of peptic ulcer, in which case there may have been ingestion of large amounts of calcium (milk) and absorbable antacids.

Hypercalcemia with a significant elevation of alkaline phosphatase may suggest Paget's disease of bone.

Other causes of hypercalcemia are severe thyrotoxicosis, malignant tumors with or without bone metastasis, and bone fractures, especially during bedrest. Hypercalcemia may also be found in idiopathic hypercalcemia, acute bone atrophy, hypervitaminosis D, polycythemia vera, some cases of acromegaly, Cushing's syndrome with osteoporosis, and in patients taking thiazide diuretics.

Hypocalcemia

Whenever hypocalcemia is encountered, it is advisable to perform a serum protein electrophoresis. If there is significant diminution of the albumin fraction, the hypocalcemia may not reflect true hypocalcemia and may not be significant in terms of calcium metabolism. This is termed pseudohypocalcemia. In such a situation, a reduction of albumin would also cause the serum calcium to be low.

The causes of hypocalcemia, after ruling out pseudohypocalcemia, are:

1. Hypoparathyroidism, especially if the patient has undergone thyroid or parathyroid surgery
2. Osteomalacia in adults and rickets in children resulting from vitamin D deficiency
3. Chronic steatorrhea, resulting from pancreatic insufficiency, sprue, celiac disease, or biliary obstruction, all of which cause decreased absorption of calcium from the gastrointestinal tract (malabsorption syndrome); in this case as well as in acute pancreatitis, fatty acids form calcium soaps, which precipitate, causing calcium to be lost in the feces
4. Pregnancy
5. Diuretic intake if there is a history of such intake, particularly "loop" diuretics such as furosemide or ethacrynic acid
6. Respiratory alkalosis and hyperventilation; since alkalosis causes calcium ions to bind to protein, there is a decrease in the ionized calcium fraction
7. Hypomagnesemia, possibly secondary to suppression of release of parathyroid hormone

Certain types of hypocalcemias in the newborn respond to magnesium administration, indicating a primary etiology of hypomagnesemia.

Effect of calcium on the electrocardiogram

The S-T segment changes of the ECG may be very helpful in case of doubt as to laboratory error or in situations where a quick evaluation of the serum calcium level is desirable, particularly in the hyperventilation syndrome. Usually, hypocalcemia causes significant prolongation of the S-T segment of the Q-T interval. Hypercalcemia causes shortening of the Q-T interval and perhaps a widening and rounding of the T waves.

PHOSPHORUS (PO_4)

The phosphorus level is usually determined in the phosphate form. It is always correlated with the calcium level. The optimal ratio is 1:1, with adequate vitamin D intake. Calcium and phosphorus determinations are always ordered together because of their close relationship. As mentioned in the discussion of calcium, the parathyroid hormone causes an increased rate of absorption of calcium and phosphorus, and causes phosphate to be lost in the urine and calcium to be saved as a result of its effect on renal tubular reabsorption. Phosphate is a threshold substance, and as such its loss in the urine is dependent upon both its level in the serum and the level of calcium, since if either element is in excess the other will be excreted.

Of the total phosphorus, 85% is combined with calcium in the skeleton. It is found abundantly in all tissues and is involved in almost all metabolic processes.

With these principles in mind, it is evident that, in the absence of significant glomerular disease (with normal BUN and normal creatinine), phosphate abnormalities should direct attention toward some kind of abnormality associated with the endocrine system or bone metabolism.

NORMAL SERUM PHOSPHORUS

Adults:	1.8-2.6 mEq/L
	3.0-4.5 mg/dl
Children:	2.3-4.1 mEq/L
	4.0-7.0 mg/dl

Hyperphosphatemia

Probably the most common cause of elevated phosphate is chronic glomerular disease with elevated BUN and creatinine. However, the importance of measuring blood phosphate and calcium levels lies in its value in diagnosing hypoparathyroidism, the hallmark of which is hyperphosphatemia in association with hypocalcemia and normal renal function.

The phosphate level may be normal or increased in both milk-alkali syndrome and sarcoidosis when normal renal function is associated with primary abnormal calcium metabolism. In the former there will be a history of peptic ulcer disease; the latter may be suggested by hyperglobulinemia and the clinical picture.

Other endocrine conditions associated with elevated phosphates include hyperthyroidism and increased growth hormone secretion. Other causes may be pseudohypoparathyroidism, fractures in the healing stage, malignant hyperpyrexia (following anesthesia), feeding newborns on unadapted cow's milk, which has a much higher phosphate content than human milk, and hypervitaminosis D.

Hypophosphatemia

Hypophosphatemia may be the result of one of the following:

1. Hyperparathyroidism, the hallmark of which is hypophosphatemia in association with hypercalcemia. Although possibly not the most common cause of decreased phosphate, this combination in the absence of significant renal disease is clinically characteristic of hyperparathyroidism.
2. Childhood rickets or adult osteomalacia, particularly if there is elevation of

the alkaline phosphatase. In either of these conditions, the serum calcium may be low or normal.

3. Certain types of renal tubular acidosis, which is relatively rare and may be a single defect of phosphate reabsorption from the distal tubules (that is, phosphate diabetes) or multiple defects (De Fanconi syndrome and the aminoacidurias). These diseases may be associated with other abnormalities of amino acid metabolism, distal tubular acidosis, and acid-base abnormalities.
4. Rapid correction of hyperglycemia and diabetic ketoacidosis.
5. Chronic use of antacids containing aluminum hydroxide, which binds phosphate.
6. In the absence of the above conditions, hypophosphatemia may be an indication of such conditions as malabsorption syndromes and hyperinsulinism.

BLOOD GLUCOSE (Gluc)

Most carbohydrates in the diet are digested to form glucose or fructose and are taken by the portal vein to the liver, where fructose is converted to glucose. The utilization of glucose by the body cells is intimately related to insulin, the hormone secreted from the islets of Langerhans in the pancreas.

Assuming that the patient was in a fasting state when the blood for the analysis was drawn, one usually sees the following order of frequency and range for blood glucose:

1. Normal, between 80 and 100 mg/100 ml
2. Mild elevation, between 120 and 130 mg/100 ml
3. Moderate elevation, between 300 and 500 mg/100 ml
4. Marked elevation, greater than 500 mg/100 ml, associated with ketoacidosis, which is reflected by decreased CO_2 combining power
5. Marked elevation with hyperosmolar state, without ketoacidosis
6. Below the normal accepted ranges

The normal range for fasting blood sugar varies among laboratories and with the type of procedure used. One should consult the particular laboratory as to the normal range and the method used.

Since the implications of each of the above classifications are different, consideration of the blood sugar determination in these categories is advantageous.

NORMAL BLOOD GLUCOSE

Serum or plasma: 70-110 mg/100 ml
Whole blood: 60-100 mg/100 ml

Although the most commonly encountered category is a fasting blood glucose that is within normal limits, it should be remembered that a normal value rules out any significant diabetic problem, but that it does not rule out diabetes as such. Patients who have latent diabetes or prediabetes will have normal fasting blood sugars even though they are, by definition, diabetic. This is certain if both parents are known to be diabetic, if an identical twin is a known diabetic, or if the patient has diabetic vascular changes without an elevated blood sugar.

Hyperglycemia

Hyperglycemia is usually equated with diabetes. In most cases any degree of elevated blood sugar does indicate diabetes, whether the elevation is transient or permanent. However, in always equating hyperglycemia with diabetes, one runs the risk of forgetting other diseases that may be associated with hyperglycemia. For example, hyperglycemia is present in Cushing's disease and in patients being treated with steroids. It is uncertain whether the hyperglycemia in the latter situation is latent diabetes manifested as a clinical diabetes by excess steroids, or whether this kind of an elevated blood sugar is an altogether different pathophysiologic entity from the well-known inherited form of diabetes mellitus. The uncertainty is compounded by the fact that one of the tests employed in the diagnosis of latent diabetes is the steroid stimulation test.

It is probably best to simply define diabetes mellitus as the hereditary disease associated with fasting hyperglycemia and found in the majority of hyperglycemic patients. However, it bears repeating that hyperglycemia may not necessarily mean diabetes. A reasonably diligent search for other possible causes of hyperglycemia may produce the correct diagnosis. A glucose tolerance test is indicated when blood glucose levels are borderline or there is clinical evidence of hereditary diabetes.

Mild hyperglycemia (120-130 mg/100 ml)

Entities (other than diabetes) associated with mild hyperglycemia are:

1. Conditions causing elevation of blood catecholamines and steroids. The most frequent cause of this is acute stress (acute infection, myocardial infarction, and the like) which may herald the onset of hereditary diabetes.
2. Pheochromocytoma, a tumor producing epinephrine (adrenaline) and norepinephrine (noradrenaline).
3. Cushing's syndrome and Cushing's disease, both of which cause hyperglycemia because of elevated glucocorticoids. In Cushing's syndrome, which may be caused by a pituitary adenoma, growth hormones may be involved, which definitely elevate the blood sugar.
4. Hyperthyroidism, which is suggested when mild hyperglycemia is associated with hypocholesterolemia. The increase in blood sugar is probably mediated through an increase in catecholamines.
5. Adenoma of the pancreas, producing only glucagon that antagonizes insulin, causing hyperglycemia.

6. Diuretics, mainly the thiazide diuretics and the "loop" diuretics, most likely by inducing hypokalemia, which is known to suppress the release of insulin.
7. Acute or chonic pancreatic insufficiency, the mechanism of which may be the destruction of islet cells.

Moderate hyperglycemia (300-500 mg/100 ml)

A moderate elevation in blood sugar usually leaves no doubt as to the diagnosis of diabetes mellitus. Depending on the age of the patient and other findings, a moderate hyperglycemia usually becomes a management problem.

Marked hyperglycemia (>500 mg/100 ml)

When a marked elevation in blood sugar is encountered, attention should immediately be directed to the CO_2 content. This is extremely important, because if the CO_2 content is low, the patient has uncontrolled diabetes associated with ketoacidosis, a potentially dangerous situation.

The second possibility, which is relatively rare, is a marked hyperglycemia without ketoacidosis (reflected by a normal CO_2 content). This entity, also serious, is called nonketotic and nonacidotic hyperglycemia; it is not necessarily associated with diabetes. The patient is usually very ill, with significant abnormal intermediary carbohydrate metabolism, caused by the uncoupling of oxidative phosphorylation. It is usually found in elderly patients with advanced vascular disease and anoxemia. There is associated dehydration with hypernatremia.

Hypoglycemia

The finding of a fasting hypoglycemia is quite unusual. However, once it is encountered the following conditions should be considered:

1. Pancreatic islet cell tumor, which independently secretes insulin without the associated check and balance of a normal metabolism
2. Large tumors of nonpancreatic origin, particularly large retroperitoneal sarcomas or large hepatomas
3. Pituitary hypofunction
4. Adrenocortical hypofunction (Addison's disease); if this is the cause the patient will also have slight hyperkalemia and hyponatremia and a slightly elevated BUN
5. Acquired extensive liver disease

Other relatively rare conditions associated with hypoglycemia include glycogen storage disease; postnatal hypoglycemia in infants of diabetic mothers; and alcoholic hypoglycemia, which is usually associated with a substantial alcohol ingestion after a period of fasting.

Rarer still is hypoglycemia caused by certain amino acids (leucine hypoglycemia). One should also be aware of patients who are taking oral hypoglycemics or insulin and who may have a fasting hypoglycemia in the morning.

Reactive hypoglycemia

In functional reactive hypoglycemia, a rising blood sugar level stimulates excessive insulin secretion. In this syndrome the insulin continues to act after most of the carbohydrate has been stored or metabolized, and hypoglycemia results. A 5-hour glucose tolerance test usually detects a lowering of the blood sugar between 3 and 5 hours. Preferably, samples should be drawn every half hour. For the 5-hour glucose tolerance test to be diagnostic, the blood sugar must drop below 40 mg/100 ml with symptoms of hypoglycemia.

URIC ACID

Uric acid is the end product of purine metabolism and is cleared from the plasma by glomerular filtration and perhaps by tubular secretion. One very rarely encounters a uric acid level significantly below expressed ranges. Therefore, we will not consider hypouricemia except to state that in very rare conditions, such as Wilson's disease or Fanconi syndrome, the uric acid level may be low. It may also be low in malabsorption states.

NORMAL SERUM URIC ACID

Male: 2.1-7.8 mg/dl
Female: 2.0-6.4 mg/dl

In most instances a normal uric acid value is given no further attention. However, a normal uric acid level does not rule out gout, although it makes such a diagnosis unlikely.

Hyperuricemia

Hyperuricemia is usually equated with gout, in which there is a clinical picture of either tophi or acute arthritis with significant hyperuricemia.

However, mild hyperuricemia is most commonly idiopathic, in which case the patient is asymptomatic. It would be an unfortunate mistake to label every hyperuricemia "gout" and treat the hyperuricemia rather than the patient. Usually the blood uric acid reflects the balance of uric acid production and excretion.

The association of idiopathic hyperuricemia with hyperlipidemia and coronary artery disease is of clinical importance, although the reason for the association is unclear.

Another common cause of hyperuricemia is chronic renal failure. This can be ascertained relatively quickly by correlating the uric acid elevation with the creatinine and BUN, both of which will be elevated.

A differential diagnosis is necessary between hyperuricemia caused by chronic renal failure and that caused by gouty nephropathy with secondary chronic renal failure. In the latter condition, which is relatively rare, it would be impossible to determine through laboratory tests which came first, the gouty nephropathy or the renal failure. In this situation the clinical picture is extremely helpful.

Other causes of hyperuricemia are congestive heart failure with decreased creatinine clearance, starvation (particularly absolute starvation of obese persons for weight reduction purposes), and certain glycogen storage diseases (Von Gierke's disease or Lesch-Nyhan syndrome).

Most of the conditions associated with the excessive production of uric acid belong to the lympho- and myeloproliferative diseases, such as acute or chronic leukemia, both leukocytic and granulocytic, multiple myeloma, or any other malignancy associated with rapid destruction of nucleic acid and purine products. Chemotherapy or radiotherapy in these disorders may further elevate the uric acid level.

Several drugs are associated with hyperuricemia. The most common of these are the diuretics, particularly the thiazide diuretics, which impair uric acid clearance by the kidneys.

In addition, hyperuricemia may be found in Tangier disease (alpha lipoprotein deficiency), hypoparathyroidism, primary hyperoxaluria, lead poisoning resulting from ingestion of moonshine whiskey (saturnine gout), and excessive ethyl alcohol intake.

CHOLESTEROL (Chol)

Cholesterol exists in the body in both a free and an esterified form (combined with a fatty acid). Most of the ingested cholesterol is esterified in the intestine and absorbed as such into the lymph. The liver synthesizes cholesterol from acetate. This synthesis is presumably inhibited by a high level of circulating cholesterol.

Cholesterol is used in the body to form cholic acid in the liver, which in turn forms bile salts, important for fat digestion. A small quantity of cholesterol is used in the formation of hormones by the adrenal glands, ovaries, and testes. A large amount is used to make the skin highly resistant to the absorption of water-soluble substances.

The concentration of cholesterol in the blood is influenced by thyroid hormones and estrogens, both of which cause a decrease. Plasma cholesterol is elevated when biliary flow is obstructed, and also in hereditary hypercholesterolemia and untreated diabetes mellitus, in spite of a decrease in cholesterol synthesis in diabetes.

There is popular interest in cholesterol values since hypercholesterolemia is a much publicized risk factor for coronary artery disease. This is discussed in Chapter 4. It is important to keep in mind that normal values for cholesterol are arbitrarily defined and show much variation in different populations and age groups.

NORMAL SERUM CHOLESTEROL

150-250 mg/dl (varies with diet and age, and from country to country)

Marked hypercholesterolemia (>400 mg/dl)

Marked hypercholesterolemia is seen in:

1. Liver disease associated with biliary obstruction; in this condition elevated alkaline phosphatase and bilirubin levels accompany hypercholesterolemia
2. Nephrotic stage of glomerulonephritis; elevated BUN and creatinine may be present
3. Familial hypercholesterolemia, a genetically transmitted disorder, more pronounced if homozygous

Other causes of hypercholesterolemia are hypothyroidism, pancreatectomy, and pancreatic dysfunction such as that in diabetes mellitus and chronic pancreatitis.

Significant hypocholesterolemia (<150 mg/dl)

A significantly low blood cholesterol may reflect dietary habits, malnutrition, extensive liver disease, and possibly hyperthyroidism, which does produce a low normal serum cholesterol.

In liver disease it is advisable to fractionate the cholesterol to the esterified form, since esterification is affected by liver damage much more than is the total cholesterol.

Other conditions that may be associated with hypocholesterolemia are severe sepsis, anemia (megaloblastic and hypochromic), serum α and β lipoprotein deficiency, and certain enzyme deficiencies associated with cholesterol metabolism.

TOTAL PROTEIN AND ALBUMIN/GLOBULIN RATIO (tot prot and A/G ratio)

Plasma proteins serve as a source of rapid replacement of tissue proteins during tissue depletion, as buffers in acid-base balance, and as transporters of constituents of the blood, such as lipids, vitamins, hormones, iron, copper, and certain enzymes. The antibodies of the body are contained in the gamma globulins, and a number of the plasma proteins participate in blood coagulation. Of the total protein, between 52% and 68% is albumin. This fraction is responsible for about 80% of the colloid oncotic pressure in the serum. The capillary walls are impermeable to the proteins in plasma. The proteins, therefore, exert an osmotic force across the capillary wall (oncotic pressure) that tends to pull water into the blood.

Although the total protein and A/G ratio is still a commonly employed test, it is gradually being replaced by serum protein electrophoresis, which more clearly delineates the different albumin and globulin fractions.

Electrophoresis is the migration of charged particles in an electrolyte solution in response to an electrical current passed through the solution. The proteins move at different rates because each is different in electrical charge, size, and shape. Thus the proteins tend to separate into distinct layers.

Immunoelectrophoresis is a combination of electrophoresis and immunodiffusion to permit analysis of the various immunoglobulin fractions.

NORMAL TOTAL PROTEIN AND ALBUMIN/GLOBULIN RATIO

Total: 6.0-7.8 gm/dl
Albumin: 3.2-4.5 gm/dl
Globulin: 2.3-3.5 gm/dl

Hypoalbuminemia

A depressed albumin with a slightly elevated globulin is a reversal of the A/G ratio and suggests chronic liver disease. Thus an albumin of 2.5 gm and below, with a globulin of 3 gm/100 ml and a total protein in the range of 5.5 gm/100 ml is extremely suggestive of chronic liver disease.

Other conditions associated with hypoalbuminemia are significant malnutrition (especially protein), nephrotic syndrome, and malabsorption syndromes, particularly protein-losing enteropathies.

Normal total protein, low albumin, and elevated globulin

When a normal total protein is associated with a low normal albumin and an elevated globulin the A/G ratio is reversed. This type of laboratory picture is suggestive of diseases with hypergammaglobulinemia and includes the myeloproliferative diseases such as multiple myeloma, Hodgkin's disease, and leukemias; the chronic granulomatous infectious diseases such as tuberculosis, brucellosis, collagen disease, chronic active hepatitis, and sarcoidosis.

Under the above circumstances one is obliged to use serum protein electrophoresis to determine if one is dealing with a broad band of gamma globulin or a sharp peak in the gamma, alpha I, alpha II, or beta range. The latter would be indicative of variants of multiple myeloma and macroglobulinemias.

THE ENZYMES

A usual analysis includes the following enzymes: alkaline phosphatase (alk phos), lactic dehydrogenase (LDH), and serum glutamic oxaloacetic transaminase (SGOT).

Enzymes are found in all tissues. They are complex, naturally occurring compounds that catalyze the biochemical reactions of the body; that is, they speed up reactions that might otherwise proceed very slowly. Each tissue has its own specific enzyme, with one enzyme being common to more than one type of tissue. For example, alkaline phosphatase is found mainly in bone and liver and in small amounts in kidneys and the gastrointestinal tract. SGOT is found mainly in heart and skeletal muscle and in the liver, kidneys, and red blood cells.

One looks for elevation of these enzymes in the laboratory examination, the implication being that the particular tissue is damaged enough to release significant quantities of the enzyme into the blood.

Alkaline phosphatase (alk phos)

Alkaline phosphatase is an enzyme that mediates some of the complex reactions of bone formation. When the osteoblasts are actively depositing bone matrix, they secrete large quantities of alkaline phosphatase.

The two main sources of alkaline phosphatase are bone and liver. Consequently, an elevation of alkaline phosphatase immediately directs attention to either liver problems or bone disease that will correlate with clinical findings, such as jaundice indicating liver disease. The chemical composition of the enzyme from each of these sources is slightly different, so that if the enzyme is fractionated one of the fractions (isoenzymes) is specific to the particular organ or tissue from which it came. For clinical purposes, the isoenzymes are not separated, although in highly specialized laboratories the different isoenzymes can be isolated by the process of electrophoresis (pp. 12 and 13).

NORMAL ALKALINE PHOSPHATASE (TOTAL SERUM)

Adults:	1.5-4.5 U/dl (Bodansky)
	4-13 U/dl (King-Armstrong)
	0.8-2.3 U/ml (Bessey-Lowry)
	15-35 U/ml (Shinowara-Jones-Reinhart)
Children:	5.0-14.0 U/dl (Bodansky)
	3.4-9.0 U/ml (Bessey-Lowry)
	15-30 U/dl (King-Armstrong)

Extreme elevation of alkaline phosphatase with liver disease

When an extremely high level of alkaline phosphatase (15 U/dl or more, Bodansky) is associated with liver disease (abnormal liver function tests) the following are indicated:

1. Early phases of obstructive jaundice, with obstruction at the level of the major biliary ducts (gallstone or carcinoma of the head of the pancreas). In this case the patient initially has a slight bilirubinemia; it gradually increases and is accompanied by the extremely high alkaline phosphatase.
2. Space-occupying lesions of the liver, either widespread metastatic liver disease or an obstructive tumor of the biliary ducts. The alkaline phosphatase in the latter case is presumed to come from the cells lining the bile ducts. The obstruction and the damage cause the enzyme to leak from the cells and appear in the bloodstream.

Extreme elevation of alkaline phosphatase without liver disease

In the absence of any indication of liver disease (normal liver function tests), extreme elevation of alkaline phosphatase along with some indication of bone pathology suggests Paget's disease of bone, in which the highest level of this enzyme is found, especially if osteogenic sarcoma develops.

Extreme elevations of alkaline phosphatase can also be found in carcinomas metastatic to bone.

Moderate and slight elevation of alkaline phosphatase with liver disease

In the presence of liver disease, moderate elevation (8-12 U/dl, Bodansky) of alkaline phosphatase is usually associated with cholangiolitic hepatitis.

A slight elevation of alkaline phosphatase in the presence of liver disease usually indicates cirrhosis of the liver with some active hepatitis.

Moderate and slight elevation of alkaline phosphatase without liver disease

In the absence of liver involvement (normal liver function tests) and in the presence of hypercalcemia an elevated alkaline phosphatase level indicates the possibility of hyperparathyroidism. In this situation there is a slight elevation of the enzyme in the initial stage. At a later stage there may be significant elevations. In secondary and tertiary hyperparathyroidism, borderline elevations may be encountered.

If other indicators of bone pathology (bone scan revealing evidence of bone disease) are present, mild to moderate elevations of alkaline phosphatase suggest osteomalacia. Usually such elevation will supply the differential diagnosis between osteomalacia and osteoporosis. In the latter condition the alkaline phosphatase is normal.

A slight elevation of alkaline phosphatase also occurs in childhood and during the growth period, in pregnancy, and in rickets.

Low alkaline phosphatase

A low alkaline phosphatase level is usually not of much clinical significance. However, if a low value of this enzyme persists, one should consider some of the extremely rare entities such as hypophosphatasia, achondroplasia, cretinism, and vitamin C deficiency.

Lactic dehydrogenase (LDH)

Lactic dehydrogenase is an enzyme that catalyzes the reversible oxidation of lactic acid to pyruvic acid. It is present in nearly all metabolizing cells, with highest concentrations in heart, liver, kidney, brain, skeletal muscle, and erythrocytes. Damage to nearly any tissue can cause this enzyme to be released into the bloodstream. The origin of the release cannot be determined by routine examination. However, LDH can be separated into five isoenzymes, thus sharpening its diagnostic value. Electrophoresis is used to separate the isoenzymes of LDH, thus determining the source of an elevation of this enzyme.

One should be aware of the possibility of falsely elevated LDH levels because of hemolyzed blood specimens. Thus when all other parameters are normal except the LDH, the test should be repeated before any further investigations are undertaken.

NORMAL LDH (SERUM)

80-120 Wacker units
71-207 IU/L
150-450 Wroblewski units

Extreme elevation of LDH (>1500 Wroblewski units)

The highest values of this enzyme are seen in patients with myocardial infarction, hemolytic disorders, and pernicious anemia.

Slight elevation of LDH (500-700 Wroblewski units)

Slight elevations that are persistent should direct attention to the following disease entities: chornic viral hepatitis; malignancies of skeletal mucles, liver, kidney, brain, blood, and heart; destruction of pulmonary tissue (pneumonia and pulmonary emboli); generalized viral infection involving multiple organs (infectious mononucleosis); low grade hemolytic disorders; cerebrovascular accidents with brain damage; and renal tissue destruction (renal infarcts, infections, or malignancies).

Serum glutamic oxaloacetic transaminase (SGOT)

The transaminase enzymes catalyze the conversion of one amino acid to the corresponding keto acid with simultaneous conversion of another keto acid to an amino acid. Transamination reactions occur in many tissues.

Glutamic oxaloacetic transaminase is found mainly in heart muscle and the liver and to a certain degree in skeletal muscle, kidney, and red blood cells. Normally, almost all of this enzyme is intracellular. Following injury or death of physiologically active cells, the enzyme is released into the circulation. Elevated values may be found 8 hours after injury and should peak in 24 to 36 hours if the original episode is not repeated. It usually falls to normal in 4 to 6 days. The amount of SGOT is in direct proportion to the number of cells damaged and the interval of time between tissue injury and the test.

NORMAL SGOT (SERUM)

8-33 U/ml

Extreme elevation of SGOT (>1000 U/ml)

There are extremely high levels of this enzyme in the acute stages of severe fulminating hepatitis in which there is massive destruction of liver tissue, in severe liver necrosis, and in skeletal muscle damage.

High values of SGOT also occur in acute myocardial infarction. The level found following infarction depends on the size of the infarct and the time relationship between the onset of the infarct and the drawing of the blood.

Minor elevation of SGOT (40-100 U/ml)

Minor elevations of SGOT can be seen in congestive heart failure, tachyarrhythmias in the presence of shock, pericarditis, pulmonary infarction, and dissecting aneurysm, as well as in cirrhosis, cholangiolitic jaundice, metastatic liver disease, skeletal muscle disease, posttraumatic states, and generalized infections such as infectious mononucleosis.

Serum glutamic pyruvic transaminase (SGPT)

This enzyme is found mainly in liver cells; thus an elevated SGPT is a sensitive index of acute hepatocellular injury. In the presence of elevated SGOT and LDH, a normal SGPT rules out hepatic origin of the enzymes. On the other hand, markedly elevated SGPT in the presence of a mild to moderate elevation of SGOT definitely suggests either hepatic disease or hepatic disease combined with other conditions.

NORMAL SGPT

1-36 U/ml

BILIRUBIN (total serum)

Bilirubin is formed from the hemoglobin of destroyed erythrocytes by the reticuloendothelial system and is the predominant pigment of the bile. Being a by-product of hemoglobin metabolism, it is a waste product and thus must be excreted.

Bilirubin exists in two forms in the body, soluble (conjugated or direct-reacting) and protein bound (unconjugated or "indirect-reacting"). The routine examination does not differentiate between the two, and further tests are run if the total bilirubin level is elevated. These tests and normal bilirubin physiology are discussed in Chapter 7 on pp. 154 and 155.

NORMAL BILIRUBIN (SERUM)

Total:	0.1-1.2 mg/dl
Newborn total:	1-12 mg/dl

A normal level of total bilirubin rules out any significant impairment of the excretory function of the liver or hemolysis.

Greatly elevated total bilirubin (>12 mg/dl)

A markedly elevated total bilirubin level along with a significant drop in hemoglobin and significant reticulocytosis is highly indicative of the possibility of massive hemolysis. Further tests show the bilirubin to be of the indirect-reacting type (Chapter 7, pp. 154 and 155).

Significant elevation of direct-reacting bilirubin (Chapter 7, p. 155) indicates obstructive jaundice in the form of obstructive phase of hepatitis, cholangiolitis, and lower bilary tree obstruction by either calculus or carcinoma.

BLOOD UREA NITROGEN (BUN)

Urea, formed in the liver by the deamination of amino acids, is the primary method of nitrogen excretion. Urea, then, is the end product of protein metabolism and is formed in the liver. After synthesis, urea travels through the blood and is excreted in the urine.

NORMAL BUN

8-18 mg/dl

Elevated BUN

Acute or chronic renal failure is the most common cause of high BUN levels. In prerenal failure, a low renal blood supply, such as occurs with congestive heart failure, leads to reduced glomerular filtration and therefore an elevated BUN. In renal failure, damage to the nephrons, particularly such as occurs with glomerular nephritis or pyelonephritis, leads to decreased glomerular filtration and excretion. As a result, the blood urea nitrogen begins to rise when the glomerular filtration rate falls below 50 ml/min (the normal in an average-size man is approximately 125 ml/min).

Postrenal failure resulting from urinary tract obstructions can also cause uremia. Prostatic enlargement is probably the most common cause of urinary tract obstruction.

Other causes of borderline elevated levels of BUN are unusually high protein intake and excessive body protein catabolism such as occurs with sepsis or fever and gastrointestinal bleeding.

SERUM CREATININE (Creat)

Creatinine is a waste product of creatine, which is present in skeletal muscle as creatine phosphate, a high energy compound.

Serum creatinine determination is another test of renal function, reflecting the balance between its production (proportional to the body's muscle mass) and filtration by the renal glomerulus.

NORMAL CREATININE (SERUM)

0.6-1.2 mg/dl

Elevated serum creatinine

Serum creatinine is elevated in all diseases of the kidney in which 50% or more of the nephrons are destroyed.

Nonrenal causes of elevation or fluctuation in serum creatinine levels are few, making this a more specific test of renal failure. People with large muscle mass or patients with acromegaly may have values slightly over the normal range in the presence of normal kidney function.

ELECTROLYTES

The serum electrolyte analysis includes sodium (Na), potassium (K), chloride (Cl), and CO_2 content. The levels of these electrolytes in the blood are the outcome of fine regulatory mechanisms of ionic charges and the osmotic balance of the extracellular fluid. This is accomplished by the marvelous adaptation of the kidneys, lungs, and endocrine system to varying and multidirectional forces. The kidneys and the lungs are involved in acid-base balance, while osmotic balance is finely governed by the endocrine system, with the hypothalamus, posterior pituitary gland, and kidneys being intricately interrelated.

It is apparent, then, that the determination of the serum level of a single electrolyte is insufficient for an overall evaluation of the patient's metabolic state. When one wishes to determine the serum level of any electrolyte, the whole series should be ordered. This approach will have a profound bearing on the correct interpretation and evaluation of the patient's electrolyte status.

The following example is given to emphasize the importance of a complete electrolyte analysis. A serum potassium level of 4.5 mEq/L means one thing if the CO_2 content is 35 mEq/L and means something altogether different if the CO_2 content is 10 mEq/L. In the first case, the patient probably has a metabolic alkalosis. This would cause the potassium to migrate into the cell and be excreted in the urine. A serum potassium of 4.5 mEq/L does not, then, really reflect a true potassium homeostasis, since when the alkalosis is corrected the potassium will return to its extracellular position with a possible decrease in total body potassium.

In the second case (CO_2 content of 10 mEq/L), the patient probably has a metabolic acidosis. This would then cause the potassium to leave the cell. A serum potassium of 4.5 mEq/L would, then, reflect a much lower potassium level when acidosis is corrected, since the available potassium will migrate back into the cell when the acidosis is corrected.

In addition to electrolyte determination, it is extremely important that the blood urea nitrogen (BUN) or creatinine be determined as well. This serves two purposes. First, serum electrolyte values have one implication in the presence of an elevated BUN level with the associated metabolic acidosis, whereas when the BUN level is normal the implication changes. In addition, the BUN is a relatively good indication of the patient's overall water metabolism and hydration status, which has a pronounced effect on the different electrolytes. Second, if therapy must be instituted, particularly potassium replacement, it is essential to know kidney function. Preferably a creatinine clearance is ordered. However, if this is not available, at least one BUN determination is ordered so that the patient's condition may be managed safely.

It is preferable to measure the arterial pH, Po_2, and Pco_2 directly because the pH affects and is affected by the serum electrolyte level. This is particularly true in complex metabolic and/or respiratory acid-base problems, in which it is extremely difficult to evaluate the patient's electrolytes without knowing the arterial blood gases and pH.

Serum eletrolyte levels may vary from moment to moment and are, therefore, only a rough indicator of the total body concentration of the ions. For example, in the condition known as dilutional hyponatremia the serum sodium level is below normal, but the total body sodium is increased.

There is no direct way of measuring intracellular levels of electrolytes. It is known, however, that the Q-T interval and U wave of the electrocardiogram reflect the ratio of intracellular and extracellular electrolytes. Initial information about the patient's overall electrolyte and acid-base state, therefore, may be drawn from this source.

Keeping in mind the above principles and problems, one can evaluate the electrolytes much more rationally and obtain a more significant insight into the patient's overall metabolic state. At the present time electrolyte determinations are usually performed in critical care units and in hospital environments. However, the value of electrolyte determination is being appreciated more and more in the daily office practice of physicians, particularly in view of the large number of medications employed that alter electrolytes and body water metabolism.

Collecting and handling the specimen

When blood is being drawn for electrolyte determination, the procedure should be as atraumatic as possible, and the blood obtained should be centrifuged quickly. If there is any hemolysis this fact should be noted, because tissue breakdown or hemolysis will cause a false elevation of serum potassium levels.

Serum sodium (Na)

Sodium is the major cation of the extracellular fluid. It plays an important part in regulating acid-base equilibrium, protecting the body against excessive fluid loss, and preserving the normal function of muscle tissue.

NORMAL SERUM SODIUM

136-142 mEq/L

Hypernatremia

Hypernatremia in the normally functioning individual is very uncommon. Hypernatremia most frequently occurs in the critical care unit, where excess intravenous sodium is given to an unconscious patient whose thirst mechanism is absent. Serum sodium levels have a strong influence on the body's osmoreceptors, and in the healthy individual this initiates the thirst mechanism. The individual then drinks water until the serum sodium level is back to normal.

Hyperglycemia is associated with hypernatremia in some rare hypothalamic lesions, head trauma, and hyperosmolar states. Other causes of hypernatremia are dehydration and steroid (mineralocorticoid) administration or excess.

Hyponatremia

Hyponatremia is more frequently encountered clinically than is hypernatremia. In the ambulatory patient and in those seen in the physician's office, hyponatremia may reflect or be associated with diminution of total body sodium, normal body sodium, or excess body sodium.

Hyponatremia associated with an absolute sodium loss. Hyponatremia is associated with absolute sodium loss in the following conditions:

1. Addison's disease; in the absence of adrenal steroids, sodium reabsorption is impaired and the clinical picture is that of hyponatremia, hyperkalemia, and mild dehydration, reflected by a slight BUN elevation
2. Chronic sodium-losing nephropathy; this is probably a more frequent cause than Addison's disease, and may be a stage in chronic glomerulonephritis, pyelonephritis, manifested by abnormal renal function tests and an elevated BUN
3. Loss of gastrointestinal secretions by vomiting, diarrhea, or tube drainage, with replacement of fluid but not electrolytes
4. Loss of sodium from the skin through diaphoresis or burns, with replacement of fluids but not electrolytes
5. Loss of sodium from the kidneys through the use of diuretics (mercurial, chlorothiazide) and in chronic renal insufficiency with acidosis
6. Metabolic loss of sodium through starvation with acidosis and diabetic acidosis
7. Loss of sodium from serous cavities through paracentesis or thoracentesis

Dilutional hyponatremia. Excessive water, or dilutional hyponatremia, is associated with either normal or even excess total body sodium concentrations and is found in the following conditions: chronic diuretic use with sodium restriction, secondary hyperaldosteronemia, hepatic failure with ascites, congestive heart failure, excessive water administration, acute or chronic renal insufficiency (oliguria), and diabetic acidosis (therapy without adequate sodium replacement).

Hyponatremia associated with inappropriate antidiuretic hormone syndrome. In this condition the patient continues reabsorbing water from the distal tubules and excreting a concentrated urine in spite of serum hypoosmolarity. Inappropriate antidiuretic hormone syndrome has been described in association with various other diseases such as bronchogenic carcinoma (releasing ADH-like chemicals), pulmonary infections, metabolic diseases such as porphyria, and diuretic-induced hypokalemia.

Hyponatremia associated with intracellular potassium depletion. An impairment of the sodium-potassium pump mechanism results in an excessive intracellular sodium influx and potassium efflux. The potassium is then lost in the urine, leaving the patient with a normal serum potassium level and low serum sodium level, which reflects the quantity of intracellular sodium influx and equivalent potassium loss.

Serum potassium (K)

Potassium is the major cation of the intracellular fluid, functioning as sodium does in the extracellular fluid, by influencing acid-base balance, osmotic pressure, and cellular membrane potential.

Serum potassium levels are profoundly affected by momentary acid-base changes. A discussion of serum potassium can be divided into three major categories: the hyperkalemias, normokalemia with normal or decreased total body potassium, and hypokalemia, which is usually associated with decreased total body potassium levels.

NORMAL SERUM POTASSIUM

3.8-5.0 mEq/L

Hyperkalemia

Hyperkalemia is encountered most frequently in renal failure. It is rarely developed by oral potassium chloride ingestion with normal kidneys and with normal creatinine clearance.

Addison's disease, accompanied by hypovolemia and retention of blood urea nitrogen, is the second most common clinical condition associated with hyperkalemia.

Massive tissue destruction, particularly of muscle tissue, will result in hyperkalemia caused by cellular trauma and leakage of intracellular potassium into the serum. Also, any causes of significant metabolic acidosis, such as lactic acidosis and diabetic ketoacidosis, can produce initial hyperkalemia.

A relatively rare condition, called pseudohyperkalemia, is suspected when one encounters hyperkalemia without electrocardiographic evidence. Once documented, pseudohyperkalemia should suggest a myeloproliferative disease such as thrombocytosis. In such cases, the plasma potassium should be checked instead of serum potassium in order to obtain a true potassium level.

Normokalemia with decreased total body potassium

The most commonly encountered clinical cause of normal potassium serum levels with decreased total body potassium levels is chronic diuretic use with inadequate potassium chloride supplementation. Other causes will be discussed under hypokalemia.

The following are a few clues that may be helpful in determining total body potassium depletion with normokalemia:

1. Alkalosis; this can be verified either directly or by arterial blood pH measurement or indirectly by the elevation of the CO_2 content in the absence of chronic obstructive lung disease.
2. In the presence of significant hypochloremia and alkalosis, significant total body potassium depletion, not reflected in the serum, may exist.
3. A cellular level aberration of Na-K dependent ATPase and the Na-K pump may cause gradual cellular potassium depletion and may be reflected by hyponatremia rather than hypokalemia.
4. The presence of a U wave or an apparent Q-T prolongation on the ECG should suggest cellular potassium depletion.

Hypokalemia

Most often, significant hypokalemia reflects total body depletion of potassium, which may have profound metabolic consequences.

Causes of hypokalemia are as follows:

1. Iatrogenic causes
   a. Diuretic therapy that depletes the body of potassium and chloride
   b. Diuretic therapy with supplementation of potassium and not chloride, causing a continual alkalosis with only a partial correction of the hypokalemia
2. Hypomagnesemia is quite frequently associated with hypokalemia. In such a situation, there will be continuous renal loss of potassium until the hypomagnesemia is corrected.
3. Endocrine causes
   a. Cushing's syndrome
   b. Primary or secondary hyperaldosteronism resulting from secondary hyperaldosteronemia
   c. Liver disease with ascites
   d. Excessive ingestion of licorice, which contains a chemical very similar to aldosterone; the symptoms are, therefore, those of primary aldosteronism
   e. Antiinflammatory drugs, indomethacin, phenylbutazone, and steroids and sex hormones, particularly estrogens
   f. Conditions associated with hyperreninemia, when an elevated renin introduced into the system can cause a secondary aldosteronemia; such conditions include malignant hypertension, hypertensive disease, and occasionally unilateral renal vascular hypertension
4. Poor dietary habits and crash diets with inadequate intake of potassium
5. Chronic stress

6. Excessive loss of potassium without adequate replacement
   a. Gastrointestinal tract (chronic diarrhea, malabsorption syndrome)
   b. Perspiration and chronic fever
7. Renal losses of potassium associated with either potassium-losing nephropathy or other kinds of renal tubular acidosis typically involving hypokalemia in association with acidosis and hyperchloremia and usually also associated with aminoacidurias

Electrocardiographic recognition of hyperkalemia and hypokalemia

The electrocardiogram is a very sensitive indicator of the ratio of intracellular to extracellular potassium and shows signs of hypokalemia even when the serum potassium level is still within normal limits. Hypokalemia and hyperkalemia threaten cardiac safety. It is, therefore, important to know the changes that a potassium deficit or excess will initiate on the ECG. This is discussed in Chapter 4 of Unit Two.

Serum chloride (Cl)

Chloride, chiefly an extracellular ion, is present in large quantities in the serum, exerting an important influence on acid-base balance and osmotic pressure.

NORMAL SERUM CHLORIDE

95-103 mEq/L

Hyperchloremia

Hyperchloremia is most frequently associated with renal tubular acidosis, decreased CO_2 content, and hypokalemia.

Hypochloremia

Most often, hypochloremia is associated with hypokalemia and alkalosis and has been termed hypokalemic-chloremic alkalosis. In such a situation the electrolyte analysis reflects low potassium, low chloride, and elevated CO_2 content. Most of the conditions associated with hypokalemia and alkalosis are also associated with hypochloremia.

Hypochloremia may also be associated with a normal serum potassium if the patient's potassium deficiency is being corrected with potassium preparations that do not contain chloride, or if the patient is receiving potassium-saving diuretics. These facts bring into focus two points of clinical importance: (1) potassium replacement therapy should be accompanied by a one-to-one ratio of potassium to chloride and (2) when potassium-saving diuretics are used one should watch very closely for the possible development of hypochloremia and hypochloremic alkalosis.

The development of hypochloremic alkalosis may occur when chronic respiratory acidosis is very rapidly corrected, precipitating significant chloride attrition from the kidneys.

Carbon dioxide (CO_2) content

Total CO_2 content determination is the usual laboratory test done for the detection of acid-base abnormalities. Since direct determination of the pH of the blood is not clinically practical in ordinary circumstances, the CO_2 content is used instead. This test measures the total carbonic acid (H_2CO_3) and bicarbonate (HCO_3) in the plasma.

NORMAL CO_2 CONTENT

24-30 mM/L

Elevated CO_2 content

In the absence of chronic obstructive lung disease, elevated CO_2 content indicates serum alkalosis and intracellular acidosis, which are most frequently associated with hypokalemia and hypochloremia.

For practical and therapeutic consideration, metabolic alkalosis can be divided into two groups, chloride responsive and chloride nonresponsive. The chloride responsive category constitutes 90% of all hypochloremic alkalosis and can easily be corrected with potassium chloride administration. The usual causes of this category of metabolic alkalosis are gastrointestinal losses and diuretics.

The chloride nonresponsive category makes up the remaining 10% of all metabolic alkalosis and occurs with Cushing syndrome (particularly resulting from the ectopic ACTH production syndrome), primary aldosteronism, Bartter syndrome, and licorice ingestion.

The two groups of metabolic alkalosis can be differentiated from each other by a 24-hour urine chloride measurement. In chloride-responsive alkalosis, the urinary chloride excretion is less than 10 mEq/L.

Low CO_2 content

A low CO_2 content occurs in conditions associated with metabolic acidosis such as uremic acidosis, diabetic ketoacidosis, lactic acidosis, and renal tubular acidosis. However, if the arterial blood pH is determined and found to be elevated (alkalosis), a low CO_2 content would indicate respiratory alkalosis as seen in the hyperventilation syndrome.

Metabolic acidosis and the anion gap. In the serum the cations and anions should be more or less equal for a neutral pH. The measurable electrolytes contributing to this anion-cation electroneutrality are sodium, chloride, and bicarbonate. Potassium, being an intracellular ion, contributes minimally and is usually not considered. The term "anion gap" refers to the number of unmeasured anions, which is calculated by subtracting chloride and bicarbonate from the sodium concentration. With normal electrolytes, there is usually an anion gap of approximately 12.

Metabolic acidosis is commonly divided into two groups, normal anion gap and increased anion gap.

Metabolic acidosis with a normal anion gap is usually caused by diarrhea with loss of bicarbonate, chronic interstitial nephritis, mild renal failure, renal tubular acidosis with hyperchloremia, urethrosigmoidostomy, therapeutic ammonium chloride, or acetazolamide.

Metabolic acidosis with an increased anion gap is usually caused by diabetic ketoacidosis, lactic acidosis, azotemic renal failure, and ingestion of toxins such as salicylates, ethylene glycol, paraldehyde, and methyl alcohol.

2

ROUTINE HEMATOLOGY SCREENING

In a complete blood count (CBC) a routine hematology screening includes the following determinations: white blood cell count (WBC), red blood cell count (RBC), hematocrit (Hct), hemoglobin (Hgb), and differential white cell count (Diff). The differential states the neutrophils, lymphocytes, monocytes, eosinophils, basophils, and any abnormal cells as a percent of the total WBC count.

A complete hematologic examination also includes the indices, which are mean cell volume (MCV), mean cell hemoglobin (MCH), and mean cell hemoglobin concentration (NCHC). In addition, a careful inspection of the peripheral blood smear is important, as is a sedimentation rate (Sed rate or ESR).

With an accurate determination of these values, approximately 70% to 80% of the hematologic diagnosis can be made, as well as a significant amount of information gathered for the purpose either of evaluating the stages of a particular disease or of diagnosing some disease entities not directly related to the hematopoietic system.

Each hematologic measurement will be discussed separately. However, it should be emphasized that since the elements of the blood are closely interrelated, absolute values can be meaningless if the whole hematologic examination is not taken into consideration. For example, a WBC count without a differential may be normal, even in the presence of severe sepsis. In this case, a differential would reveal an extreme increase in the percentage of segmented bands.

WHITE BLOOD CELL COUNT (WBC)

The white blood cell count expresses the number of WBCs in 1 microliter of whole blood. The correct WBC count can be obtained by multiplying the figure obtained from the automated Coulter counter by 1000. For example, a

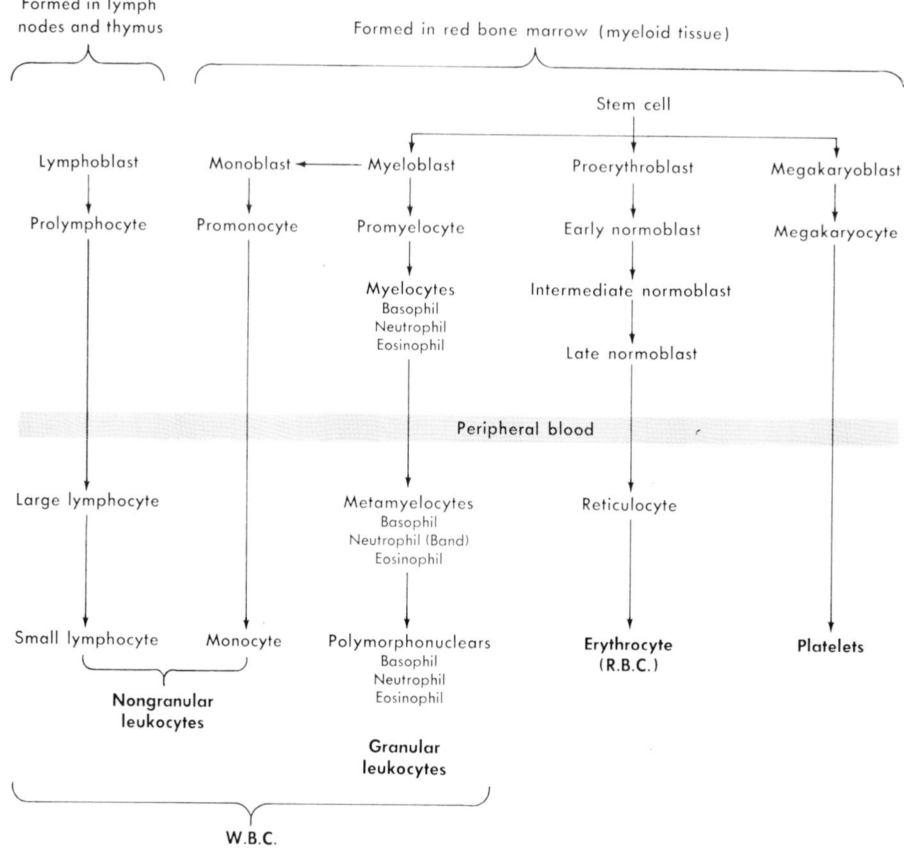

FIG. 2-1
The development of the various formed elements of the blood. In the adult, red blood cells, the granular white blood cells, monocytes, and platelets are formed in the bone marrow. The lymphocytes are formed mainly in the lymph nodes and thymus.

WBC count reported to be 7.25 should be interpreted as 7250 WBCs per microliter of whole blood.

Absolute determination of the leukocytes (total white blood cells) gives only partial information. Unless an accurate differential white cell count is done, significant pathology or information can be missed, as in the case cited above.

White blood cells (leukocytes) are either granular or nongranular. The granular leukocytes are the basophils, neutrophils, and eosinophils. The nongranular leukocytes are the lymphocytes and monocytes. (See Fig. 2-1.)

Granulocytes

Neutrophils, eosinophils, and basophils are formed from stem cells in the bone marrow. Their nuclei have two to five or more lobes, and they are therefore called polymorphonuclear. Neutrophils are so named because they stain with neutral dyes. Eosinophils stain with acid dye and basophils stain with basic dyes.

In a healthy person, the number of granulocytes is regulated at a constant level. However, when infection occurs, the number in the blood rises dramatically. When bacteria invade the body, the bone marrow is stimulated to produce and release large numbers of neutrophils, which are phagocytic. The basophils contain heparin, but their role is uncertain. Eosinophils phagocytize antigen-antibody complexes. Therefore, in patients with allergic diseases the circulating eosinophil level is often elevated.

Nongranular leukocytes

Monocytes arise in the bone marrow and migrate into inflammatory exudates, but not as rapidly as the neutrophils. Monocytosis is seen in chronic inflammatory disorders.

Lymphocytes are formed in the thymus, in lymph nodes, and in bone marrow. Lymphocytes derived from the thymus (T cell lymphocytes) are longer-lived than those derived from the lymph nodes and bone marrow (M cell lymphocytes). The small lymphocytes are capable of producing a specific antibody in response to an antigenic challenge.

Normal WBC count

The normal WBC count is usually between 4500 and 11,000/cu mm and may vary in a particular individual at different times of the day. A minor variation outside the normal range is not significant as long as the differential count and the peripheral blood smear are both normal. However, some early disorder, whether infectious or myeloproliferative, is not necessarily ruled out.

Mild to moderate leukocytosis (11,000-17,000/cu mm)

Mild to moderate elevation of the WBC count usually indicates infectious disease, mainly of bacterial etiology. Usually, the leukocytosis increases with the severity of the infection. However, there are exceptions to this rule, particularly in elderly patients in whom severe sepsis can coexist with only a modest leukocytosis. As mentioned previously, the differential WBC count is of additional help.

Leukemoid reaction

Occasionally such massive leukocytosis accompanies a systemic disease that the blood picture of leukemia is simulated. When a blood picture looks like leukemia but is not, the term "leukemoid reaction" is used. Severe sepsis, miliary tuberculosis, and other nonmalignant infectious conditions are among the more common causes.

In the differentiation of myelogenous leukemia versus leukemoid reaction determination of the leukocyte alkaline phosphatase is helpful. This enzyme is high in leukemoid reaction and is decreased in myelogenous leukemia. Also, the presence of Philadelphia antigen is specific for the majority of cases of chronic myeloid leukemia.

Leukopenia

A decreased absolute WBC count (leukopenia) can be mild (3000-5000/cu mm), moderate (1500-3000/cu mm), or extremely severe (<1500/cu mm), and may be associated with diminution of the WBC count as a whole, decreases in neutrophils, or diminution of all the blood particles (pancytopenia).

Leukopenia associated with neutropenia

The most common causes of a mild to moderate decrease in neutrophils are:

1. Familial benign neutropenia, usually accompanied by moderate monocytosis up to 50%
2. Acute viral infections
3. Starvation neutropenia (anorexia nervosa)
4. Primary and secondary splenic neutropenia associated with Felty's syndrome, portal hypertension, lymphoma, and some specific bacterial and protozoal infections
5. Drug-induced neutropenia, with the following drugs implicated: phenothiazines (Thorazine group), antithyroid drugs, sulfonamides, phenylbutazone, chloramphenicol, phenindione, and aminophylline, or their derivatives
6. Excessive ingestion of alcohol

Leukopenia associated with eosinopenia

The most common causes of mild to moderate decrease in eosinophils are acute and chronic stress, either emotional or somatic; and endocrine causes such as excess ACTH, cortisone, or epinephrine, intermenstrual period, certain diurnal variations, and acromegaly.

Granulocytopenia

From a practical point of view, one determination of neutrophenia in the absence of any other indication of disease should be regarded as benign, possibly diurnal, or maybe stress related. However, granulocytopenia associated with any other disease states should be evaluated according to the following causes:

1. Acute hypersensitive reactions
2. Steroids (ACTH, thyroxine, epinephrine, estrogen)
3. Diurnal changes

4. Hyperthyroidism
5. Pituitary basophilism
6. Radiation therapy
7. Acute and chronic infection
8. Ovulation
9. Pregnancy
10. Aging
11. Megaloblastic anemia

The differential count

The differential count is performed on a peripheral blood smear for the purpose of identifying the different types of leukocytes. Red blood cell and platelet morphology can also be evaluated in this way.

Among the leukocytes, the neutrophils are usually the most abundant cells seen on the peripheral smear, comprising 56% of the total white blood cell count. Normally, 2.7% will be eosinophils, 0.3% will be basophils, and 34% will be lymphocytes.

When an extremely high leukocytosis is reported, one should very carefully inspect the peripheral smear. An accurate differential count may be enough to make the diagnosis of myelocytic leukemia or lymphocytic leukemia.

A thorough examination of the peripheral blood smear should routinely include the following:

1. A diligent search should be made for abnormal lymphocytes and monocytes that may indicate some specific disease such as infectious mononucleosis. This disease is diagnosed by the Downey cells found in the peripheral smear.
2. An extreme shift to the left implies a significant number of early neutrophils and band forms rather than lobulations. This shift will indicate some kind of acute stress on the bone marrow or severe bacterial disease causing the release of an early granulocytic series and will, at the same time, give the interpreter some indication of the stage and severity of the disease.
3. Abnormal granulations in the leukocytes may give an index of toxicity generated by a specific disease (toxic granulation).
4. In examining the leukocytes, one may gain significant information by counting the lobulations of hypersegmented neutrophils. Hyperlobulation (from three to six) or segmentation of neutrophils is suggestive of vitamin B_{12} deficiency or folic acid deficiency.

Neutrophilic leukocytosis

The most commonly encountered conditions that manifest a mild to moderate leukocytosis of neutrophilic origin are the bacterial infections, inflammatory disorders, tumors, physical and emotional stimuli, stresses, and drugs.

The bacterial infections are usually moderately severe bacterial pneumonias or systemic infections, which are sometimes coccal.

The inflammatory but noninfectious diseases causing neutrophilic leukocytosis are rheumatic fever, collagen disease, rheumatoid arthritis, vasculitis, pancreatitis, thyroiditis, and tumors and carcinomas, particularly gastric, bronchogenic, uterine, pancreatic, squamous cell, lymphatic, and those of Hodgkin's disease. Additional conditions are burns, crush injury, infarctions, and poisoning with carbon monoxide or lead.

Stresses that produce neutrophilic leukocytosis can be extreme cold, heat, exercise, electroshock therapy, and the emotional stimuli of fear, panic, and anxiety.

Drugs that can cause neutrophilia are catecholamines, corticosteroids, lithium, methysergide, niacine, niacinamide, and others.

The catabolic disorders causing neutrophilia are diabetic acidosis, acute gout, thyroiditis, uremia, Cushing's syndrome, and a few hereditary conditions such as familial neutrophilia.

Eosinophilic leukocytosis

In eosinophilic leukocytosis most of the cells causing the elevated WBC count are eosinophils. Anywhere from 5% to 90% can be seen, although the most frequently encountered pattern in eosinophilic leukocytosis is an eosinophil count of approximately 10% to 20%. The associated diseases are the following:

1. The most common causes of an increase in eosinophils are allergic disorders of nearly any kind, such as hay fever, asthma, angioneurotic edema, and serum sickness.
2. Parasitic diseases should be considered second in commonality to allergic conditions. *Trichinella* predominates in the United States. Malaria and amebiasis are also possibilities, particularly in view of widespread travel. *Ascaris* is the most common parasite in Middle Eastern countries. Other parasites associated with eosinophilia are ameba, hookworm, *Schistosoma*, and *Toxoplasma*. In making the differential diagnosis of eosinophilic leukocytosis, particularly when parasites are a consideration, the epidemiology of the suspected disease and the area in which the patient has traveled become of prime importance.
3. Other rarer conditions associated with mild to moderate eosinophilia are malignant conditions such as mycosis fungoides, brain tumors, Hodgkin's disease, and other lymphomas. Gastrointestinal causes include colitis and protein-losing enteropathy. In hypoadrenocorticism, eosinophilia may be found and may suggest the diagnosis of Addison's disease if other features of the disease are found.

4. An extremely high eosinophil count in the range of 80% to 90% usually indicates eosinophilic granulomatosis or eosinophilic leukemia.

Basophilic leukocytosis

An elevated WBC count associated with basophilia is uncommon and most frequently suggests some kind of myeloproliferative disease such as myelofibrosis, agnogenic myeloid metaplasia, and polycythemia vera. A rapid fall in the basophil count may be heralded an anaphylactic reaction.

Lymphocytosis

Lymphocytosis may be mild to severe and occurs in two varieties: relative, in which the total number of circulating lymphocytes is unchanged but the WBC count is low because of neutropenia; and absolute, in which the number of circulating lymphocytes increases. Relative lymphocytosis accompanies most conditions mentioned in the section on leukopenia associated with neutropenia.

The most common cause of severe lymphocytosis (80% to 90% mature lymphocytes) is chronic lymphocytic leukemia. This is associated with a marked elevation of the leukocyte count.

Marked lymphocytosis with moderate leukocytosis is found in infectious diseases, particularly pertussis, infectious mononucleosis, and acute infectious lymphocytosis.

Mild to moderate relative lymphocytosis is seen mainly in viral infections with exanthema such as measles, rubella, chicken pox, and roseola infantum.

In bacterial infections, mild to moderate lymphocytosis associated with mild to moderate leukocytosis usually indicates a chronic infectious state. Depending on the overall presenting picture other considerations are brucellosis, typhoid and paratyphoid fever, and chronic granulomatous diseases such as tuberculosis.

In noninfectious disorders and nonmyeloproliferative diseases, thyrotoxicosis and adrenal insufficiency (Addison's disease) are associated with mild to moderate lymphocytosis.

Relative lymphocytosis is a normal occurrence in infants and children between 4 months and 4 years of age.

RED BLOOD CELL COUNT (RBC)

Red blood cells (erythrocytes) are formed in the red bone marrow. Their production (erythropoiesis) is inhibited by a rise in the circulating red cell level and stimulated by anemia and hypoxia. The hormone erythropoietin mediates the responses to these normal and abnormal situations. (Tissue hypoxia is the ultimate stimulus for erythropoietin production.)

The red blood cells contain a complex compound called hemoglobin, which is made up of heme, a pigmented compound containing iron, and globin, a colorless protein. Hemoglobin binds with oxygen (a reversible reaction) and can also combine with carbon dioxide. Thus the red blood cell functions primarily to transport oxygen to the tissues and to carry carbon dioxide to the lungs.

The red blood cell (RBC) count represents the number of RBCs in 1 microliter of whole blood. The correct RBC count can be obtained by multiplying the figure obtained from the automated Coulter counter by 1 million. For example, an RBC count reported to be 5.11 should be interpreted as 5,110,000 RBCs in 1 microliter of blood.

In the past, the determination of the red blood cell count was tedious and occasionally erroneous. Thus the determination of the hematocrit and hemoglobin were adopted for routine use. However, because of the development of automated methods, particularly the Coulter counter, routine hematologic determinations are now quick and accurate. The RBC count is, however, still not used as much as the hemoglobin and hematocrit determinations, which are also part of the Coulter panel.

Normal RBC count

The normal RBC count is between 4.6 and 6.2 $\times$ 10^6 per microliter for men, 4.2 and 5.4 $\times$ 10^6 per microliter for women, 5.0 and 5.1 $\times$ 10^6 for infants, and 4.6 to 4.8 $\times$ 10^6 in children.

The main value of the RBC count in a routine screening examination lies in the gross evaluation of the indices, which are also obtained through automated means, either directly through a writeout from the Coulter counter or through the automatic analyzer.

The erythrocyte indices

The relationship between the number, size, and hemoglobin content of the RBCs is important in accurately describing anemias. An index of these elements may be obtained from an inspection of the stained peripheral blood smear.

Terminology (the peripheral blood smear)

hematocrit (Hct) is the volume of packed red blood cells found in 100 ml of blood. For example, a value of 46% implies that there are 46 ml of red blood cells in 100 ml of blood. The normal Hct in the male is 40% to 54%; in the female it is 38% to 47%.

hemoglobin (Hgb) is the oxygen-carrying pigment of the red blood cells and is reported in grams per 100 ml. For example, a value of 15.5 implies that there are 15.5 gm of hemoglobin in each 100 ml of blood. The normal hemoglobin in the male is 13.5 to 18.0 gm/100 ml; in the female it is 12.0 to 16.0 gm/100 ml. In infants the normal hemoglobin is 12.2 to 20.0 gm/100 ml, and in children it is 11.2 to 13.4 gm/100 ml.

mean cell volume (MCV) describes the red cells in terms of individual cell size. It is given usually as a direct writeout from the automated system. However, it can also be calculated by dividing the volume of packed cells (hematocrit) by the number of RBCs. The result is expressed as microcubic millimeters per red cell. The normal MCV is 82 to 98 cu microns.

mean cell hemoglobin concentration (MCHC) measures the concentration of hemoglobin in grams per 100 ml of RBCs. This can be done by dividing the hemoglobin in grams by the hematocrit. The percentage is obtained by multiplying this figure by 100. The normal MCHC is 32% to 36%.

mean cell hemoglobin (MCH) is the hemoglobin content of each individual red blood cell and is calculated by dividing the hemoglobin by the red blood cell count. It is expressed as micromicrograms or picograms of hemoglobin per red blood cell. The normal MCH is 27 to 31 pg.

Examining the peripheral smear

Platelets. Platelets are important in blood coagulation and are visible on stained blood smears. Their absolute absence from the peripheral smear is extremely significant indicating an aplastic bone marrow. Decreased numbers of platelets (thrombocytopenia) may be caused by various conditions.

Sometimes a careful observation of the peripheral smear is a better indication of the platelet status than is an absolute platelet count. This observation is easy to do, quick, and accurate. The shape and character of the platelets are also important. When an abnormality is noted it is termed thrombocytopathy (abnormal-looking thrombocytes). Thrombocytosis is the term used when there is an unusually large number of platelets in the blood. This will be seen most often in the blood smear of polycythemia, in essential thrombocytosis, and in persons who have had splenectomies.

Polycythemia

Polycythemia is any condition in which the number of circulating erythrocytes rises above normal. When the red cell mass increases in response to an identifiable physiologic or pathologic stimulus, the condition is called secondary polycythemia. If no etiology can be documented, the change is considered primary, and is described as polycythemia vera (true polycythemia).

Polycythemia vera, according to some authorities, is equivalent to leukemia and in some cases does progress into one of the myeloproliferative diseases.

Secondary polycythemia has been found in erythropoietin-secreting tumors, hypernephroma, renal cysts, and hepatic carcinoma. It has also been associated with chronic obstructive pulmonary disease and cyanotic congenital heart disease with hypoxemia, and is accompanied by an elevated erythrpoietin level.

Erythropoietin, a hormone thought to be formed by the action of a renal factor on a plasma globulin, stimulates the proliferation and release of RBCs from the bone marrow into the peripheral circulation. One of the most sensitive ways of differentiating between primary and secondary polycythemia is the determination of the erythropoietin level. This level is diminished in polycythemia vera because the excess number of RBCs produced in this disease suppresses the production of the hormone. The level is elevated in secondary polycythemia.

In the differential diagnosis of polycythemia vera versus other polycythemias, the most important diagnostic test is the total red cell volume measured by the chromium tagging technique. In this test the red cell volume is increased in polycythemia vera but not in other polycythemic states.

Normal absolute RBC count and the peripheral smear

Findings on the blood film may suggest a disorder when the absolute RBC count is within normal limits, such as may occur in the following.

1. Significant spherocytosis, polychromatophilia, and erythrocyte agglutination suggest compensated, acquired hemolytic anemia.
2. Spherocytosis with polychromatophilia is very suggestive of hereditary spherocytosis.
3. Target cells are found mainly in hemoglobin C disease and liver disease.
4. Marked hypochromia associated with target cells is suggestive of thalassemia major or thalassemia minor.
5. Erythrocytes with basophilic stipplings are characteristic of lead poisoning.
6. Macrocytosis in association with hypersegmented neutrophils suggests vitamin B_{12} and/or folic acid deficiency.
7. Rouleaux formation suggests multiple myeloma or macroglobulinemia.
8. Parasites in RBCs are the distinguishing characteristic of malaria.
9. Schistocytes and "burr" cells in association with a decreased platelet count suggest consumption coagulopathy.
10. Mechanical hemolysis is suggested by schistocytes and "burr" cells.
11. A relative increase in neutrophils with increased band forms and toxic granulations suggests severe infection.
12. Atypical lymphocytes indicate the possibility of infectious mononucleosis.
13. Decreased neutrophils and increased lymphocytes suggest agranulocytosis.
14. Eosinophilia usually suggests an allergic reaction.
15. Blast (primitive) forms indicate the possibility of acute leukemia.

Anemia

Anemia is a deficiency of the total hemoglobin red cell mass is the result of many disorders. Usually anemias are classified into three broad categories:

1. Hypochromic microcytic anemia
2. Normochromic normocytic anemia
3. Macrocytic normochromic, hypochromic, or hyperchromic anemia

Terminology

normochromic normal color (normal hemoglobin content)
hypochromic less than normal color (decreased hemoglobin content)
hyperchromic more than normal color (increased hemoglobin content)
normocytic normal cell size
microcytic smaller than normal cell size
macrocytic larger than normal cell size

Hypochromic microcytic anemia

Iron deficiency. The most frequent cause of hypochromic microcytic anemia is iron deficiency. The patient may or may not have an overt anemia. However, a borderline low hematocrit and hemoglobin, even though the RBC count is normal, should suggest the possibility of hypochromic microcytic anemia. Although the number of cells may be within normal limits, there is a definite diminution in the size of the RBCs as well as in the hemoglobin concentration.

For a more definitive diagnosis of iron deficiency the serum iron level is checked. In an iron deficient state the serum iron will be low with an elevated iron binding capacity. Additionally, serum ferritin levels seem to correlate well with total body iron stores and thus may obviate the need for either bone marrow studies for determination of total body iron levels or for liver biopsy for iron stain evaluations. A low serum ferritin level associated with a low serum iron and a low binding capacity may indicate a decrease in total body iron levels.

Diseases associated with hypochromia and microcytosis, with low iron and increased iron body stores, are chronic infections, malignancies, and chronic kidney disease.

NORMAL SERUM IRON

50-150 μg/dl

NORMAL IRON-BINDING CAPACITY

250-450 μg/dl

NORMAL SERUM FERRITIN

Female: 5-280 μg/dl
Male: 10-270 μg/dl

The hemoglobinopathies. This term is used to describe the clinical syndromes produced in persons having production of abnormal types of hemoglobin resulting from genetic reasons. The most important of these syndromes are thalassemia major and thalassemia minor (Mediterranean anemia), sickle cell anemia, and hemoglobin C disease. The blood picture of the hemoglobinopathies simulate that of iron deficiency anemia on the peripheral smear. However,the bone marrow stores, serum iron level, and iron binding capacity will differentiate between the two.

Normochromic normocytic anemia

The most common cause of normocytic normochromic anemia is an acute loss of red blood cell mass such as occurs in hemorrhage or hemolysis.

Hypoplastic anemia. Another major group of normochromic normocytic anemias are the aplastic or hypoplastic anemias. In some very rare situations a combination of macrocytic and microcytic anemia may produce a normal index. Such a situation will occur in vitamin B_{12} deficiency anemia associated with carcinoma of the stomach and chronic blood loss. However, the overall clinical picture and other clues on the blood smear (multisegmented leukocytes and mild hemolysis) will suggest the correct pathology.

Macrocytic anemia

In macrocytic anemia there is a decreased absolute number of RBCs per cubic micrometer. However, the individual cells are larger in diameter and volume and contain more hemoglobin than normal. Consequently, there will be an elevated MCV and MCHC.

The two most common diseases associated with macrocytosis with significant anemia are folic acid deficiency and vitamin B_{12} deficiency, which is also known as Addisonian or pernicious anemia. These two conditions are also associated with megaloblastic changes in the bone marrow.

Some macrocytosis is also observed in the anemia of myxedema, as well as in the anemias following acute blood loss, either through bleeding or hemolysis. The latter two conditions are not accompanied by megaloblastic changes in the bone marrow since the macrocytosis reflects increased reticulocytes, which are slightly larger than normal RBCs.

Macrocytic normochromic anemia is also seen in some cases of chronic liver disease, hypothyroidism, and aplastic anemia.

In the differential diagnosis among folic acid deficiency, macrocytic or megaloblastic anemia, and Addisonian or pernicious anemias, the determination of the levels of B_{12} and folic acid in the blood and the Schilling test are the most widely used. The Schilling test is described on p. 147.

Sedimentation rate (sed rate or ESR)

The sedimentation rate is the speed with which RBCs settle in uncoagulated blood. This rate is affected by many factors too numerous to mention in this book. It is, therefore, a nonspecific test, having neither organ nor disease specificity. Its chief value lies in the fact that a normal value does diminish the probability of a significant disease process, giving some reassurance to the investigator. An abnormal result indicates that a more extensive search is necessary.

In addition to its general screening value, the sed rate is useful in following the progress of certain diseases such as rheumatic fever. A gradually diminishing sed rate indicates a better prognosis, whereas a gradually increasing rate indicates a poorer prognosis.

NORMAL SEDIMENTATION RATE (WESTERGREN)

Men under 50 yrs:	<15 mm/hr
Men over 50 yrs:	<20 mm/hr
Women under 50 yrs.:	<20 mm/hr
Women over 50 yrs:	<30 mm/hr

3

URINALYSIS

The urine examination, properly performed, may give valuable information.

The urine that is to be analyzed should be a clean catch (midstream) specimen collected in a clean, dry container and examined as quickly as possible, preferably within 2 hours. It should be a morning specimen and the patient should not have had fluids for 12 hours preceding the collection of the urine. Urine becomes alkaline on standing, bacteria multiply, and leukocytes and casts disintegrate.

The standard urinalysis includes pH, specific gravity, the presence or absence of glucose and ketones, protein semiquantitation, and microscopic examination of the centrifuged urinary sediment.

pH (ACIDITY OR ALKALINITY)

Normal fresh urine is usually acid, with a pH of 4.6 to 8. If the specimen has not been standing too long, the pH will reflect the patient's acid-base balance.

An alkaline urine is seen in metabolic alkalosis. The exception to this is long-standing hypokalemic chloremic alkalosis, in which a potassium deficiency causes the renal tubular cells to secrete hydrogen ions in lieu of potassium. A paradoxical aciduria is the result. This situation (metabolic alkalosis with aciduria) may suggest generalized intracellular acidosis.

SPECIFIC GRAVITY (SG)

NORMAL SPECIFIC GRAVITY

1.016-1.022 (normal fluid intake)
1.001-1.035 (range)

The specific gravity of a morning urine specimen voided by a fasting patient reflects the maximum concentrating ability of the kidney. In the absence of formed elements, protein, or glycosuria, the specific gravity in a clear urine should be 1.025 to 1.030. Anything below this value reflects distal renal tubular disease and inability of the kidney to concentrate urine to the maximum. Endocrine disease associated with insufficient ADH secretions is also a possibility.

A fixed specific gravity indicates chronic glomerulopyelonephritis.

A long-standing hypokalemic and hypercalcemic nephropathy, in which the patient has symptoms of frequency, nocturia, and polyuria can be easily diagnosed by a proper examination of the urine for specific gravity and osmolality. The specimen should be collected after overnight fasting. If simultaneous serum and urine osmolality determinations are performed, the serum osmolality will be high while the urine osmolality will be relatively low.

GLUCOSE

When a urine specimen voided in the morning is free of glucose, diabetes mellitus is not ruled out because, normally, a blood sugar of 130 to 140 mg/100 ml is necessary before traces of glucose appear in the urine.

Glucosuria means one of two things: diabetes mellitus or a low renal threshold for glucose resorption if the blood glucose level is normal.

PROTEIN

The absence of protein in the urine, particularly in a concentrated urine, rules out significant renal glomerular disease. The presence of protein in the urine indicates the possibility of any one of a large number of diseases, the differential diagnosis of which will be discussed in Chapter 6, pp. 127 to 132.

When there is a trace of protein in the urine, a follow-up is indicated. However, if there is more than a trace, 24-hour urine excretion of protein should be ascertained. For a more specific diagnosis, a quantitative analysis of the kind of protein, be it albumin, one of the globulins, or Bence Jones proteins, should be performed.

MICROSCOPIC EXAMINATION OF SEDIMENT

Normally, a microscopic examination of the sediment in the urine will show fewer than one or two RBCs, one or two WBCs, and only an occasional cast. Anything more is considered pathologic. Urine microscopy is especially important in making the diagnosis of acute pyelonephritis, the classical findings of which are numerous WBCs, WBC casts, and bacteria.

Casts

Casts are formed in the kidney tubules by the agglutination of protein cells, or cellular debris. Their presence in the urine implies tubular or glomerular disorders. Because casts are cylindrical structures, their occurrence in the urine is sometimes called cylindruria. Since protein is necessary for cast formation, proteinuria often accompanies cylindruria.

WBC casts indicate pyelonephritis, and sometimes are also found in the exudative stage of acute glomerulonephritis. RBC casts may appear colorless if only a few RBCs are present. However, they are often yellow. Their presence indicates glomerulonephritis.

Epithelial casts may be difficult to distinguish from leukocyte or mixed-cell casts. When they are seen together with red blood cells and lipids in the casts, glomerulonephritis is suggested.

A coarsely granular cast is the result of the first step in the disintegration of the WBC or epithelial cell cast. If disintegration continues, the coarse granules break down to small granules, forming the finely granular cast. The next step is the formation of what is known as the waxy cast, which is translucent and shaped by the tubule where it was formed.

Hyaline casts are clear, colorless cylinders made up of protein. They pass almost unchanged down the tubules. They may be coarsely or finely granular depending upon the degenerative changes that took place in the tubules. The appearance of hyaline casts alone is usually a sudden, mild, and temporary phenomenon and must be correlated with other clinical findings.

Urine that is loaded with hyaline casts and protein is suggestive of the nephrotic syndrome, since they are seen in concentrated acid urine high in protein.

Red blood cells

The appearance of red blood cells in the urine is an indication of bleeding after the blood has passed through the glomeruli and tubules, such as would occur with hemorrhagic cystitis or calculi in the renal pelvis. Another possibility is disease of the renal collecting and tubular systems, such as tuberculosis or tumors.

Telescoping

Urine sediment that shows different stages of glomerular nephritis (acute and subacute) and that also has the findings of the nephrotic syndrome is called "telescoping" of the urine. Such a sediment is seen in lupus nephritis.

Crystals

The type of crystals found in normal urine varies with the pH of the specimen. Calcium oxalate, uric acid, and urate crystals may be seen in acid urine. Phosphate and carbonate crystals and amorphous phosphates are often seen in alkaline urine.

Calcium oxalate crystals, if numerous, may suggest hypercalcemia.

APPEARANCE

The color of the urine is not usually reported in the routine urinalysis and should be specifically requested if a rare diagnosis is suspected.

The normal urine is golden yellow. A darker color suggests hematuria, hemoglobinuria, bilirubinuria, urobilinuria, or porphyria. Tests specifically directed toward the cause of these entities should be ordered.

A urine that changes to a bright burgundy red when exposed to the light is highly suggestive of porphyria.

Tea-colored urine that stains the underwear indicates the possibility of obstructive jaundice with urobilinogen in the urine.

The fruity aroma of a diabetic urine and the red discoloration of the urine in patients taking pyridium are two well-known diagnostic clues commonly encountered in the emergency room.

APPENDIX TO UNIT ONE

Common variances in the routine screening panel and clinical implications

This appendix contains some of the most common variances found in the routine screening examination and the clinical implications or potential disease condition that may exist. Generally speaking, a variance in one value has more significance when compared with the results of the total examination.

This appendix has been provided so that the reader can more easily determine what further action is indicated when there is a variance from a normal value. The last column refers the reader to the page on which are found additional tests for the evaluation or confirmation of a suspected disease condition.

Text continued on p. 59.

Test	Abbreviation	Normal value	Variance	Clinical implication	Subsequent laboratory studies, comments, and/or conclusive symptoms
Alkaline phosphatase (total serum)	alk phos	Adults: 1.5-4.5 U/dl (Bodansky) 4-13 U/ml (King-Armstrong) 0.8-2.3 U/ml (Bessey-Lowry) 15-35 U/ml (Shinowara-Jones-Reinhart) Children: 5.0-14.0 U/dl (Bodanksy) 3.4-9.0 U/ml (Bessey-Lowry) 15-30 U/dl (King-Armstrong)	↑ (marked) with liver disease (bilirubinemia)	Early obstructive jaundice	pp. 153-160
			↑ (marked) without liver disease	Paget's disease of bone	Bone x ray
			↑ (marked)	Carcinoma with bone metastasis	Bone scan
			↑ (moderate) with liver disease	Cholangeolitic hepatitis	p. 154
			↑ (mild) with liver disease	Liver cirrhosis with active hepatitis	pp. 159-160
			↑ (mild) without liver disease and with hypercalcemia	Hyperparathyroidism	p. 172
			↑ (mild to moderate) with N or ↓ Ca	Osteomalacia	History, physical, and x rays
Bilirubin (serum)		Up to 0.3 mg/dl (direct or conjugated) 0.1-1.0 mg/dl (indirect or unconjugated) Total: 0.1-1.2 mg/dl Newborn total: 1-12 mg/dl	↑ indirect or unconjugated, with reticulocytes, absent urine bilirubin	Low grade hemolytic disease	p. 188
			↑ indirect or unconjugated with normal liver function	Gilbert's disease	p. 155
			↑ direct or conjugated with abnormal albumin, globulin and enzymes	Parenchymal liver disease, obstructive liver disease	pp. 153-160
			↑ (marked) indirect or unconjugated	Massive hemolysis	p. 194
			↑ (marked) direct or conjugated	Obstructive jaundice: obstructive phase of hepatitis, cholangeitis, lower biliary tract obstruction (carcinoma or calculus)	pp. 153-160

N = normal
↑ = elevated
↓ = depressed

Continued.

Test	Abbreviation	Normal value	Variance	Clinical implication	Subsequent laboratory studies, comments, and/or conclusive symptoms
Calcium (serum)	Ca	Ionized: 4.2-5.2 mg/dl; 2.1-2.6 mEq/L or 50-58% of total; Total: 9.0-10.6 mg/dl; 4.5-5.3 mEq/L; Infants: 11-13 mg/dl	N with marked ↓ albumin	Hypercalcemia	See hypercalcemia
			N with ↑ BUN	Primary hyperparathyroidism, secondary hyperparathyroidism	p. 172
			↑ with ↓ phosphorus and N BUN	Hyperparathyroidism	p. 172
			↑ with ↑ gamma globulin	Sarcoidosis, multiple myeloma, malignancies with possible metastasis to bone	Biopsy
			↑ with metabolic alkalosis	Milk-alkali syndrome	History of peptic ulcer disease
			↑	Severe thyrotoxicosis	p. 167
			↑	Malignant tumors with or without bone metastasis	X-ray; alkaline phosphatase
			↑	Bone fractures	History, physical, and x rays
			↑ with ↑ alk phos	Paget's disease of bone	X-ray
			↓ with ↓ albumin fraction of serum protein	Pseudohypocalcemia	X-ray
			↓ with ↑ phosphorus, N BUN, N creat	Hypoparathyroidism	p. 173
			↓	Osteomalacia (adults), rickets (children)	History, physical, and x-rays
			↓	Malabsorption syndrome	p. 148
			↓	Acute pancreatitis	p. 161
			↓	Pregnancy	History and physical
			↓	Diuretics	History
			↓	Respiratory alkalosis	Blood gases, p. 108
Carbon dioxide content (plasma serum, venous)	CO_2 content	24-30 mM/L	↑ without chronic obstructive lung disease and frequently with ↓ K and ↓ Cl	Hypokalemic-chloremic alkalosis (serum alkalosis and intracellular acidosis)	24 hr Cl

			↓	Uremic acidosis	Blood gases, p. 108
			↓	Diabetic ketoacidosis	Glucose tolerance test
			↓	Lactic acidosis	Serum lactic acid levels
			↓ with ↓ K and ↑ Cl	Renal tubular acidosis	Anion gap, p. 25
			↓	Respiratory alkalosis (hyperventilation syndrome)	p. 108 (blood pH)
Chloride	Cl	95-103 mEq/L	↑ with ↓ CO_2 content and ↓ K	Renal tubular acidosis, iatrogenic (tube feeding and inappropriate IV fluids)	Anion gap, p. 25
			↓ with ↑ CO_2 content, and NK	Potassium-saving diuretics	History
			↓ with ↓ K and ↑ CO_2 content	Hypokalemic-chloremic alkalosis	24 hr Cl
Cholesterol (total serum)	Chol	150-250 mg/dl (varies with diet and age)	↑ (marked) with ↑ alk phos and ↑ bilirubin	Liver disease with biliary obstruction	pp. 153-160
			↑ (marked) with ↑ BUN and ↑ creat	Nephrotic stage of glomerulonephritis	p. 127
			↑ (marked)	Familial hypercholesterolemia	p. 82
			↓ (marked)	Diet and malnutrition	History and physical
			↓ (marked)	Extensive liver disease	p. 154
			↓ (marked)	Hyperthyroidism	p. 171
Creatinine	Creat	0.6-1.2 mg/dl	↑	Kidney disease with $>$50% destruction of nephrons	p. 129
Blood glucose	Gluc	70-110 mg/dl	↑	Diabetes mellitus	History and glucose tolerance test
		60-100 mg/dl	↑ mild with ↑ blood catecholamines	Acute stress, pheochromocytoma	History, p. 180

Continued.

BLOOD CHEMISTRY—cont'd

Test	Abbreviation	Normal value	Variance	Clinical implication	Subsequent laboratory studies, comments, and/or conclusive symptoms
Blood glucose—cont'd			↑ (mild) with ↑ glucocorticoids	Cushing's syndrome (hyperadrenalism), Cushing's disease (secondary hyperadrenalism)	p. 181
			↑ (mild) with ↓ cholesterolemia	Hyperthyroidism	p. 167
			↑ (mild)	Diuretics	History
			↑ (mild)	Acute and chronic pancreatic insufficiency	Malabsorption, p. 145
			↑ (moderate)	Diabetes mellitus	History and glucose tolerance test
			↑ (marked) with ↓ CO_2 content	Uncontrolled diabetes and ketoacidosis	Electrolytes
			↑ (marked) with N CO_2 content and hypernatremia	Nonketotic, nonacidotic hyperglycemia	Electrolytes
			↓	Pancreatic islet cell tumor	p. 161
			↓	Large nonpancreatic tumor	IVP and laminograms
			↓	Pituitary hypofunction	p. 186
			↓ with hyperkalemia, hyponatremia, and ↑ BUN	Addison's disease (adrenocortical hypofunction)	p. 177
			↓	Extensive liver disease	pp. 153-160
			↓	Reactive hypoglycemia	5-hour glucose tolerance test, p. 83
Lactic dehydrogenase (serum)	LDH	80-120 Wacker units 150-450 Wroblewski units 71-207 IU/L	↑ (marked)	Myocardial infarction	p. 63
			↑ (marked)	Hemolytic disorders (pernicious anemia)	p. 194
			↑ (mild)	Chronic viral hepatitis	p. 159
			↑ (mild)	Pneumonia, pulmonary emboli	Chest x ray, pp. 106, 111
			↑ (mild)	Generalized viral infections	p. 236

			↑ (mild)	Low grade hemolytic disorders	p. 194
			↑ (mild)	Cerebral vascular accident	p. 202 (spinal tap)
			↑ (mild)	Renal tissue destruction	p. 121
Phosphorus (serum)	PO_4	Adults: 1.8-2.6 mEq/L 3-0-4.5 mg/dl Children: 2.3-4.1 mEq/L 4.0-7.0 mg/dl	↑ with ↑ BUN, ↑ creat	Chronic glomerular disease	p. 121
			↑ with ↓ Ca, N BUN, N creat	Hypoparathyroidism	p. 173
			N or ↑ with N BUN, N creat	Milk-alkali syndrome	History of peptic ulcer disease
			N with ↑ Ca and ↑ gamma globulin	Sarcoidosis	Biopsy
			↓ with ↑ Ca, N BUN N creat	Hyperparathyroidism	p. 172
			↓ with N or ↓ Ca and ↑ alk phos	Rickets (children), osteomalacia (adults)	History, physical, and x rays
			↓	Renal tubular acidosis	Anion gap, p. 25
			↓	Malabsorption syndrome	p. 148
Potassium (plasma)	K	3.8-5.0 mEq/L	↑	Renal failure	p. 121
			↑ with hypovolemia and ↑ BUN	Addison's disease	p. 182
			N with ↓ total body K and ↑ CO_2 combining power	Chronic diuretic use, alkalosis	History, p. 108
			↓ with ↑ CO_2 combining power	Cushing's syndrome	p. 181
			↓	Primary and secondary hyper-aldosteronism with chronic congestive heart failure	History and physical, p. 131
			↓	Liver disease with ascites	History and physical, pp. 153-160
			↓	Excessive licorice ingestion (hypertension)	History

Continued.

BLOOD CHEMISTRY—cont'd

Test	Abbreviation	Normal value	Variance	Clinical implication	Subsequent laboratory studies, comments, and/or conclusive symptoms
Potassium (plasma)—cont'd			↓	Antiinflammatory drugs	History
			↓	Malignant hypertension, hypertensive disease, unilateral renal vascular hypertension	↑ reninemia, p. 131
			↓	Poor diet	History
			↓	Chronic stress	History
			↓	Chronic diarrhea	History
			↓	Malabsorption syndrome	p. 148
			↓	Diaphoresis	History
			↓	Chronic fever	History and physical
			↓ with ↑ Cl and ↓ CO_2 combining power	Renal tubular acidosis	Anion gap, p. 25
Total protein and albumin/globulin ratio (serum)	Tot prot and A/G ratio	Total: 6.0-7.8 gm/dl Albumin: 3.2-4.5 gm/dl Globulin: 2.3-3.5 gm/dl	↓ with ↓ albumin (<2.5 gm) and ↑ globulin (3 gm) (reversed A/G ratio)	Chronic liver disease	pp. 153-160
			N with ↓ albumin and ↑ globulin (reversed A/G ratio)	Myeloproliferative diseases, chronic granulomatous infectious diseases	Serum protein electrophoresis, pp. 12-13
Sodium (serum)	Na	136-142 mEq/L	↑	Iatrogenic	History
			↑ with hyperglycemia	Hypothalamic lesion, head trauma, and hyperosmolar states	History and physical
			↓ with dehydration (slight ↑ BUN)	Addison's disease (primary adrenocortical deficiency)	p. 182
			↓ with N or ↑ BUN	Chronic sodium-losing nephropathy	24 hr urine Na
			↓ with ↓ Cl	Vomiting, diarrhea, or tube drainage	History
			↓	Diaphoresis, burns	History and physical

			↓	Diuretics (mercurial and chlorothiazide)	History
			↓ with ↑ BUN, ↑ creat	Chronic renal insufficiency with acidosis	p. 121
			↓	Starvation with acidosis, diabetic acidosis	pH
			↓	Paracentesis, thoracentesis	History
			↓	Dilution hyponatremia: diuretics with Na restriction, secondary hyperaldosteronism, hepatic failure with ascites, congestive heart failure, excessive water administration, acute or chronic renal insufficiency (oliguria), hypothermia, lobar pneumonia	History and physical, p. 179
			↓ with inappropriate ADH syndrome (↑ S. G. and ↓ Na)	Bronchogenic carcinoma, pulmonary infections, and porphyria	Chest x ray
Serum glutamic oxaloacetic transaminase	SGOT	8-33 U/ml	↑ (marked)	Acute severe fulminating hepatitis, severe liver necrosis, and acute myocardial infarction	pp. 63, 159
			↑ (moderate)	Myocarditis, cardiomyopathies	Chapter 4
			↑ (mild)	Cirrhosis, cholangiolitic jaundice, metastatic liver disease, skeletal muscle disease, posttrauma, and generalized infections, dissecting aneurysm, pulmonary infarction, shock, pericarditis	pp. 61, 114-115, 153-160; history and physical
Blood urea nitrogen	BUN	8-18 mg/dl	↑	Acute or chronic renal failure, congestive heart failure with decreased renal blood supply, and obstructive uropathy	p. 121

Continued.

BLOOD CHEMISTRY—cont'd

Test	Abbreviation	Normal value	Variance	Clinical implication	Subsequent laboratory studies, comments, and/or conclusive symptoms
Uric acid (serum)		Male: 2.1-7.8 mg/dl Female: 2.0-6.4 mg/dl	↑ with acute arthritis	Gout	X ray and 24-hour urine excretion of uric acid
			↑ (mild)	Idiopathic	
			↑ with ↑ BUN, ↑ creat	Chronic renal failure	p. 121
			↑	Starvation	History and physical
			↑	Glycogen storage disease	Liver biopsy or bone marrow biopsy
			↑	Diuretics	History

N = normal
↑ = elevated
↓ = depressed

HEMATOLOGY

Test	Abbreviation	Normal value	Variance	Clinical implication	Subsequent laboratory studies, comments, and/or conclusive symptoms
White blood cell count	WBC	4500-11,000/microliter	↑ (mild to moderate)	Infectious disease, mainly bacterial and moderate	History, physical, and differential
			↑ (mild to moderate)	Severe sepsis in elderly patients	History, physical, and differential
			↑ (marked)	Severe sepsis	History, physical, and differential
Red blood cell count	RBC	Male: 4.6-6.2 × 10^6/microliter	↑ (primary)	Polycythemia vera (leukemia)	↓ erythropoietin level
		Female: 4.2-5.4 × 10^6/microliter	↑ (secondary)	Chronic obstructive lung disease, cyanotic congenital heart diseases with hypoxemia	p. 112 and ↑ erythropoietin level
THE DIFFERENTIAL WBC COUNT					
Neutrophils		Mean %: 56% Range of absolute counts: 1800-7000/microliter	↑ (mild to moderate)	Bacterial infections, inflammatory disorders, tumors, physical and emotional stimuli, stresses (heat, extreme cold, exercise, electroshock therapy, emotional stimuli), and drugs (catecholamines, corticosteroids)	History and physical, and cultures
			↓ (mild to moderate) with monocytosis (up to 50%)	Familial benign neutropenia	History
			↓ (mild to moderate)	Acute viral infections, anorexia nervosa (starvation), primary and secondary splenic neutropenia, drug induced, and excessive ingestion of alcohol	History and physical

N = normal
↑ = elevated
↓ = depressed

Continued.

HEMATOLOGY—cont'd

Test	Abbreviation	Normal value	Variance	Clinical implication	Subsequent laboratory studies, comments, and/or conclusive symptoms
Eosinophils		Mean %: 2.7%	↑	Allergic disorders, parasitic diseases	History and physical, pp. 238-240
		Range of absolute counts: 0-450/microliter	↑ (90%)	Eosinophilic leukemia	p. 188
			↓	Acute and chronic stress (emotional or somatic), Endocrine causes (excess ACTH, cortisone, epinephrine, intermenstrual period, diurnal variations, and acromegaly)	History, p. 179
Basophils		Mean %: 3%	↑	Myeloproliferative disease	p. 188 (bone marrow, serum protein electrophoresis)
		Range of absolute counts: 0-200/microliter	↓	Anaphylactic reaction	Serology
			↓ with granulocytopenia	Acute hypersensitive reactions, steroids, diurnal changes, hyperthyroidism, pituitary basophilism, radiation therapy, acute and chronic infection, ovulation, pregnancy, and aging	History and physical, p. 171
Lymphocytes		Mean %: 34% Range of absolute counts: 1000-4800/microliter	↑ (80%-90%) with ↑ (marked) leukocytes	Chronic lymphocytic leukemia	p. 188
			↑ (marked) with ↑ (moderate) leukocytes	Infectious diseases: pertussis, infectious mononucleosis, and acute infectious lymphocytosis	p. 236 (bone marrow, peripheral smear)
			↑ (mild to moderate relative)	Viral infections with eczemas	History and physical
			In bacterial infections: ↑ (mild to moderate) with ↑ (mild to moderate) leukocytes	Chronic infectious state	History and physical

			↑ (mild to moderate) in noninfectious and nonmyeloproliferative disease	Thyrotoxicosis, adrenal insufficiency (Addison's disease)	p. 182
THE PERIPHERAL SMEAR					
Platelets		290,000/mm (140,000-440,000) Brecher-Cronkite method)	Absolute absence	Aplastic bone marrow, thrombocytopenia (various etiologies)	p. 188
			↑	Polycythemia, essential thrombocytosis, persons who have had splenectomies	↓ hemopoietin, history
Hemoglobin	Hgb	Male: 13.5-18.0 gm/dl	↓	Anemia	p. 188
		Female: 12.0-16.0 gm/dl	↓ (borderline) with ↓ (borderline) Hct and N RBC count	Hypochromic microcytic anemia: iron deficiency, thalassemia major and minor, sickle cell anemia, and hemoglobin C disease	p. 188 (bone marrow), ↓ serum iron level, Hgb electrophoresis, p. 197
			↓	Normochromic normocytic anemia	History, reticulocyte count
			↓ with ↑ MCV and ↑ MCHC	Macrocytic anemia: folic acid deficiency, vitamin B_{12} deficiency (pernicious anemia)	p. 38
ADDITIONAL FINDINGS ON THE PERIPHERAL SMEAR					
			Spherocytosis, polychromatophilia, and erythrocyte agglutination	Compensated, acquired hemolytic anemia	p. 197
			Spherocytosis with polychromatophilia	Hereditary spherocytosis	Fragility test
			Basophilic stipplings	Lead poisoning	Peripheral smear for lead
			Macrocytosis and hypersegmental neutrophils	Vitamin B_{12} and/or folic acid deficiency	Serum folate, RBC folate

Continued.

HEMATOLOGY—cont'd

Test	Abbreviation	Normal value	Variance	Clinical implication	Subsequent laboratory studies, comments, and/or conclusive symptoms
			Rouleaux formation	Multiple myeloma or macro-globulinemia	p. 188 (bone marrow, serum protein electro-phoresis)
			Parasites in RBCs	Malaria	p. 238
			Schistocytes and "burr" cells with ↓ platelet count	Consumption coagulopathy	Fibrinogen degradation product
			Schistocytes and "burr" cells	Mechanical hemolysis (prostatic valves)	History
			↑ neutrophils, ↑ band forms and toxic granulations	Severe infection	History and physical
			Atypical lymphocytes	Infectious mononucleosis	p. 238
			↓ neutrophils and in-creased lymphocytes	Agranulocytosis	p. 188
			Eosinophilia	Allergy reaction	History
			Blast (primitive) forms	Acute leukemia	p. 188

N = normal
↑ = elevated
↓ = depressed

URINALYSIS

Test	Abbreviation	Normal value	Variance	Clinical implication	Subsequent laboratory studies, comments, and/or conclusive symptoms
pH (acidity or alkalinity)		4.6-8.0	↑ (alkaline) with CO_2 combining power	Metabolic alkalosis	p. 108
			↓ (aciduria) with metabolic alkalosis, ↓ K, ↓ Cl	Generalized intracellular acidosis	p. 108
Specific gravity	SG	1.016-1.022 (normal fluid intake)	↓ with ↓ K, ↓ Ca, ↑ Cl	Distal renal tubular disease	p. 122
			Fixed SG (isosthenuria)	Chronic renal disease	p. 122
		1.001-1.035 (range)	↓ with ↑ Ca, ↓ K	Hypokalemic and hypercalcemic nephropathy	pp. 123-124, osmolality
Glucose (qualitative)	Gluc	Negative	Glycosuria with ↑ blood glucose	Diabetes mellitus	Gluc tolerance test
			Glycosuria with ↓ blood glucose	Low renal threshold for glucose resorption	Gluc tolerance test
Protein (qualitative)		Negative	Proteinuria (trace)	Follow-up indicated	p. 121
			Proteinuria (more than a trace)	Twenty-four hour urine quantitative analysis indicated	
MICROSCOPIC EXAMINATION					
Casts		Negative	WBC casts	Pyelonephritis	p. 224
			RBC casts	Glomerulonephritis	p. 127
			Hyaline casts with proteinuria	Nephrotic syndrome	pp. 128-129
Red blood cells	RBCs	Negative	Hematuria	Hemorrhagic cystitis or calculi in the renal pelvis, tuberculosis or tumors of the renal collecting and tubular system	pp. 124-127
Crystals		Negative	Present with amorphous substances and ↑ uric acid	Possible gouty nephropathy	p. 10
			Calcium oxalate crystals with ↑ serum calcium	Suggests hypercalcemia	p. 4

N = normal
↑ = elevated
↓ = depressed

Continued.

URINALYSIS—cont'd

Test	Abbreviation	Normal value	Variance	Clinical implication	Subsequent laboratory studies, comments, and/or conclusive symptoms
Color		Golden yellow	Darker color	Hematuria, bilirubinuria, hemoglobinuria, urobilinuria, and porphyria	p. 132
			Color changes when exposed to light	Porphyria	Measurement of porphyrins
			Tea-colored and staining (urobilinogen in urine)	Possible obstructive jaundice	pp. 153-160

UNIT TWO

EVALUATIVE AND DIAGNOSTIC LABORATORY TESTS FOR SPECIFIC DISEASES

Unit One dealt with the routine screening of the patient through laboratory tests. In Unit Two additional tests are discussed to provide guidelines in ordering and understanding the tests that will lead to a more definitive diagnosis when an abnormality is detected in the screening examination.

The anatomy and physiology of the organ or system that is involved in the disease process are developed before the specific laboratory tests are discussed so that the rationale behind the test, the nomenclature, and the limitations of the specific test may be better understood.

4

DIAGNOSTIC TESTS FOR CARDIOVASCULAR DISORDERS

ANATOMY AND PHYSIOLOGY

The heart is a muscular pump with four chambers guarded by four valves. It is innervated by the autonomic nervous system, receives its blood supply from the coronary arteries, and possesses a marvelous conductive system, which stimulates it to beat and assures adequate conduction velocity.

The course of the blood through the four chambers of the heart and the great vessels is shown in Fig. 4-1. The blood enters the two atria simultaneously, unimpeded by valves. The right atrium receives venous blood through the inferior and superior venae cavae. The left atrium receives arterial blood through the four pulmonary veins. During diastole both the atria and the ventricles fill. During atrial systole an extra complement of blood is pushed into the ventricles. When the ventricular systole begins the two valves (mitral and tricuspid) guarding the atria close (S_1), and blood is pumped to the lungs from the right ventricle via the pulmonary artery and to the systemic circulation from the left ventricle via the aorta. When diastole begins the valves (pulmonary and aortic) guarding the two ventricles close (S_2).

The two coronary arteries (right and left) spring from the root of the aorta. During diastole the coronary arteries fill, supplying the myocardium with oxygenated blood.

The conductive system of the heart is shown in Fig. 4-2. The sinus node paces the heart and lies in the superior portion of the right atrium. The atrioventricular (A-V) node lies in the lower part of the right atrium. Its function is to receive the impulse from the sinus node and delay it slightly so that the atria will have time to pump their contents into the ventricles before they contract, thus complementing cardiac output. The internodal tracts connect the two nodes and ensure rapid conduction velocity between them. The interatrial tract (Bachmann's bundle) speeds the impulse to the left atrium.

Since there is a fibrous ring separating the atria from the ventricles, the

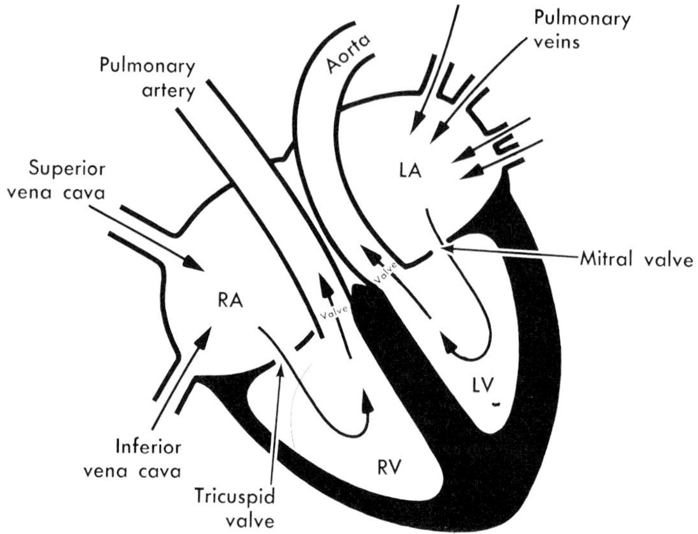

FIG. 4-1
The course of blood flow through the heart chambers and great vessels. (From Conover, M. H., and Zalis, E. G.: Understanding electrocardiography: physiological and interpretive concepts, ed. 2, St. Louis, 1976, The C. V. Mosby Co.)

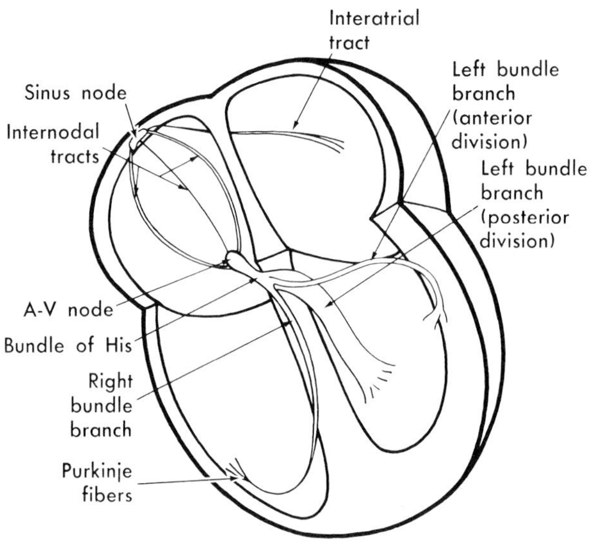

FIG. 4-2
The conductive system.

bundle of His is the sole muscular connection between these two parts of the heart. The impulse, then, enters the A-V node and is passed down the bundle of His and rapidly completes its journey through the ventricles via the bundle branches and the Purkinje fibers. The right bundle branch serves the right side of the heart and the left bundle branch, which is divided into an anterior and a posterior division, serves the left side.

The conductive system of the heart enables the impulse to travel six times faster than would be possible without it.

ROUTINE TESTS

The electrocardiogram (ECG)

This brief section on electrocardiography will not teach the performance or interpretation of electrocardiograms. It is hoped that it will increase appreciation of the value and the limits of this diagnostic test and will provide the motivation for a further study of the subject. Subsequent sections will assume a working knowledge of the vocabulary used in electrocardiography. Although the electrocardiogram is used in almost all types of heart disease, this section will emphasize those areas in which the test has been found most useful.

Coronary artery disease

The electrocardiogram is indispensable in the proper diagnosis and treatment of coronary artery disease, and valuable information can be obtained on both the asymptomatic person with a normal resting electrocardiogram (by means of stress electrocardiography, see the section on exercise electrocardiography) and the patient with acute myocardial infarction.

Electrocardiographic changes in coronary artery disease include the following.

ST-T abnormalities. "Nonspecific ST-T abnormalities" is one of the most common electrocardiographic interpretations made. This vague and nonspecific interpretation can frustrate the beginner or one who expects a diagnostic label from every ECG. This is not always possible. Nonspecific ST-T abnormalities are what the term says they are. They are changes of the S-T segment and the T waves that are outside the range of what is considered normal, and this renders the electrocardiogram abnormal. They can be seen in a variety of disorders, cardiac or noncardiac, and do not necessarily signify heart disease. Still, these deviations may be the earliest manifestations of coronary artery disease.

S-T depressions. These may indicate myocardial ischemia and are more specific changes, being flat or downsloping of 1 mm or more. Although not diagnostic of coronary artery disease, they are quite characteristic. Digitalis and electrolyte abnormalities can accentuate or even mimic these changes.

S-T elevations. Marked S-T elevations in well localized leads in a 45-year-old man clutching his chest in the emergency room is the hallmark of acute myocardial infarction. But an unqualified diagnosis of acute myocardial infarction would be incorrect. Such a tracing from the person may reflect early changes in acute myocardial infarction ("hyperacute") or may revert to normal in a matter of minutes, at which time they would be characteristic of variant (Prinzmetal's) angina, reflecting massive but totally reversible myocardial ischemia. Thus an unqualified diagnosis of myocardial infarction, either acute or chronic, cannot be based upon an abnormality of ST-T waves, regardless of the severity of the changes. Abnormal Q waves (see the section on QRS changes) are necessary before such a diagnosis is made. S-T elevations that remain unchanged over many weeks following an acute myocardial infarction may point to a ventricular aneurysm.

T inversions. Prominent or giant T inversions may reflect diffuse myocardial ischemia or possibly subendocardial infarction but are by no means specific. Central nervous system lesions, usually caused by massive damage or subarachnoid hemorrhage, can produce marked T wave inversions that can easily be confused with those of severe coronary artery disease.

QRS changes. Changes of the QRS complex are commonly seen in coronary artery disease. Abnormal Q waves are the hallmark of myocardial infarction. By also observing the associated changes in the ST-T segment, one can make a reasonable estimate of the age of the infarction as to acute, subacute, or chronic. It is generally accepted that the more leads in which the Q waves are seen, the larger the infarction. Also, most Q waves persist indefinitely, but it is not uncommon for an electrocardiogram with diagnostic Q waves to lose the Q waves or even revert to normal months or years following an infarction.

Pathologic Q waves do not necessarily signify coronary artery disease or myocardial infarction. They can also be seen in infiltrative myocardial disorders, such as amyloidosis.

P waves. Diagnostic usefulness of the P waves in coronary artery disease is limited. In patients with atrial infarctions or heart failure with elevated pressures in the left atrium, P waves may become abnormal.

U waves. These are seen in normal people, become more prominent in electrolyte disorders (hypokalemia), and may be inverted in myocardial ischemia.

P-R segment. The P-R segment is commonly normal in coronary artery disease. Prolonged P-R segment (first degree heart block) is frequently seen in patients with myocardial infarction, especially of the inferior wall. Prolonged P-R segment also can result from digitalis excess.

Q-T interval. The Q-T interval in coronary artery disease with myocardial ischemia may be prolonged. This fact is helpful in differentiating the ST-T abnormalities caused by ischemia (which is accompanied by Q-T prolongation) from those changes caused by digitalis (which is commonly accompanied by Q-T shortening).

Other clinical uses for the ECG

Besides the diagnosis of coronary artery disease, the electrocardiogram is invaluable in the diagnosis of rhythm disorders caused by coronary artery disease and in valvular heart disease, in which stenosis or regurgitation of various valves can cause hypertrophy or enlargement of the respective chambers.

Valvular heart disease. Valvular heart disease is commonly reflected in the electrocardiogram by either increased voltage or ST-T abnormalities of the leads reflecting those chambers. Common examples include the following: *Aortic stenosis* or *aortic insufficiency* gives evidence of left ventricular hypertrophy on the electrocardiogram by the time the patients are symptomatic or in need of surgical correction. Exceptions do occur. *Mitral stenosis* produces increased pressure in the left atrium, causing this chamber to hypertrophy and dilate, and the result is reflected as a broad notched P wave in leads II and III, indicating left atrial enlargement, otherwise called P mitrale. Similar examples can be extended to all other valvular lesions. *Hypertension* acts similarly to aortic stenosis, since it also causes a pressure overload of the left ventricle, producing left ventricular hypertrophy. It should be noted that left ventricular hypertrophy identified by electrocardiogram does not necessarily mean a fixed increase of the muscle mass of the left ventricle, since treating the hypertension may improve the electrocardiogram, and in some cases may cause it to revert to normal.

Arrhythmias. Although an astute examiner can make a specific diagnosis of a rhythm disorder by examining the radial pulse, the jugular venous pulsations, and the quality of the heart sound, the simplest and most accurate method of arrhythmia diagnosis is by electrocardiogram. In selected cases, further investigations by intracardiac electrocardiography (see p. 96) may be necessary before a definite diagnosis can be established. Any deviation of the rhythm from the arbitrarily set sinus rhythm of 60 to 100/min is considered to be an arrhythmia; some are trivial and considered to be usual elements of a normal heart, such as sinus arrhythmia or sinus tachycardia.

Extrasystoles. *Premature atrial contractions (PACs)* can be seen in an otherwise normal heart. If frequent, they may indicate atrial disease and herald the onset of atrial fibrillation. *Premature ventricular contractions (PVCs)* may be considered benign if seen in a healthy young individual without other evidence of cardiac disease. They may herald ventricular tachycardia or fibrillation, especially if seen in a setting of myocardial ischemia, severe heart disease, or acute myocardial infarction, in which the ventricular fibrillatory threshold is lowered. Premature ventricular contractions in the presence of organic heart disease are thought to be malignant if they are multiform, appear in pairs, or are early and appear on the T wave of the preceding complex. Three or more PVCs are commonly designated as ventricular tachycardia. In the presence of organic heart disease, usually coronary artery disease, these arrhythmias increase the risk of sudden death.

Ectopic tachycardia. *Atrial fibrillation* is the most common sustained atrial arrhythmia. Its presence frequently indicates organic heart disease, usually mitral valve disease or coronary artery disease. Although the diagnosis can be suspected because of an irregular pulse, an electrocardiogram is essential for an accurate diagnosis. Frequent premature beats can mimic the pulse of atrial fibrillation, while a regular pulse may be seen in atrial fibrillation with a high degree of A-V block. This may indicate digitalis excess.

Paroxysmal atrial tachycardia (PAT). This disorder implies functional abnormality of the A-V node and is commonly seen in otherwise healthy, young people free of significant heart disease.

Atrial flutter. This is another common atrial arrhythmia that usually indicates the presence of organic heart disease. It is frequently seen in acute pericarditis.

Ventricular tachycardia. Ventricular tachycardia is rarely seen in an otherwise normal heart, usually indicates severe heart disease, and dictates prompt and accurate diagnosis and treatment. Occasionally, the surface electrocardiogram is inadequate in a definitive diagnosis of this disorder because of the difficulty in distinguishing it from a supraventricular tachycardia with aberrant conduction. In such a situation, if permitted by the clinical setting, an intracardiac electrocardiogram can settle the diagnosis.

Ventricular fibrillation. This arrhythmia is the end stage of severe organic heart disease, but it can also be induced by drugs (such as digitalis), electrolyte abnormalities (marked hypokalemia and marked hypomagnesemia), or electrocution. It is thought to be the most common cause of sudden death. This extreme rhythm disorder permits no effective cardiac output. Irreversible brain damage and subsequent death follow if effective resuscitative measures are not instituted in 3 to 5 miutes. As a rule, one should not wait to make an electrocardiographic diagnosis of ventricular fibrillation before instituting such measures.

Wolff-Parkinson-White syndrome (WPW). In this syndrome there are frequent supraventricular tachycardias with an increased risk of sudden death. The diagnosis is made only by electrocardiography, in which the characteristic features are a short P-R (or P-Q) interval measuring 0.10 seconds or less, widened QRS complexes of 0.11 to 0.14 seconds, and a slurred onset of the QRS complex, commonly known as the delta wave. The QRS complexes resemble those of bundle branch block with associated ST-T abnormalities. In the presence of this disorder, diagnosis of acute myocardial infarction or ventricular hypertrophy may be difficult or impossible to make.

Heart block. Heart block is commonly classified as first degree heart block, which indicates P-R prolongation; second degree heart block, which indicates occasionally nonconducted P waves; and complete or third degree heart block, which indicates nonconducted P waves.

First degree heart block may be secondary to increased parasympathetic tone, or may reflect digitalis excess, myocarditis, or infiltration of the myocardium by tumor or amyloid. By itself it causes no hemodynamic compromise and warrants no treatment.

Second degree heart block can be of two types. In type I (Wenckebach) there is progressive prolongation of the P-R interval preceding a nonconducted P wave; in type II the P-R interval is constant.

Type I second degree heart block can result from a marked increase in parasympathetic tone. When seen in trained athletes or only during sleep, it may not signifiy cardiac disease. Digitalis excess and diaphragmatic myocardial infarction are common pathologic causes.

Type II second degree heart block is always indicative of organic heart disease and frequently indicates involvement of the His-Purkinje system. Common causes are anteroseptal myocardial infarction and degenerative or infiltrative disease of the myocardium. Pacemakers are commonly necessary.

Third degree (complete) heart block is usually caused by degenerative disease of the conduction system. Coronary artery disease is the second most common cause. This arrhythmia can also be seen in traumatic or inflammatory disease or drug toxicity. Occurring in adults it usually causes significant hemodynamic impairment and can cause syncope (Stokes-Adams syndrome) or death. As a rule, permanent demand ventricular pacing is used in all adult patients. In congenital complete heart block with stable, narrow QRS complexes and an adequate ventricular rate, a pacemaker may not be necessary if close follow-up is available.

Bundle branch block is classically viewed as right bundle branch block (RBBB) or left bundle branch block (LBBB), but in recent years recognition of anterior and posterior branches of the left bundle have been recognized. In the presence of left bundle branch block, diagnosis of myocardial infarction or ventricular hypertrophy may be difficult or impossible to make. Right bundle branch block does not mask a diagnosis of myocardial infarction and may be the clue to silent coronary artery disease. It is commonly seen postoperatively, especially after repair of ventricular septal defects or in the presence of atrial septal defect. Bifascicular block (right bundle branch block and left anterior hemiblock or left posterior hemiblock) in the presence of acute myocardial infarction usually indicates massive myocardial damage with a poor prognosis. Although pacemakers have been used electively (or prophylactically) in these patients, their use is controversial and the salvage rate has been low. In chronic bifascicular block pacemakers are effective in preventing recurrences of syncope caused by intermittent second degree or complete heart block.

Congenital heart disease. Congenital heart disease in infants, as well as in adults, is commonly accompanied by an abnormal electrocardiogram. The electrocardiogram is characteristic and can lead to an exact diagnosis in a few conditions, such as endocardial cushion defect, atrial septal defect of the ostium primum type, and transposition of the great vessels with ventricular inversion. More frequently, the abnormality helps in localizing the disease to the right or the left side of the heart. Of course, in infants and children a different set of criteria for normals must be used.

The effects of drugs and electrolytes on the electrocardiogram

Digitalis is commonly used in patients with heart disease and can mimic many of the diagnostic changes of the electrocardiogram. It is important to be familiar with the usual electrocardiographic abnormalities produced by this drug. In normal therapeutic doses digitalis causes sagging of the S-T segment with flattening of the T waves, shortened Q-T interval, and slight prolongation of the P-R interval (Table 4-1). In the presence of atrial fibrillation it also slows

TABLE 4-1
Effect of drugs and electrolytes on the electrocardiogram

Drug or electrolyte	QRS complex	S-T segment	P wave	T wave	U wave	P-R segment	Q-T interval
Digitalis		Sagging		Flattens		Prolongs	Shortens
Quinidine	Widens (toxic)	Depresses	Widens and notches (toxic)	Flattens or inverts			Prolongs
Propranolol				Normal or slightly higher		Prolongs	Shortens
Phenytoin						Shortens	Shortens
Disopyramide	Widens		Widens			Prolongs	
Potassium							
Hyperkalemia	Widens	Depresses (>6.5 mEq/L)	Widens (>7.5 mEq/L)	Tall and peaked (5.5-6.5 mEq/L)		Prolongs (>7.5 mEq/L)	
Hypokalemia		Sagging		Notching, then inversion	Prominent		Prolongs (due to U wave)
Calcium							
Hypercalcemia				Widens and rounds			Shortens
Hypocalcemia							Prolongs
Magnesium	Widens (toxic)			Flattens		Prolongs (toxic)	
Lithium				Flattens			

the ventricular rate, or it may produce a reversion to normal sinus rhythm. In digitalis excess the following arrhythmias are commonly noted: marked P-R prolongation, second and third degree heart block, and paroxysmal atrial tachycardia with A-V block. Digitalis toxicity should be strongly suspected in the presence of ventricular premature beats with bigeminy, multifocal premature beats, pairs of PVCs, or runs of ventricular tachycardia. In the presence of atrial fibrillation, digitalis excess or toxicity may produce a regular pulse because of high degree of A-V block and an accelerated junctional focus.

Quinidine in therapeutic doses produces prolongation of the Q-T interval, with widening and notching of the P waves. There could be some S-T segment depression and flattening or inversion of the T waves. When therapeutic levels in the blood are exceeded, the toxic effects noted are varying degrees of A-V block, widening of the QRS complexes over 50% of normal, and ventricular arrhythmias, including ventricular tachycardia or fibrillation—thus the term "quinidine syncope."

Occasionally, ventricular tachycardia or fibrillation is precipitated in the absence of drug toxicity. Usually, marked Q-T prolongation or U waves precede the onset of these arrhythmias.

Propranolol (Inderal) predictably slows the sinus rate and produces sinus bradycardia with slight prolongation of the P-R interval. The Q-T interval is shortened and the T waves may remain normal or be slightly higher (Table 4-1). In atrial fibrillation propranolol will slow the ventricular response.

Phenytoin (Dilantin) is used in the treatment of digitalis toxicity. It tends to shorten the P-R interval and the Q-T interval without having a significant effect on the QRS complex (Table 4-1). This characteristic of phenytoin is considered to make it the drug of choice in the treatment of digitalis toxicity in the presence of prolongation of the P-R segment or first or second degree heart block.

Disopyramide (Norpace) is a new antiarrhythmic agent effective in atrial and ventricular arrhythmias. Like quinidine, in high doses it may cause prolongation of the P wave, the QRS complex, and the P-R interval.

Lidocaine has little effect on the electrocardiogram. Some studies have shown increased intraventricular conduction delay, while other studies have refuted this. For practical purposes no significant change on the surface electrocardiogram is recorded.

Hyperkalemia is reflected in the electrocardiogram in the following manner: The first electrocardiographic manifestation of hyperkalemia occurs with blood concentrations in the range of 5.5 to 6.5 mEq/L. At this level the T waves become characteristically tall and peaked. With further elevations in the plasma potassium concentration, there is a decreased amplitude of the R waves with increased S waves, S-T depressions, and prolongation of the QRS duration and the P-R interval. When the plasma potassium concentration exceeds 7.5 mEq/L intra-atrial conduction disturbances develop and are reflected in broad, low amplitude P waves and P-R interval prolongation (Table 4-1). At higher potassium levels, the P wave disappears altogether, and the QRS becomes markedly widened and moves into a smooth diphasic (sine) wave. The final stage, if untreated, is ventricular tachycardia, flutter, fibrillation, and standstill.

Hypokalemia initially causes an apparent prolongation of the Q-T interval. This results from the appearance of a U wave that merges with the T wave and may cause notching of the T wave. T wave inversion follows a then sagging of the S-T segment. The administration of potassium rapidly reverses these changes.

Hypercalcemia characteristically shortens the S-T segment of the Q-T interval and may also widen and cause a rounding of the T waves. Hypocalcemia causes a prolongation of the Q-T interval (Table 4-1).

Hypermagnesemia may cause T wave flattening. Very toxic levels cause P-R and QRS widening. The effects of hypomagnesemia on the electrocardiogram are poorly understood. This condition usually accompanies hypokalemia.

Lithium in therapeutic doses can cause flattening and inversion of the T waves.

Important points to remember

A normal electrocardiogram does not rule out severe organic heart disease. Severe obstructive disease of all major coronary arteries without myocardial infarction or active ischemia of the heart is a common situation that could produce a perfectly normal electrocardiogram.

A definitely abnormal electrocardiogram does not necessarily signify heart disease. Many abnormalities, even pronounced, can result from CNS lesions, autonomic influences, or be produced by drugs, electrolytes, or other causes.

Electrocardiographic interpretations should be made in the context of the clinical situation. Serious errors will be made if the clinical data are not used in interpreting an electrocardiogram.

The limitations of the standard resting electrocardiogram should be recognized. It is at most a 1 minute record of the heart's electrical activity, and it is recorded at rest, without stressing the heart. Whenever necessary further tests should be used, such as the Holter monitor for arrhythmia diagnosis or stress electrocardiography for diagnosis of coronary artery disease. These will be discussed in the following sections.

Ambulatory electrocardiography (Holter monitoring)

Ambulatory electrocardiography is an extension of the resting electrocardiogram. A portable recorder is worn by the patient and the electrocardiogram is recorded continuously on magnetic tape during unrestricted activity. The tapes are scanned rapidly by electrocardioscanners, and abnormalities or selected areas of interest are printed out in real time. Computers are utilized in the rapid processing of tapes have vastly expanded the ability to process a large number of tapes, and provide quantitative data.

Clinical value

The clinical uses of ambulatory electrocardiography are many. It enables a much larger sample of the electrocardiogram to be recorded; instead of 60 to 100 complexes noted on the usual resting electrocardiogram, this samples 50,000 to 100,000 beats on a 10- to 24-hour record. Resting, unrestricted activity, and sleep recordings are made. Many abnormalities of the electrocardiogram that have in the past gone undetected during the patient's sleep are now being recognized.

Indications for the use of ambulatory monitoring

1. *Diagnosis of arrhythmias.* In patients complaining of dizziness or palpitations or actually having episodes of syncope, the ambulatory electrocardiogram is an invaluable diagnostic tool. If the rhythm disorder *and* the symptoms are shown to be coincident, then an exact diagnosis of an elusive disorder can be made.
2. *Monitoring of high risk patients.* Holter monitoring is especially useful when the patient is discharged from the hospital soon after a myocardial infarction.
3. *Evaluation of the effectiveness of drug treatment of arrhythmias.*
4. *Diagnosis of ischemic heart disease.* Not uncommonly, ischemic S-T depressions can be noted on the ambulatory electrocardiogram during periods of stress, be it exertion, emotional stress, heavy meals, or cigarette smoking. Sometimes ischemic changes are recorded during the patient's sleep; these are commonly associated with periods of rapid eye movement sleep with dreams, associated sinus tachycardia, and possibly a rise in the blood pressure.

Prinzmetal's angina manifests S-T elevation during angina and is associated with proximal high grade coronary artery obstructive lesions and/or coronary spasm. The exercise electrocardiogram may be negative and show no ischemic S-T changes or pain. In such a case the ambulatory electrocardiogram can be very useful in detecting the S-T abnormalities that may occur during rest.

Contraindications and limitations

There are no absolute or relative contraindications for ambulatory electrocardiography; however, the limitations are several. It is a costly procedure, ranging from $100 to $200 for a 10- to 24-hour tape, recording, and analysis. Further use of computerization may overcome this hurdle. Another limitation is availability; but as the value of ambulatory electrocardiography becomes more widely recognized, it will be available on a larger scale. The commonly used one-lead system limits the diagnostic usefulness, especially if the search is for S-T depression or elevation. But as newer systems increase the number of recording leads available, this limitation also will be overcome.

Ambulatory electrocardiography is an invaluable extension of the resting electrocardiogram and should be a part of any complete hospital cardiac laboratory. It remains a totally noninvasive method, free of risks except that of misdiagnosis (inability to recognize artifacts) and overdiagnosis (detection of benign arrhythmias) with the subsequent risk of unnecessary treatment.

Exercise electrocardiography

The exercise electrocardiogram was initially a twelve-lead electrocardiogram performed after the patient had stepped up and down a set of stairs of a standard height a certain number of times (Master's test). Today the test consists of a gradually increasing level of exercise on a motorized treadmill or bicycle ergometer while the electrocardiogram is being monitored. All twelve leads can be monitored. Newer models incorporate automatic rate meter and S-T segment analyzing computers. Various investigators have proposed different protocols for the gradually increasing work load, and the most widely used is that proposed by Robert Bruce. Valuable information obtained includes (1) the minutes of exercise—given a standard load, the maximum oxygen consumption can be derived; (2) the heart rate achieved at the peak of exercise—if blood pressure is obtained at the same time, a heart rate × blood pressure "double product" is obtained that is a good approximation of myocardial or heart work; (3) the degree of S-T depression that relates to myocardial ischemia; and (4) arrhythmias provoked during exercise or, more often, during early recovery.

Clinical value

The values of exercise electrocardiography are many. In coronary artery disease, the resting electrocardiogram, may be normal, or show nonspecific changes. In this situation the stress electrocardiogram is commonly abnormal and frequently quite diagnostic, by indicating flat or down-sloping ischemic S-T depression.

Another value of treadmill testing is in diagnosis of arrhythmias. Although ambulatory monitoring remains the method of choice in detecting suspected arrhythmias, the ease of performing exercise electrocardiography has caused more interest to be shown in its use for this purpose. This is especially the case if the arrhythmias are suspected to occur during exercise, and to be major arrhythmias of a life-threatening nature. In such patients one is reluctant to advise ambulatory monitoring during exercise; however, these arrhythmias could be provoked during an exercise electrocardiogram in a controlled setting with facilities for immediate treatment.

This test is also a useful adjunct in the evaluation of the patient's functional capacity or "physical fitness." It is useful in evaluating methods of therapy, including drugs or surgery, such as coronary artery bypass surgery, as well as in obtaining an objective evaluation of the patient's disability in situations where a history is confusing or difficult to obtain. The exercise ECG is useful in exercise prescription for the rehabilitiation of patients following myocardial infarction or cardiac surgery.

Limitations

The major limitation of stress electrocardiography is the high level of false positive and false negative results in the diagnosis of ischemic heart disease. False negative tests, even when a maximal heart rate is achieved, may be seen in as many as 25% of patients with coronary artery disease. Massive coronary occlusion with myocardial infarction can be seen in patients with normal maximal exercise electrocardiograms performed days or weeks prior to the insult. False positive tests, i.e., ischemic S-T depression in the absence of coronary artery disease, can also occur. Causes for this could be digitalis administration, electrolyte abnormalities, or cardiomyopathies. This test costs approximately $100 to $125.

Indications

The indications for stress electrocardiography are many. Like the resting electrocardiogram, it can be considered an extension of the physical examination. Specific indications were discussed in the section on the value of the test.

Contraindications

This test, unlike the resting electrocardiogram, does have some contraindications. Among these are any severe acute illnesses, specifically acute myocardial infarction, myocarditis, or severe arrhythmias. Other contraindications would be uncompensated congestive heart failure and drug toxicity.

Pitfalls

In stress electrocardiography, confusion can arise in diagnosing ischemic S-T depression. Junctional S-T depression, which is not flat or downsloping of 1 mm or more, can be misdiagnosed as positive for ischemia. As already mentioned, digitalis can produce or accentuate ischemic S-T changes as can electrolyte abnormalities, specifically hypokalemia.

Nitroglycerin enables the patient with coronary artery disease to perform a higher level of exercise and possibly produce fewer arrhythmias. Thus a patient's drug history immediately prior to testing should be noted.

If careful attention is not given to details of the testing and the patient uses the handrail for support, standardization of the test will be ruined and conclusions can be erroneous.

Another pitfall is that patients do learn how to perform the test and very commonly perform better on a second test, compared with a first test, without any intervention. Usually this learning does not progress from a second to third test and so on.

Risks

Risks include mortality of one in 10,000 tests performed, which is usually from ventricular fibrillation that was not successfully resuscitated. Complications necessitating hospitalization are in the range of 0.2% and include myocardial infarction, prolonged bouts of chest pain, severe arrhythmias, and hypertensive episodes. These risks can be minimized by screening patients by means of a history and physical examination, a resting electrocardiogram prior to testing, and availability and familiarity with resuscitative equipment.

Informed consent is not routinely obtained for this test, but is advisable in high risk patients.

Vectorcardiography (VCG)

The vectorcardiogram (VCG) was introduced by Frank Wilson in 1938. Whereas the ECG displays local electrical forces of the heart at a given time and point, the vectorcardiogram displays the balance of these forces at any instant. It is a plot of voltage against voltage in three-dimensional space and is a useful addition to the scalar ECG, reinforcing and making the understanding of scalar electrocardiography more complete.

Clinical value

The diagnostic advantages of the VCG over the ECG are as follows:

1. In determining the cause of slowing of electrical waveforms, specifically; it is helpful in the diagnosis of the initial slowing of W-P-W syndrome (Wolff-Parkinson-White syndrome) and the differentiation of the bundle branch blocks from other causes of widened QRS complexes.
2. In establishing the differential diagnosis between inferior wall myocardial infarction and left anterior hemiblock when there are S waves with embryonic r waves in leads II, III, and aV_F
3. In the differential diagnosis of RBBB from right ventricular hypertrophy
4. In detecting left ventricular hypertrophy in the presence of LBBB; analysis of the vector angle and magnitude can be helpful
5. As an adjunct to scalar electrocardiography, increasing the diagnostic yield by approximately 10%

The vectorcardiogram at present has not gained as wide an acceptance or use as the scalar electrocardiogram in most community hospitals. Recent introduction of standardized techniques in obtaining and interpreting vectorcardiograms may help in popularizing this diagnostic tool.

Routine radiographic examination of the heart

The chest x-ray examination in two projections, posterior-anterior (PA) and lateral, provides valuable information about the size and contour of the heart. Anatomic changes of individual chambers are seen in the right and left anterior oblique projections. These projections are illustrated in Figs. 4-3 to 4-6. Before the advent of echocardiography, radiographic examination was the simplest, most accurate way of assessing cardiac size, a fact that has made percussion of the chest for heart size in the physical examination of the patient almost a lost art.

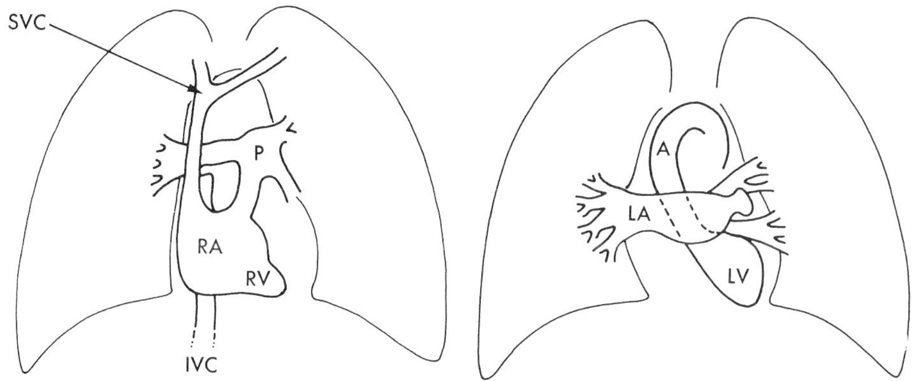

FIG. 4-3
The x-ray film of the chest in the posterior-anterior projection. *SVC*, superior vena cava; *IVC*, inferior vena cava; *RA*, right atrium; *RV*, right ventricle; *P*, pulmonary artery; *LA*, left atrium; *LV*, left ventricle; *A*, aorta.

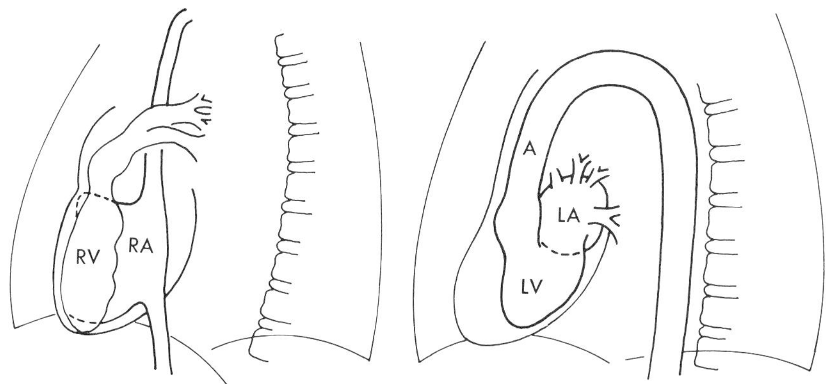

FIG. 4-4
The x-ray film of the chest in the left lateral projection.

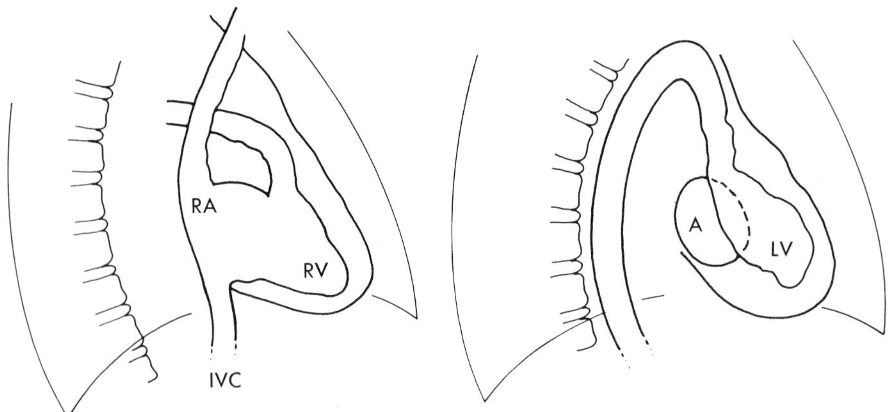

FIG. 4-5
The x-ray film of the chest in the right anterior oblique projection.

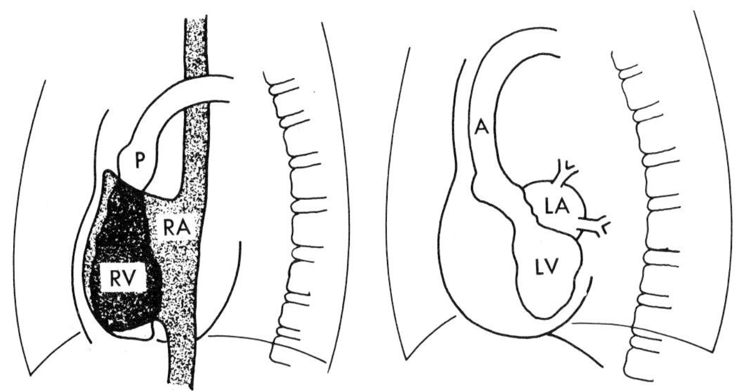

FIG. 4-6
The x-ray film of the chest in the left anterior oblique projection.

Clinical value

The simplest and most frequently used measurement is the cardiothoracic ratio. This measurement is achieved by adding the longest distance from the midline of the chest to the right and left sides of the heart (Fig. 4-7). The transverse diameter of the heart equals the sum of the longest mid-to-right and the longest mid-to-left measurements from a line drawn in the midline of the chest. This transverse diameter is divided by the longest transverse diameter of the chest to arrive at a cardiothoracic ratio. This is a relatively crude way of assessing cardiac size, but because it is easily obtained, it is commonly used. Generally, a cardiothoracic ratio over 50% is considered cardiac enlargement. Some reasonable assessment of individual chamber enlargement can be made from inspection of the plain chest film in the PA and lateral projections.

Inspection of the lung fields. Overcirculation or undercirculation of the

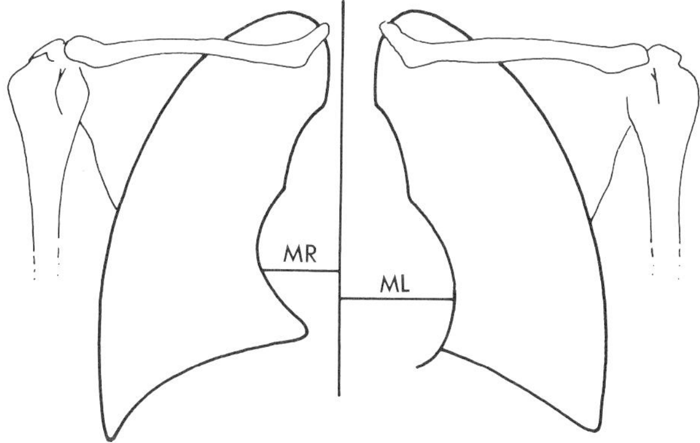

FIG. 4-7
The cardiothoracic ratio derived by adding the midright *(MR)* and midleft *(ML)* measurements. The sum is then divided by the longest transverse diameter of the chest.

lung fields as compared with normal circulation is most helpful in the differential diagnosis of congenital heart diseases. In the presence of a left-to-right shunt there are signs of increased circulation in the pulmonary vessels; in the presence of a right-to-left shunt there is evidence of uncercirculation. Patterns of pulmonary veins, their size and prominence, as well as the presence or absence of pulmonary lymphatic markings help in the diagnosis of elevated pulmonary venous pressure, which is a common sign of congestive heart failure.

Pulmonary edema can be of two kinds, alveolar and interstitial. Alveolar edema is characteristic of acute left-sided heart failure and is manifested by bilateral confluent densities that start centrally and spread peripherally. This is commonly referred to as the butterfly-wing pattern. In interstitial edema, fluid accumulates in the interstitial tissues of the lungs and produces a generalized haziness and clouding of the vascular shadows. When such fluid collects in the interlobular septa of the lung, septal lines are formed that are referred to as Kerley's lines.

Inspection of the pleural spaces. Approximately 250 ml of pleural effusion is necessary for an accurate radiologic diagnosis. This is usually manifested as blunting of the costophrenic angle. Larger effusions, approximately 1 liter, can also accumulate, and may be an accompaniment of congestive heart failure or be independent of heart disease and indicate the presence of lung disease. Pleural fluid examination is discussed on p. 109. Occasionally, pleural effusions are hidden under the lung (subpulmonic effusion) and therefore do not obliterate the costophrenic angle. These effusions can be detected by obtaining the film with the patient in the lateral position (lateral decubitus film).

Inspection of the rib cage. Inspection may provide a clue for coarctation of

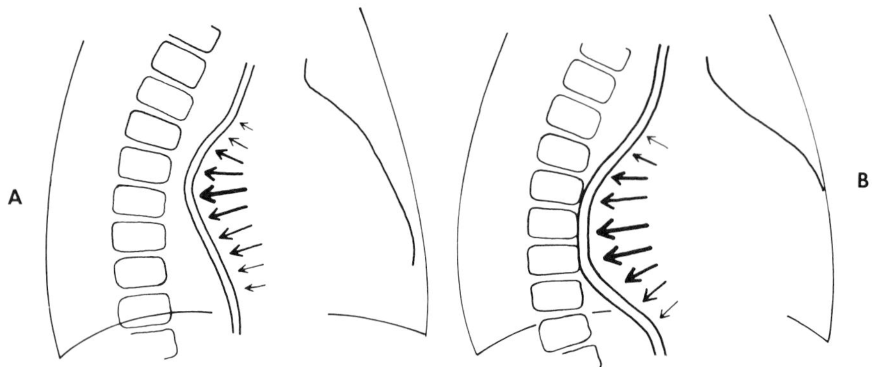

FIG. 4-8
The x-ray film of the chest obtained after the patient has swallowed barium (a "cardiac series"). Note the moderate, **A**, and marked, **B**, degrees of left atrial enlargement reflected in the displacement of the atrium by the barium-filled esophagus. This is a right anterior oblique projection.

the aorta where collateral circulation from enlarged intercostal arteries would produce characteristic deformity or notching of the rib margins.

Cardiac series. The ability to make a more accurate diagnosis of specific chamber enlargement is enhanced by obtaining a cardiac series, in which a bolus of barium is swallowed by the patient, opacifying the posterior-lying esophagus. In addition to the PA and lateral films two oblique films are obtained. In the cardiac series an enlarged left atrium or even an enlarged aorta could be noted displacing the barium-filled esophagus (Fig. 4-8). This, along with the additional projections, would aid in the diagnosis of left or right ventricular enlargement.

CO_2 injection and cardiac fluoroscopy. Carbon dioxide (CO_2) may be injected into a peripheral vein for the diagnosis of pericardial effusion. After a brief period, x-ray films are taken with the patient in the left lateral position. The carbon dioxide acts as a contrast material within the right atrial chamber, defining the thickness of the right atrial and pericardial walls. At present this technique is not commonly used and is being replaced by the echocardiogram because of the latter's diagnostic simplicity and accuracy.

Cardiac fluoroscopy is most useful in detecting calcifications of various parts of the heart. Introduction of image intensifiers has decreased the overall radiation hazard of this test and has improved the quality of the images seen. Cardiac fluoroscopy is useful in detecting calcification in the coronary artery system. Although the diagnostic method of choice for detection and semiquantitation of coronary artery disease is by selective coronary angiography (see p. 95), cardiac fluoroscopy is a useful screening tool for this purpose. Approximately 75% of the patients with coronary artery disease have calcification of the coronary artery system, but 20% of the patients (especially older patients) with no obstructive coronary disease also reveal calcification of the coronary arteries. Calcification of the various valves of the heart, specifically the aortic and mitral valves, is unequivocal evidence of disease of these valves. Although heavy calcification suggests more advanced disease of the valves (usually narrowing), an exact correlation cannot be made. Other cardiac diseases in which calcification is helpful in the diagnosis are tumors of the heart, calcification of the pericardium in constrictive pericarditis, and calcification of the myocardium secondary to old myocardial infarction.

Limitations

The chest x-ray examination of the heart can be perfectly normal in the presence of severe organic disease of the heart. The information revealed is mainly of a static nature, with the dynamic aspects of the working heart not detected.

Variations of heart size in systole as compared with diastole also diminish the accuracy of detection of cardiac enlargement.

Indications

The chest x-ray examination and cardiac series are used almost as an extension of the physical examination and are performed on patients with all kinds of cardiac disease as well as in screening of the normal population. As discussed, cardiac fluoroscopy is indicated when calcification of various parts of the heart is suspected.

Contraindications

There is no absolute contraindication, since the risk is limited to a minimal exposure to ionizing radiation, a risk that increases with exposure. This becomes more important in young children and in pregnant women in whom studies should be performed only when necessary and the gonads or the fetus should routinely be shielded.

Pitfalls

In the use of radiographic examination of the heart, diagnostic errors can originate either from the recording technique or during the interpretation of the information.

Technical errors. Films exposed during expiration may produce a false impression of an enlarged heart and pulmonary vascular congestion. This also becomes exaggerated in the patient who is obese with a high diaphragm and enlarged pericardial fat. Overpenetration may produce disappearance of pulmonary vascular markings. Rotation of the patient may produce a false appearance of enlargement or may produce magnification of various vessels.

Errors of interpretation. In the presence of a pectus excavatum deformity of the chest, the heart may be displaced posteriorly and produce a false impression of cardiomegaly. In pectus carinatum deformity of the chest, the anterior-posterior diameter is increased and possible enlargement of the right ventricle may go undetected. Patients with a straight dorsal spine may simulate cardiomegaly, especially on the lateral projection. In patients with severe kyphoscoliosis, accurate assessment of cardiac size and pulmonary vasculature may be impossible. A portable chest x-ray examination cannot be used to assess cardiac size, although it can be helpful in assessing the degree of pulmonary congestion.

Further pitfalls in the interpretation of x-ray films of the chest are many, but discussion of them would be beyond the scope of this book.

Use of blood tests in cardiac disease

A multitude of blood tests are used in evaluation of the cardiac patient. Like the electrocardiogram and the chest x ray, they are an extension of the physical examination and constitute an integral part of a complete evaluation. Automation has further popularized these tests by making them easily available and also reducing the cost.

Cardiac enzymes

These have been discussed in Chapter 1 and are briefly mentioned here. Normal blood levels for these enzymes as well as the organs in which the content is high can be found in Fig. 4-9 and Table 4-2.

SGOT (serum glutamic oxaloacetic transaminase). Levels of this enzyme begin to rise in about 8 hours, peak in 24 to 48 hours (Fig. 4-9), and return to normal in 4 to 8 days following a myocardial infarction. Damage to other tissues besides the heart may elevate this enzyme and cause a false diagnosis of myocardial infarction.

LDH (lactic dehydrogenase). Elevated LDH levels usually persist longer than SGOT levels and can be helpful if the patient is seen several days after the onset of myocardial infarction (Fig. 4-9).

Fractionation of LDH into its five isoenzymes further adds to the specificity of the test. Myocardial LDH is predominantly in fraction No. 1.

CPK (creatine phosphokinase). This enzyme is found in the heart as well as in skeletal muscle and the brain, but is not elevated appreciably in damage to red blood cells or the liver. There are many causes for elevated CPK, including vigorous exercise, skeletal muscle disease, intramuscular injections, cerebral infarctions, and myocardial infarction. People with an unusually large muscle mass, such as athletes, have a higher CPK value than the general population. CPK is separated into three isoenzymes, labeled as CPK-MM, CPK-BB, and CPK-MB. The myocardium contains MB fraction as well as some MM fraction. In myocardial injury the elevated fraction is of the MB type. In skeletal muscle injury, CPK elevation is of the MM fraction. Recently, at-

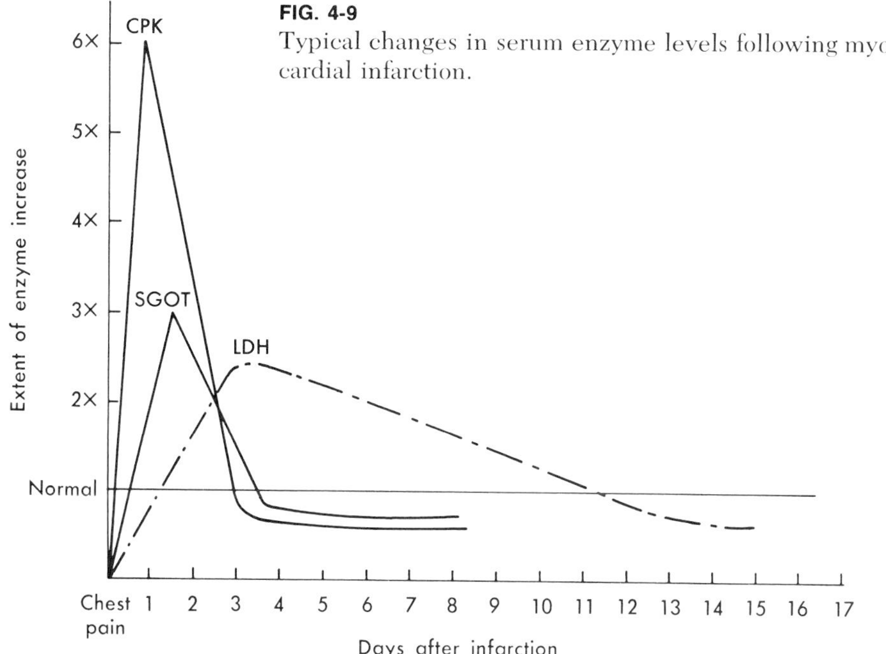

FIG. 4-9
Typical changes in serum enzyme levels following myocardial infarction.

TABLE 4-2
Normal blood levels and enzyme distribution in cells*

Enzyme	Tissue	Normal blood levels
Creatine phosphokinase (CPK)	Heart Brain Skeletal muscle	Female 5-25 U/ml Male 5-35 U/ml Female 55-170 U/L at 37° C Male 30-135 U/L at 37° C
Serum glutamic oxaloacetic transaminase (SGOT)	Heart Kidney Red cells Brain Pancreas Lung Liver Skeletal muscle	10-40 Karmen units 6-18 IU/L
Lactic dehydrogenase (LDH)	Heart Kidney Red cells Brain Lymph nodes Spleen Leukocytes Pancreas Lung Liver Skeletal muscle	80-120 Wacker units 150-450 Wroblewski units 71-207 IU/L

*The normal levels vary from laboratory to laboratory according to the test used.

tempts have been made to quantitate the total CPK rise, to relate this to the amount of muscle necrosis in myocardial infarction, and, in turn, to relate this to the prognosis of the patient. In general the larger the CPK rise, the larger the infarct area and the poorer the prognosis for the patient.

Clinical value. At present the value of these enzymes in diagnosis of myocardial infarction is: (1) as an adjunct to the history, physical examination, and the ECG in confirming the clinical impression of myocardial infarction and (2) in following the course of the myocardial infarction and especially in detecting extension of myocardial infarction where the electrocardiogram may not change.

Blood lipids

Elevated blood lipid as an abnormality in relation to coronary artery disease has received much attention recently. The blood lipids (cholesterol, triglycerides, and phospholipids) circulate in the plasma bound to protein, thus the term "lipoproteins." Electrophoresis is the method used to separate the lipoproteins, and from this several classifications have evolved. For practical purposes two types of hyperlipidemia are important in cardiac disease: type 2, in which the cholesterol is elevated and the triglycerides are normal or mildly elevated, and type 4, in which the cholesterol is normal and the triglycerides are elevated.

The normal designation for cholesterol and triglycerides, as discussed in Chapter 1, varies among populations and age groups (Table 4-3). The generally accepted upper limit of normal is 250 mg for cholesterol and 150 mg for triglycerides.

The association of hyperlipidemia and coronary artery disease is well established, an association that is more striking in the younger population. Although there is no conclusive proof at this time that lowering abnormally elevated lipids will hold or retard the progression of coronary artery disease, it is prudent to detect these elevations and to use dietary and, if indicated, drug measures to bring these levels to within normal range or at least to lower

TABLE 4-3

Concentrations of cholesterol, triglycerides, or low density lipoproteins, which, if exceeded, clearly indicate hyperlipidemia

Age	C*	TG*	LDL*
>29 years	240	140	170
30-39 years	270	150	190
40-49 years	310	160	190
50+	330	190	210

*C=Cholesterol; TG=Triglyceride; LDL=Low density lipoproteins.

Reproduced with permission from Frederickson, D. S.: A physician's guide to hyperlipidemia, Mod. Concepts Cardiovasc. Dis. **41**(7), 1972, American Heart Association, Inc.

them. It is generally agreed that the lower the blood lipids, the less chance for acquiring coronary artery disease.

There are two common pitfalls in the measurement of blood lipids: the patient has to be fasting if useful information is to be obtained, and there can be marked fluctuations in the same patient in day-to-day measurements. Therefore, the patient should have several measurements before a definite diagnosis of hyperlipidemia is made and dietary and/or drug therapy is instituted.

Blood glucose and glucose tolerance test (GTT)

An abnormal glucose tolerance test is commonly associated with hyperlipidemia and obesity, and is an additional risk factor for coronary artery disease. Fasting blood glucose measurements will detect the overt symptomatic diabetic patient. The value of the glucose tolerance test in detecting the asymptomatic patient with diabetes lies in defining this risk factor. Generally, no treatment is necessary except weight reduction in the obese.

Pitfalls. Two pitfalls in the measurement of the glucose tolerance test are: (1) the patient should not have a below-average carbohydrate intake before the test and (2) this test should not be done too soon (days to weeks) after a myocardial infarction, since glucose levels are elevated following infarction.

Other blood tests

Among the other blood tests commonly employed are determinations of electrolytes, blood urea nitrogen (BUN), and serum creatinine. For a complete discussion of these tests refer to Chapter 1.

Abnormalities of electrolytes are common in patients with heart disease and are either secondary to congestive heart failure or occur as side effects to drug therapy for this condition.

Chronic congestive heart failure causes total body, as well as myocardial, potassium and magnesium depletion and in severe stages, when water is not restricted, may also produce lowering of the serum sodium level (hyponatremia). Diuretics used to decrease total body sodium may also produce hyponatremia if water is not restricted. They commonly produce total body potassium depletion and this *may* be detected as a lowering of the serum potassium (hypokalemia), although significant total body potassium depletion can occur in the absence of hypokalemia.

Creatinine clearance may fall and blood urea nitrogen level may rise in severe congestive heart failure.

Measurement of drug levels in plasma

Monitoring of blood levels of various cardiac drugs is essential for successful and safe treatment. Of the commonly used drugs, assays for plasma levels are presently available for digoxin, quinidine, procainamide, diphen-

TABLE 4-4
Therapeutic and potentially toxic blood levels for cardiac drugs

Drug	Therapeutic blood level (per ml)	Potentially toxic blood level (per ml)
Digitoxin	14-30 ng	Over 30 ng
Digoxin	1- 2 ng	Over 3 ng
Propranolol (Inderal)	20-85 ng	Over 150 ng
Procainamide (Pronestyl)	4- 8 μg	Over 8 μg
Diphenylhydantoin (Dilantin)	10-18 μg	Over 18 μg
Quinidine	2.5-5 μg	Over 5 μg
Lidocaine	1.4-6 μg	Over 6 μg
Verapamil (Isoptin)	2- 4 μg	Over 5 μg
Disopyramide (Norpace)	2- 4 μg	Over 6 μg
Tocainaide	6-12 μg	Over 14 μg
Theophylline	10-20 μg	Over 20 μg

ylhydantoin, lidocaine, and propranolol. The therapeutic and toxic blood levels for these drugs are displayed in Table 4-4.

Miscellaneous blood tests

The complete blood count (CBC) is useful in detection of anemias, which may (1) present as angina in the patient with coronary artery disease, (2) aggravate congestive heart failure, (3) give a diagnostic clue in subacute bacterial endocarditis, or (4) present evidence of hemolysis in patients with prosthetic valves.

The white blood cell count (WBC) is elevated in patients with myocardial infarction, bacterial endocarditis, and the postmyocardial infarction (Dressler) syndrome.

The sedimentaiton rate is elevated in acute myocardial infarction, bacterial endocarditis, Dressler's syndrome, and in many other diseases that cause inflammation. It is considered to be characteristically low in congestive heart failure.

The C reactive protein is usually absent in normal people and is elevated in persons with acute rheumatic fever.

Antistreptolysin-O (ASO) titer is elevated after streptococcal infections and can be the clue to diagnosis of acute rheumatic fever.

The VDRL, discussed on p. 205, can be the clue to syphilitic heart disease, usually presenting as aortic insufficiency or disease of the ostia of the coronary arteries.

Prothrombin time is used in initiating and maintaining anticoagulation with oral anticoagulants (drugs such as Coumadin). Usually the prothrombin time is kept within 2 to 2.5 times the normal, and that is generally comparable to 20% to 30% of the activity of normal. The partial thromboplastin time (PTT) and the clotting time are used in following patients receiving heparin, and 2 to 2.5 times the normal is the therapeutic range.

Anticoagulation with heparin, and subsequently with Coumadin-type drugs, is used in pulmonary embolism, deep venous thrombosis, cerebral embolism, and acute peripheral arterial embolism and is felt to be beneficial in patients with acute myocardial infarction with congestive heart failure during the period of bed rest. Because multiple drugs interfere with the metabolism and reaction of the Coumadin-type anticoagulants, frequent measurements of the prothrombin time and careful checks of the interaction of other drugs are important in minimizing the risk of hemorrhage in patients receiving anticoagulant drugs.

Blood cultures are crucial in the diagnosis of infective endocarditis. It is important to obtain an adequate number of cultures. Generally six cultures are considered adequate. These should be obtained by sterile technique, preferably inoculated at the bedside, and cultured on aerobic, anaerobic, and microaerophilic media.

The common pitfalls in the diagnosis of endocarditis from blood cultures are (1) contamination, causing a false positive diagnosis and (2) the presence of antibiotics in the patient's serum or treatment with antibiotics prior to the blood culture may give false negative results.

Arterial blood gas determinations are discussed on p. 108. Patients with myocardial infarction or congestive heart failure commonly manifest abnormalities of the arterial blood gases. Patients who have hypoxemia or desaturation secondary to altered ventilation perfusion ratios usually benefit from oxygen administration in an attempt to keep their saturation 90% or higher. Patients who have myocardial infarctions, especially with pulmonary congestion or edema, commonly hyperventilate, with subsequent lowering of the P_{CO_2} and mild respiratory alkalosis. In the presence of severe pulmonary edema, hypoventilation with elevation of the P_{CO_2} and mild respiratory acidosis may occur.

Some drugs used in the treatment of myocardial infarction, especially morphine, produce a predictable drop in the rate and depth of respiration and may, in excessive doses, precipitate hypoventilation with respiratory acidosis. Therefore, in patients who are receiving larger than usual doses of morphine or morphine along with other suppressants, arterial blood gas determinations are indicated to detect and/or avoid respiratory depression.

Carbon monoxide level is elevated in moderate to heavy smokers, as well as in persons living in areas of heavy industrial pollution, and may precipitate or exacerbate angina pectoris in the presence of coronary artery disease. Measurement of carbon monoxide levels in the blood can be helpful in detecting unusually heavy industrial exposure as well as the heavy cigarette smoker with angina pectoris.

Urine examination

Measurement of the volume of urine through 24 hours is helpful, since in heart failure the night volume may be from 30% to 50% more than the day volume; such nighttime elevation is referred to as nocturia.

The presence of red cells in the urine may be the clue to evidence of infective endocarditis or embolic disease of the kidneys.

Mild proteinuria, 1 to 2 gm per day, can be seen in congestive heart failure. Patients with marked elevation of venous pressure, constrictive pericarditis, or tricuspid insufficiency may present with massive proteinuria, and even with the nephrotic syndrome.

Recently, the detection of myoglobin in the urine (myoglobinuria) has been found useful as a sensitive test in the diagnosis of myocardial infarction, but clinical experience with this test remains limited.

NONINVASIVE SPECIALIZED DIAGNOSTIC METHODS IN CARDIOLOGY

The following is a discussion of the more important tests used in the physician's office and hospital practice of cardiology. These tests are grouped together because they are noninvasive; that is, they do not break the patient's skin or interfere with or alter the events that are being observed. They also pose no risk or significant discomfort to the patient and can be repeated at frequent intervals with absolute safety. There has been increasing interest in these tests, and although presently they do not, with rare exceptions, eliminate the need for invasive (such as cardiac catheterization) tests, they complement them in many cases. Tests with proved clinical value are discussed in the order of their general importance or usefulness.

Echocardiography

Echocardiography (ultrasound cardiography) is a relatively recent tool in cardiology and has rapidly found widespread acceptance and use. Simply, it is a technique in which echoes (reflected ultrasound) from pulsed, high frequency sound waves are used to locate and study the movements and the dimensions of various cardiac structures. The technique yields direct recordings of the motion of the mitral, aortic, tricuspid and, with some experience, the pulmonic valve leaflets, the interventricular septum, and the right and left ventricular walls. It provides accurate measurement of the size of the cardiac chambers and the changes of these dimensions during the cardiac cycle. It also permits recognition of abnormal filling defects, as in atrial tumors.

Because the ultrasound beam tracks the motion of various cardiac structures over a period of time, it provides a time-motion study of the heart (M-mode echocardiography). This technique has given cardiologists the unique opportunity to visualize internal structures of the heart in a totally noninvasive manner and with a degree of sensitivity exceeding that of ordinary x-ray films. The test is usually performed in the echocardiographic laboratory with the patient supine. The transducer (the source of ultrasound as well as the receiver of the reflected ultrasound) is placed on the surface of the chest along the left sternal border, third to fifth interspace, to avoid interference from the lung, as ultrasound transmits very poorly in air.

Cross-sectional echocardiography is a newer development in this field. Whereas in M-mode echocardiography the angle of the ultrasound beam is kept stationary, in cross-sectional echocardiography this angle is changed within a sector (usually 45°-80°) producing a "sector scan." Images produced by this technique more closely resemble cardiac structures.

In acutely ill patients or others who may not be able to be transferred to the echocardiographic laboratory, portable echocardiographic equipment can be used and the complete test performed at the bedside. The echocardiogram is recorded on photographic paper (strip chart recording) or on film (Polaroid). A normal echocardiogram showing mainly the excursions of the mitral valve leaflets is shown in Fig. 4-10.

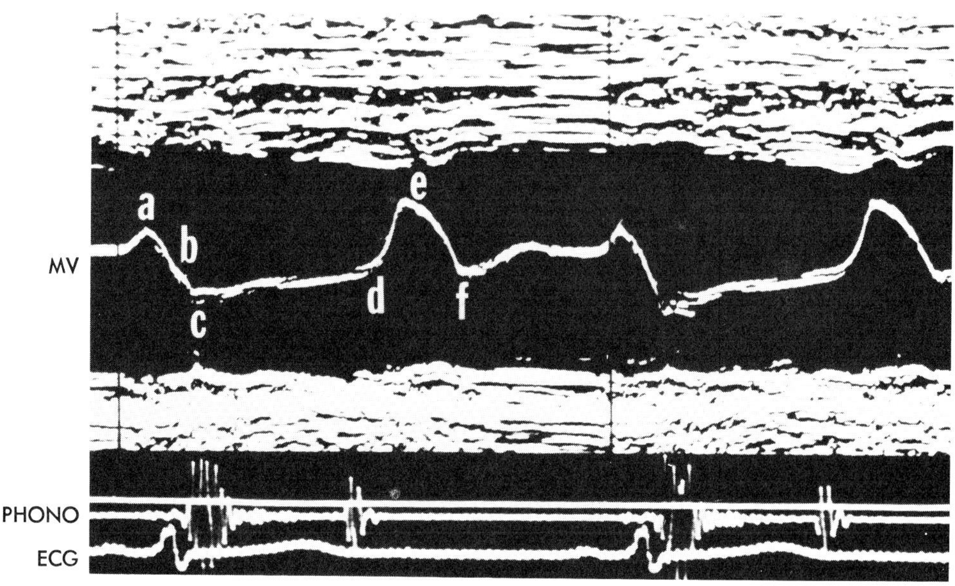

FIG. 4-10
Normal mitral valve. A normal mitral valve trace *(MV)* has been labeled to identify physiologic events. Atrial systole is followed by a peak *(a)*. Onset of ventricular systole *(b)* culminates in valve closure *(c)*. A gradual anterior motion occurs during systole. Valve opening starts at point *(d)* and the valve is fully opened at *(e)*. Posterior movement in diastole *(e-f)* is an indication of the rate of left atrial emptying. *PHONO*, Phonocardiogram; *ECG*, electrocardiogram. (From King, D. L., editor: Diagnostic ultrasound, St. Louis, 1974, The C. V. Mosby Co.)

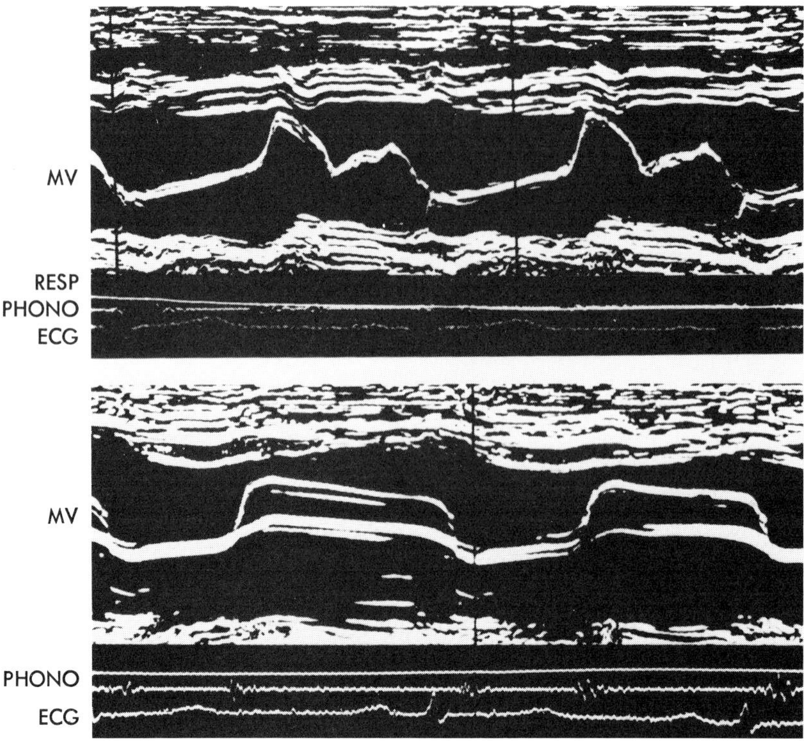

FIG. 4-11
Mitral stenosis. The upper panel is from a normal subject and shows a sharply peaked early diastolic trace, moderate sized A waves and a posterior cusp that moves in a direction opposite to the anterior cusp at the closure point. The patient with mitral stenosis (lower panel) shows a flat diastolic configuration with no visible A wave and a posterior cusp that tends to follow the anterior in diastole. *MV*, mitral valve; *RESP*, respiration; *PHONO*, phonocardiogram; *ECG*, electrocardiogram. (From King, D. L., editor: Diagnostic ultrasound, St. Louis, 1974, The C. V. Mosby Co.)

Clinical value

The echocardiogram was first employed as an aid in the diagnosis of mitral stenosis. Fig. 4-11 illustrates the abnormal movement of the mitral valve in a patient with mitral stenosis. In the past 8 to 10 years echocardiographic application has expanded very rapidly, and its indications are being continuously revised and extended.

Echocardiography is helpful in the diagnosis of the following disorders: mitral stenosis, tricuspid stenosis, pericardial effusion, atrial septal defects, prolapsing mitral leaflet syndrome, hypertrophic cardiomyopathy (obstructive or nonobstructive), atrial tumors, and multiple congenital defects in neonates and infants. It is also useful in the evaluation of aortic and pulmonic valves for stenosis or insufficiency and mitral insufficiency as well as for assessment of the function of the left ventricle (cardiac output and ejection fraction). In the large group of disorders under coronary artery disease the echocardiogram has been useful in evaluating abnormal left ventricular function secondary to coronary artery disease or myocardial infarction. Presently M-mode echocardiography is of no value in the diagnosis and evaluation of obstructive disease of the coronary arteries. Cross-sectional echocardiography has been used to visualize segments of the coronary artery tree. The clinical value of this is still unknown.

Limitations of echocardiography

Although echocardiography is an exciting and fascinating field, it has its limitations. At the present time in approximately 10% to 15% of patients, the technical quality of the results is inadequate for diagnostic purposes. Because it is a new method, technicians proficient in the performance of the test, as well as physicians able to expertly interpret the tests, are in short supply. This has been a limiting factor in both the quality of tests performed and acceptance of the techniques in a community. Because of the way echocardiography is performed, the sound wave beam samples a relatively small, select area of the cardiac structure studied or the chamber evaluated, and thus in situations where abnormalities are localized to one segment of the heart, the echocardiogram is of limited value. Cross-sectional techniques aim at overcoming some of these limitations.

Indications for echocardiography

All the disorders listed previously, or a suspicion of these disorders, would be an indication to perform an echocardiogram. The echocardiogram is indicated also in situations in which the only abnormality is a cardiac murmur heard on auscultation and the question is raised of whether or not this murmur is indicative of organic heart disease.

Pitfalls

There is no contraindication to echocardiography, since there is no inherent risk in the procedure. There are, however, pitfalls in the performance of the technique, such as difficulty in obtaining consistently high quality echocardiograms and in interpreting these records. Possible risk to the patient may be considered to be misdiagnosis or wrong therapeutic decisions that are based on poor quality echocardiograms. It can be unequivocally stated that poorly done echocardiography and inadequately interpreted echocardiography are worse than no echocardiography.

Phonocardiography and external pulse recording

Phonocardiography

This is the graphic recording of sounds that originate in the heart and the great vessels. This recording may be accomplished by placing microphones on the surface of the body or by introducing special apparatus into the heart (intracardiac phonocardiography). This discussion will be limited to the former.

Phonocardiography is an extension of auscultation of the heart as performed with the stethoscope, in that it generally records only the sounds that can be heard by the clinician. The phonocardiogram is, however, superior to the stethoscope in recording low frequency sounds (that is, gallop sounds), while the stethoscope is better in appreciating high frequency sounds, or murmurs. The phonocardiogram can record the four components of the first sound, systolic murmurs, the two components of the second sound (aortic and pulmonic), the opening snap of mitral stenosis, third and fourth gallop sounds, and clicks. It can also give information about *relative* loudness of these events. A normal phonocardiogram is displayed in Figs. 4-10 and 4-12.

The phonocardiogram is commonly recorded simultaneously with other external pulses that can serve as a reference for timing various sounds. These are carotid pulse, jugular pulse, and apexcardiogram.

Carotid pulse tracing

This is the graphic recording of the displacement of the carotid artery in the neck, produced by each heartbeat and reflecting small volume changes in a segment of this artery. This recording is obtained by applying a pressure-sensitive transducer over the point of maximal pulsation of the carotid artery in the neck. Information is thus gained about the rate of rise of this curve, its duration, and its overall contour. Although records obtained in this manner closely resemble tracings obtained by pressure transducers inside the vessels,

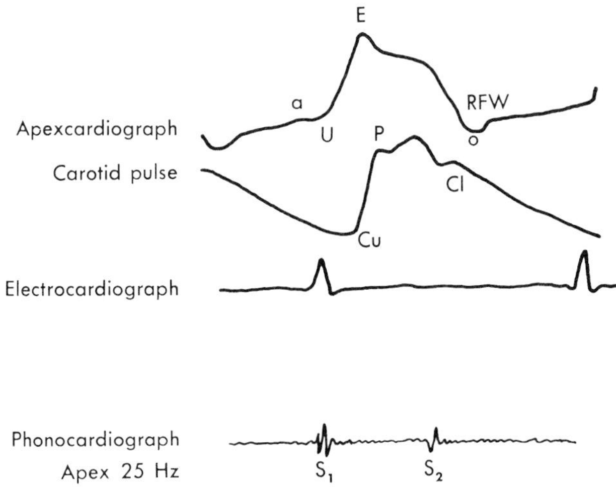

FIG. 4-12
Normal phonocardiogram and external pulse recordings displayed with the ECG.

carotid pulse tracings cannot be used to measure absolute pressures. A normal carotid pulse tracing is displayed in Fig. 4-12.

Jugular pulse tracing

This is obtained in a similar manner to the carotid pulse tracing, except that the recording is obtained over the jugular venous system and yields information about events in the right atrium and right ventricle.

Apexcardiogram

This is the graphic recording of displacement of the chest wall produced by the motion of the underlying left ventricle. Analysis of this record provides information about events in this chamber. A normal apexcardiogram is displayed in Fig. 4-12.

Clinical uses

The phonocardiogram is most useful for accurate *timing of* various sounds and murmurs. Examples are timing the opening snap of mitral stenosis, timing the closing of aortic and pulmonic valves of the second sound (A2-P2), and determining whether clicks are ejection (early in systole) or late systolic clicks. The phonocardiogram is also useful in recording the shape of various murmurs that are heard.

The carotid pulse tracing provides information about the functional state or the performance of the left ventricle. This is accomplished by measuring the various components of the curve produced on the graph. Also, general evaluation of the contour of the curve can give information about aortic stenosis, aortic insufficiency, mitral insufficiency, and idiopathic hypertrophic subaortic stenosis (IHSS).

The jugular pulse tracing serves as a reference for the phonocardiogram; it yields information about right ventricular hypertrophy, elevated pressure in the right atrium, tricuspid regurgitation, and constrictive pericarditis; and it aids in the analysis of complex arrhythmias. In complete heart block it records the cannon A wave that is observed at the bedside examination.

Apex cardiography is helpful in timing various heart sounds, especially the opening snap of mitral stenosis. It is also useful as a reference tracing for locating the fourth heart sound or the atrial gallop, and in distinguishing the origin of the gallop (right or left side). The evaluation of the contour of the tracing yields information about left ventricular hypertrophy, possible aortic or mitral stenosis, or idiopathic hypertrophic subaortic stenosis.

These four tests—the phonocardiogram, carotid pulse tracing, jugular pulse tracing, and apexcardiogram—are valuable because they provide a permanent objective record far superior to handwritten descriptive records and can be used in serial comparison in the same patient. They are also superb devices for teaching the physical examination and auscultation of the heart.

Limitations

There are limitations in the clinical use of these tests. Because they serve as an extension of the physical examination, what cannot be heard through the stethoscope usually cannot be recorded on the phonocardiogram. A specific diagnosis can rarely be made *only* by inspection of these graphic methods. Another limitation is the skill and the time necessary to perform the tests. Also, information obtained is of a qualitative nature; therefore, statements about quantitative events or abnormalities cannot be made.

Indications

These graphic methods are indicated whenever a permanent objective record is important as well as when the specific information about the pulses or timing of various auscultative findings is not otherwise available.

Equipment presently available permits the simultaneous recording and superimposition with the electrocardiogram of echocardiograms, multiple phonocardiograms, carotid pulse tracings, venous pulse tracings, and apexcardiograms. The value of the individual tests is usually enhanced when they are performed in this manner.

Nuclear cardiology

Radioactive tracer techniques are being used in cardiovascular diagnosis with increasing frequency. These tests generally qualify as "noninvasive" because they are safe and can be performed repeatedly, and the total radiation exposure is considered minimal. They do involve intravenous injection of a tracer material, but this does not involve more than the drawing of routine blood samples.

The general technique in all of these tests is the injection of a radioactive tracer material into a vein and recording the emitted radioactivity over a specific area of the body. By using various types of tracers as well as different recording techniques, vastly different types of information can be obtained. Among the diagnostic tests employing radioactive tracer techniques are lung scanning, angiocardioscan, and myocardial scanning during rest and after exercise.

Lung scanning

In lung scanning an adequate quantity of tracer is injected, which subsequently becomes trapped in the lung capillaries and provides information about the status of pulmonary perfusion.

In scanning for right-to-left shunts, the radioactive material, instead of being trapped in the pulmonary vasculature, is passed to the left side of the heart and trapped in systemic capillaries (for example, in the kidney or the spleen), where radioactivity will be seen. In such a situation an angiocardioscan (nuclear angiocardiogram) can further localize the shunt.

The lung scan is most helpful in a diagnosis of pulmonary embolus when the x-ray film of the chest is normal or near normal, and when the test is interpreted in conjunction with the ventilation scan, which would detect the presence of parenchymal lung disease. This is discussed on pp. 110 and 111.

In the presence of grossly abnormal x-ray films of the chest resulting from parenchymal lung disease, such as those normally seen in chronic obstructive lung disease or pneumonia, the diagnostic accuracy of a lung scan is markedly diminished. In questionable or doubtful cases it is necessary to use selective pulmonary angiography to obtain a definite diagnosis. Occasionally, a lung scan will reveal absolutely no perfusion on one side of the lung. This could be the manifestation of a large pulmonary embolus or may indicate a congenitally absent or atretic right or left pulmonary artery.

Nuclear angiocardiogram (angiocardioscan)

In this test a bolus of radionuclide is injected intravenously and its course through the circulatory system is followed with a scintillation camera. The size, shape, and sequence of filling of the various chambers of the heart can then be studied. This procedure is most useful in the detection of intracardiac shunt or complex congenital heart diseases. It is also helpful in evaluating a surgically performed shunt in congenital heart disease. In addition, it supplies information about cardiac size and chamber enlargement, and is helpful in diagnosis of pericardial effusion and differentiating it from cardiomegaly. Presently, the echocardiogram is superior in detecting and quantitating pericardial effusion, but in difficult or doubtful cases nuclear angiocardiography is useful. It also provides information about the contour of the left ventricle, which helps in the diagnosis of left ventricular aneurysm. Recent attempts have been made in evaluating left ventricular function by calculating volumes and ejection fractions of the left ventricle. The diagnostic accuracy of this method of scanning does not match that obtained by cardiac catheterization and angiocardiography with injection of dye, and therefore it remains a screening test.

Myocardial scanning

Recently, radioactive tracer techniques have been used in attempts to evaluate the site and extent of myocardial ischemia or infarction. This technique involves the injection of tracers, usually radioactive technetium, thalium, or potassium. The usefulness of this test is extended when performed during stress of either exercise or pacing, where a relative decrease of myocardial perfusion can be detected in patients with coronary artery disease in the absence of myocardial infarction. Thus evaluation of the size of the myocardial infarct, diagnosis of coronary artery disease, and evaluation of patency or occlusion of vein bypass grafts are making the techniques of myocardial scanning one of the most promising fields in nuclear cardiology.

Clinical value

In general, tracer techniques are inadequate or poor in the evaluation of isolated valvular lesions of mild to moderate severity or mixed valvular lesions. Although the diagnostic potential of tracer techniques is great, at the present time the main indications for tracer methods in cardiology are for the lung scan (evaluating pulmonary embolus) detecting right-to-left shunts, screening of congenital heart disease, and myocardial scanning for evaluation of ischemia or infarction.

Pacemaker evaluation

All pacemakers rely on batteries of one type or another to generate the pulse for pacing. Battery exhaustion is the most common cause of pacemaker failure. Thus the purpose of pacemaker evaluation is to obtain the longest possible use of a pacemaker pulse generator without exposing the patient to the risk of pacemaker failure. Rather than relying on the arbitrary limit set by the manufacturer to determine function, pacemaker evaluation should be used both to detect early failure of a pacemaker battery and to avoid unnecessary replacement of a well-functioning unit.

Pacemaker evaluation is performed by using an electrocardiogram equipped with an electrical interval counter, which measures the pulse interval and duration. The pulse interval or the pulse generator rate can also be transmitted over the telephone, and thus analysis can be performed without the patient leaving home.

There are several indicators of impending or actual battery exhaustion. Among these are changes in the pulse interval, a decrease in the amplitude of the pulse, a change in the duration of the pulse, and the failure of the sensing circuit. Analysis of these variables in conjunction with the standard electrocardiogram to detect loss of capture will permit detection of impending or actual pacemaker failure. Criteria as to when to replace the pacemaker have been proposed using the above variables, and although different centers may vary in their precise criteria, a loss of capture is considered an absolute indication for replacement.

INVASIVE DIAGNOSTIC METHODS IN CARDIOLOGY

Cardiac catheterization

Cardiac catheterization is the most definitive method of obtaining accurate diagnostic information of cardiac disorders and evaluating their severity. From the pioneer days of Forssmann in 1929, when he positioned a catheter in his own right atrium, to the present, this diagnostic test has been much expanded. The selective catheterization of all cardiac chambers, great vessels, and coronary arteries has been accomplished so frequently and successfully that it is now commonly performed in many hospitals with remarkable safety.

Method

Cardiac catheterization is performed by specially trained personnel (usually cardiologists and radiologists in cooperation) in a specially equipped cardiac catheterization laboratory where, besides equipment for diagnostic uses, complete resuscitative equipment is available.

In its simplest form the procedure includes introduction of cardiac catheters into the right side of the heart through an arm vein (basilic or cephalic vein) or a leg vein (the femoral vein). The catheter is advanced through the vena cava, the right atrium, the right ventricle, and pulmonary artery, and for a brief period further advanced and located in the distal pulmonary artery wedge position. On the left side of the heart the catheter is introduced through an artery, either the brachial artery in the arm or the femoral artery. It is advanced through the arterial system to the ascending aorta, through the aortic valve into the left ventricle, and if necessary to the left atrium.

Both of these routes can be approached by the cutdown technique. In this method, the veins are usually tied at the end of the procedure while the arteries are repaired. The procedure also can be performed percutaneously, a method in which the vessels are not isolated and all catheters are introduced over guide wires and needles. From the various chambers, pressures are recorded, and blood is sampled and analyzed for its oxygen content, ordinarily during rest as well as exercise. This information coupled with measurement of the patient's oxygen consumption, which is obtained by collecting gases expired by the patient, reveals (1) the patient's cardiac output (the amount of blood pumped per minute), (2) the presence and size of right-to-left or left-to-right shunt within the cardiac chambers, (3) the presence and severity of stenosis (narrowing of various valves), and (4) the calculation of the resistance of the various vascular beds. Additional information is obtained using the indicator dilution test, angiography, and selective arteriography.

Indicator dilution test. An indicator is a substance that can be harmlessly introduced into the cardiovascular system and detected with appropriate sensing apparatus. The substance commonly used for determining cardiac output is indocyanine green, which is introduced on the venous side and sampled by a densitometer (an instrument that is sensitive to optical changes of the blood). Curves that are thus obtained are used to calculate cardiac output, blood flow, and shunts. A slight modification of this principle uses hydrogen gas that is introduced into the patient's system by inhalation. The gas is diffused into the circulation at the level of the pulmonary capillaries. Left-to-right shunts at various levels within the heart chambers can be detected by specially designed platinum-tipped electrode catheters positioned at specific sites.

Angiography. Angiography is a modification of the basic catheterization technique. Here the positioning of the catheter tip in a specific area of the cardiovascular system and injection of contrast substance permit opacification of the area. Concomitant x-ray filming provides a permanent graphic record.

Injection of such contrast material into the right atrium is useful in detection of pericardial effusion and also for visualization of the tricuspid valve. Injection into the right or left ventricle gives information about the size and contraction of the respective chambers, as well as the tricuspid and the mitral valves. Injection into the pulmonary artery makes the pulmonary arterial system visible and is the most definitive way of diagnosing pulmonary embolus.

Selective coronary arteriography. Selective injection into the coronary arteries is called selective coronary arteriography. This technique was introduced in 1962 and has since served as the cornerstone for the evaluation of coronary artery disease and has enabled the development of surgical revascularization procedures. For selective coronary arteriography, various catheters are positioned at the coronary ostia, where dye is injected, and x-ray films are taken. In selected cases where variant (Prinzmetal's) angina is suspected and obstructive coronary artery disease is absent or minimal, provocative tests with intravenous ergonovine maleate are sometimes used to induce coronary artery spasm. Such spasm is promptly reversed by sublingual or intravenous administration of nitroglycerine. Results of vein bypass grafting are evaluated by injection of dye into the graft that is interposed between the aorta and the coronary arteries.

Intracardiac electrocardiography. Electrophysiologic studies can be added to standard cardiac catheterization with the use of specially designed catheters that have recording and stimulating electrodes at their tip. This technique of intracardiac electrography, sometimes referred to as His bundle recording, is useful in evaluation of atrioventricular block, supraventricular and ventricular tachyarrhythmias, and functional characteristics of the sinus node, A-V node, and any A-V bypass tracts (WPW syndrome).

Limitations

These techniques are invasive and therefore pose some discomfort as well as small but definite risks to the patient's life or well-being. In addition, the tests are costly to perform, both in manpower and equipment, and need a team of highly trained, technically capable people. Another limitation or disadvantage of the test is that the contrast medium itself can cause changes in the cardiovascular system under study.

Indications

The indications for cardiac catheterization are many but well defined. The procedure, because of its cost and inherent hazards should not be performed before careful consideration is given to the indications.

The most common indication is clinically diagnosed congenital or acquired heart disease requiring surgical therapy. In most patients noninvasive diagnostic methods are adequate in making an exact diagnosis and also in deciding on the advisability of surgery. Even in these patients, preoperative cardiac catheterization should be almost always performed to confirm the diagnosis and to evaluate cardiac function. Occasionally, cardiac catheterization will reveal an unsuspected cardiac lesion and will also be helpful in determining the type of surgical procedure for the individual patient.

Cardiac catheterization is indicated for patients with heart disease of unknown etiology where an exact diagnosis would improve or change the mode of therapy.

Evaluation of operative results, another indication, applies to both congenital cardiac disease and acquired heart disease in adults. The following could thus be evaluated: the status of prosthetic valves and of shunt procedures, the results of corrective procedures for congenital heart disease, and the adequacy and patency of grafts for coronary artery disease.

Presently, the largest number of catheterizations and angiograms are being performed on patients with coronary artery disease, first to diagnose the presence of coronary artery disease, and second to select patients for surgical revascularization.

Indications for selective coronary angiography are continuously being redefined, but at present the commonly accepted indication is the presence of symptomatic coronary artery disease with angina pectoris that has not responded well to medical therapy. Some advocates of this catheterization technique believe that all patients with suspected coronary artery disease should undergo coronary angiography. An uncommon indication for cardiac catheterization is the evaluation of the cardiac status of a patient, primarily for a nonmedical reason. This includes athletes with poorly defined murmurs who need permission for unrestricted activity, or airline pilots who have vague chest pains or mild electrocardiographic abnormalities and who need complete clearance to continue flight status.

Contraindications

There is no absolute contraindication for cardiac catheterization and angiography. Relative contraindications would be the presence of severe, uncontrolled congestive heart failure, severe arrhythmias, and a history of allergy to the dye. An essential study under this last condition can be carried out if appropriate premedication is given and precautions are taken.

Pitfalls

Individual discussion of the pitfalls in cardiac catheterization is beyond the scope of this book. To avoid serious errors, if the diagnosis from the cardiac catheterization laboratory is at variance with the clinical diagnosis, the catheterization diagnosis should not automatically be accepted without question.

The catheterization data, as well as the clinical data, should be critically reviewed.

Risks

Catheterization of the right side of the heart has essentially no mortality and a morbidity of less than 1%, which is limited to arrhythmias or minor bleeding. Catheterization of the left side of the heart, combined with cardiac angiography, is somewhat more hazardous and carries the risk of myocardial infarction, cerebrovascular accident, arterial bleeding, and arterial thrombosis with possible loss of limb. The risk of death varies among hospitals. The procedure with the highest risk of death is selective coronary angiography. In this procedure the risk of mortality varies from less than 0.1% to 1% or even higher, depending on the patient population studied and the experience of the catheterization team. It is mandatory that there be a written, informed consent in the patient's record prior to the procedure.

Patient preparation and care

The patient remains fasting prior to cardiac catheterization, since the contrast media may cause nausea and vomiting. Sedation is given, although some physicians avoid any medications because of the possible effect on hemodynamics. After the procedure vital signs are monitored and bed rest maintained for 12 to 24 hours.

The arterial puncture site should be checked for bleeding and pulses distal to the site should be checked frequently. Vascular insufficiency secondary to embolization is manifest by sudden pain and cold, white, blotchy skin. Immediate intervention is required.

A venous puncture site should be checked for warmth, pain, swelling, and redness, since thrombophlebitis may be a complication.

Diagnostic pericardiocentesis

When pericardial effusion is present in large quantities or has accumulated rapidly in smaller quantities, it causes life-threatening complications of tachycardia, hypotension, and shock with elevated venous pressure (a combination characteristic of cardiac tamponade). In such a situation, a therapeutic pericardiocentesis is performed to remove fluid and relieve pressure on the heart. In some situations in which pericardial fluid is present without causing cardiac tamponade, a diagnostic pericardiocentesis is performed to remove a small sample of the fluid for laboratory examination. This procedure is usually performed with the patient in a semisitting position, with a pericardiocentesis needle introduced via the subxiphoid approach into the pericardial space, under continuous electrocardiographic monitoring. The V lead of the ECG is connected to the needle and the ECG is monitored to prevent puncture of the heart. S-T segment elevation indicates needle contact with the epicardium and dictates withdrawal of the needle. The fluid removed is studied for chemical content (protein, sugar, LDH), malignant cells, infection (bacterial, fungal, tubercular, or viral), or other tests as indicated.

When echocardiography is being used in the evaluation of the pericardial effusion, no air should be introduced, but if x-ray films are to be used for follow-up, a volume of air equal to the volume of fluid removed may be introduced to better define the pericardial space. Monitoring right atrial pressures before and after pericardiocentesis yields hemodynamic information useful in the diagnosis of cardiac tamponade or coexistent pericardial constriction.

Clinical value

Diagnostic pericardiocentesis is useful in cardiac disorders of unknown etiology when pericardial effusion is present. This test is most helpful in diagnosing infection, tumor, or immunologic disorders such as systemic lupus erythematosus (SLE) or rheumatoid arthritis.

Limitations

Pericardiocentesis may be ineffective if pericardial effusion is loculated or mainly posterior without free-flowing anterior effusion.

Indications

The main indications for diagnostic pericardiocentesis are infective pericarditis and suspected carcinomatous infiltration of the pericardium.

Contraindications

An absolute contraindication is an uncooperative, uncontrollable patient, as this would markedly increase the risk of laceration of the heart. A bleeding disorder or anticoagulant therapy should also be considered a contraindication for elective diagnostic pericardiocentesis. Puncture of a cardiac chamber under these circumstances may precipitate uncontrollable bleeding in the pericardial sac with cardiac tamponade.

Pitfalls

Among the many pitfalls encountered in the performance of this test is the danger of puncturing and entering the right atrial chamber if the needle is directed more toward the right shoulder. In this situation elevation of the S-T segment may not be seen, but there may be elevation of the P-R interval, a clue that the right atrial chamber has been entered. Aspirated blood that clots normally and has the patient's usual hematocrit indicates that a cardiac chamber has been entered. Air should not be injected until the operator is absolutely certain that the needle is in the pericardial space and not in the cardiac chamber.

Risks

The risks of this procedure include arrhythmias (atrial or ventricular), puncture of a cardiac chamber (usually the right atrium or right ventricle), coronary arterial puncture, pneumothorax (puncture of the lung), and possible introduction of infection. With careful attention to technique and experience the risk of complications is minimal. Permission with informed consent is needed before the procedure.

Cardiac biopsy

The cardiac biopsy is probably the most invasive diagnostic test in cardiac disorders, other than open surgical exploration for diagnostic purposes. Generally, two approaches are used. Transthoracic needle biopsy of the left ventricular myocardium is the older method and is generally considered to have a higher risk of complications. Percutaneous transvenous endomyocardial biopsy is a newer and safer technique. In this procedure forceps are introduced through a vein, usually the internal jugular or the femoral, and through the right atrium into the right ventricle. The biopsy specimen is obtained from the right ventricular apex or the septum. A similar technique for biopsy of the left ventricular endomyocardium has also been developed.

Indications

Endomyocardial biopsy is indicated in the diagnosis of rejection of the transplanted heart and in diffuse infiltrative disorders of the heart (amyloidosis or tumors of the heart). It is the most specific method of evaluating the effect of cardiotoxic drugs (Adriamycin). Other conditions in which biopsy has been useful are primary myocardial disease (cardiomyopathies), hypertrophic obstructive cardiomyopathy (idiopathic hypertrophic subaortic stenosis), hypothyroidism, some of the storage diseases (glycogen storage disease), hemochromatosis, and others.

Limitations

The disease process must be diffuse to be diagnosed by the biopsy, since the sampling is very small. The transvenous endomyocardial biopsy, the more common method used, samples the right ventricle and the right ventricular septum, but does not sample the left ventricle. The risk of the procedure, although very low in initial reports, is expected to increase as the procedure is popularized and performed in more centers.

Contraindications

Bleeding disorders, anticoagulation therapy, and an uncooperative patient are among the contraindications for this procedure.

Risks

Complications of endomyocardial biopsy include right-sided pneumothorax immediately after the procedure, usually a self-limited inconsequential problem; arrhythmias, either isolated ventricular contractions, premature contractions, atrial fibrillation, flutter, or supraventricular tachycardia; and in rare cases, evidence of right ventricular puncture that presents as intrapericardial bleeding with cardiac tamponade. Permission is obtained as in cardiac catheterization.

5

DIAGNOSTIC TESTS FOR PULMONARY DISORDERS

ANATOMY AND PHYSIOLOGY

An exchange of gases between blood and air occurs within the lungs. This vital function is possible because the structure of the lungs provides open tubes (bronchi and bronchioles) that branch into millions of thin-walled air sacs (alveoli). These air sacs are in contact with the blood through the network of capillaries surrounding them. The bronchi and bronchioles are illustrated in Figs. 5-1 and 5-2. The diffusion of gases, both from the venous blood to the alveoli and from the alveoli to the capillary blood, takes place through the thin alveolar and capillary walls. Because of the tremendous number of alveoli, each well supplied with capillaries (Fig. 5-2), large amounts of oxygen diffuse very rapidly into the blood and large amounts of carbon dioxide diffuse rapidly into the alveolar spaces to be expelled during expiration.

PATHOPHYSIOLOGY (TERMINOLOGY)

Disturbances of either ventilation or perfusion can cause significant disease and incapacity in terms of pulmonary function, resulting in hypoxemia and respiratory acidosis or alkalemia. The mechanisms responsible are hyperventilation, alveolar hypoventilation, altered ventilation/perfusion ratio, arteriovenous shunt (right-to-left shunt), and diffusion block. The last three conditions are illustrated in Fig. 5-3.

Alveolar hypoventilation

A decrease in ventilation to a large number of alveoli is present in this condition. This decrease is defined by a rise in arterial carbon dioxide (Pco_2). Attendant to it will be decreased arterial, Po_2 and respiratory acidosis.

Abnormal ventilation/perfusion ratio (V/Q)

Marked decrease in ventilation/perfusion ratio (Fig. 5-4) results from marked hypoventilation in relation to perfusion. The opposite, marked de-

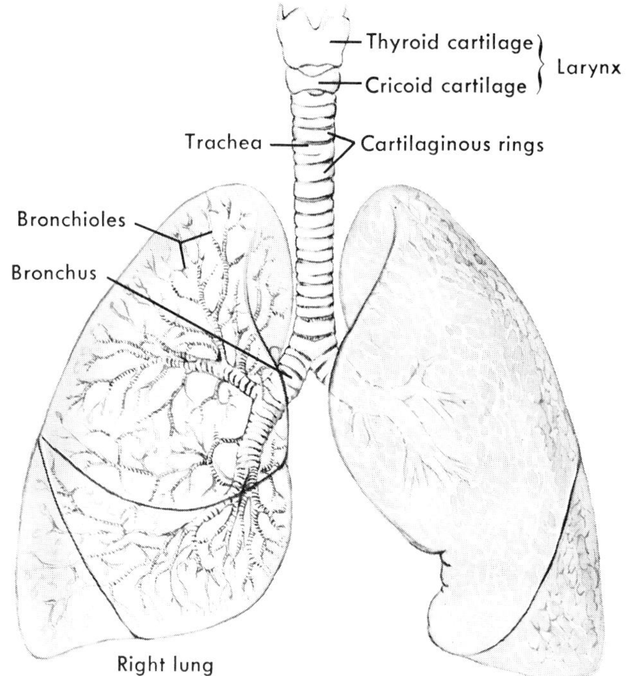

FIG. 5-1
The respiratory tract with the right lung cut away to expose bronchi and bronchioles. (From Schottelius, B. A., and Schottelius, D. D.: Textbook of physiology, ed. 17, St. Louis, 1973, The C. V. Mosby Co.)

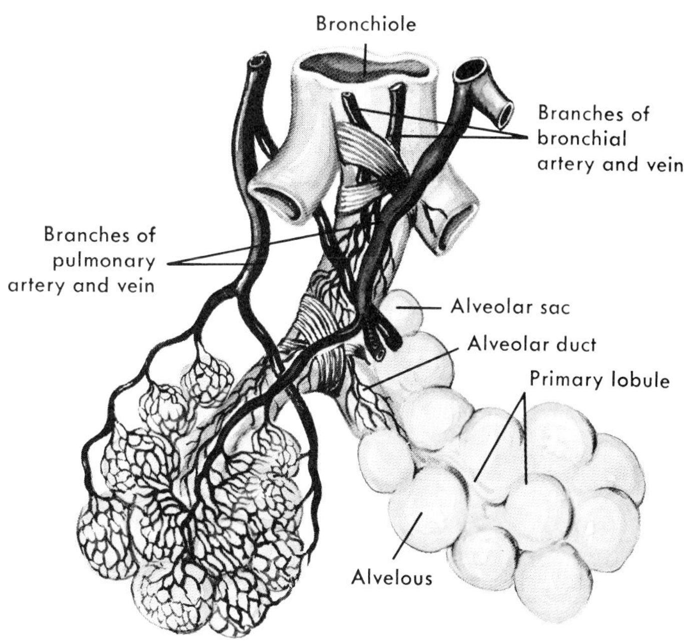

FIG. 5-2
The capillary network surrounding the alveoli. (From Schottelius, B. A., and Schottelius, D. D.: Textbook of physiology, ed. 17, St. Louis, 1973, The C. V. Mosby Co.)

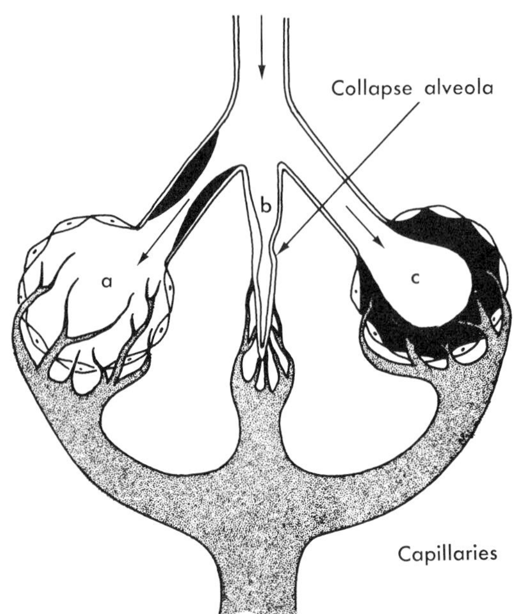

FIG. 5-3
a, Altered ventilation/perfusion ratio; *b,* arteriovenous shunt (right/left shunt); *c,* diffusion block.

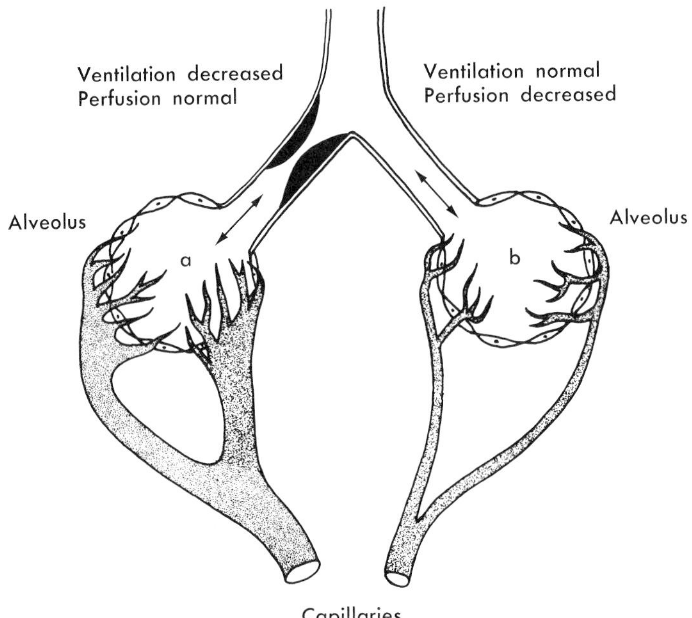

FIG. 5-4
The two possible mechanisms of altered ventilation/perfusion ratio. *a,* Increased perfusion to poorly ventilated alveoli; *b,* decreased perfusion to normally ventilated alveoli.

crease in perfusion to ventilation, causes an increased ventilation/perfusion ratio. This is mainly reflected by an increase in residual volume. Both of the above abnormalities occur in chronic obstructive lung disease. Ventilation/perfusion mismatch is an important cause of decreased arterial Po_2 (hypoxemia) in various pulmonary disorders.

Arteriovenous shunt (right-to-left shunt)

This term means that the blood from the right side of the heart will be shunted to the left side without having been oxygenated and without having given up its carbon dioxide. The mechanism of this condition is illustrated in Fig. 5-5. It will be noted when comparing Fig. 5-5 with Fig. 5-4 that the difference between ventilation/perfusion abnormalities and right-to-left shunt is determined by the size of the shunt. The mechanisms responsible are the same.

Diffusion block

This term implies a physiochemical interference with the rate of gas exchange across the alveolar-capillary membrane. Since carbon dioxide diffuses almost twenty times faster than O_2, hypoxemia is usually the result, with arterial Pco_2 unaffected. The significance of this mechanism in causing hypoxemia in disease states is debatable.

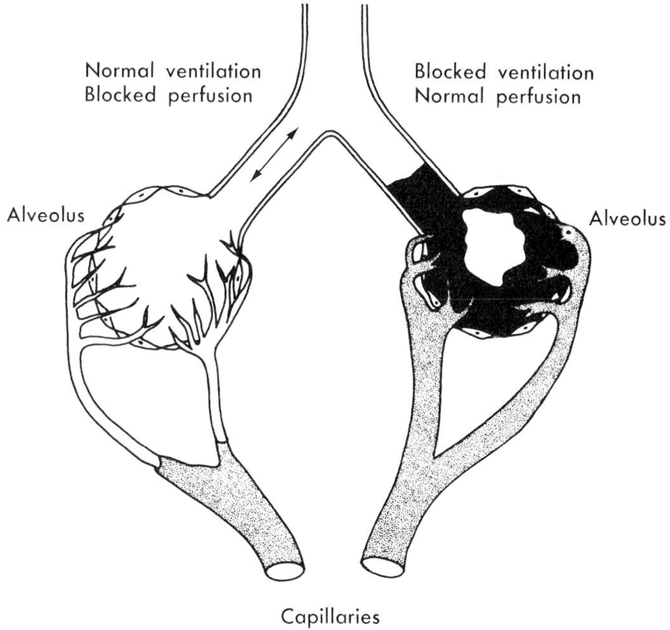

FIG. 5-5
Arteriovenous shunt (right to left shunt).

LABORATORY TESTS FOR PULMONARY DISEASE

Roentgenography

Chest roentgenography

This is a valuable extension to the physical examination. It permits visualization of the air-filled lung, as well as its vascular markings. Tumors or infiltration in the lungs are easily recognized by this test. Pleural fluid, blood (hemothorax), or air (pneumothorax) is promptly diagnosed. The roentgenographic visualization of the heart and great vessels is also very helpful in the diagnosis of lung diseases. Serial studies are particularly helpful in following the progress of a disease and evaluating the effect of therapy.

Tomography (laminography)

Tomography is an extension of the technique of simple chest roentgenography in which a series of x-ray films are exposed, each visualizing a slice of the lung at different depths (see p. 206). This procedure is useful in identifying the presence of calcium or a cavity within a lesion, the presence of hilar adenopathy, tracheal or broncheal abnormalities, and the shape of mediastinal masses.

Fluoroscopy

Fluoroscopy adds to the plain roentgenogram by permitting visualization of respiratory motion. Also, with the use of image intensifiers, small pulmonary nodular or parenchymal calcifications can be diagnosed.

Sputum examination

The sputum examination is most helpful in the diagnosis of pneumonias and suspected malignancies. In infections of the lung, a proper smear and stain of the sputum, followed by appropriate culture techniques, are needed for a specific diagnosis of the type of infection. This applies to the various bacterial pneumonias, as well as to tuberculosis and fungal infections.

Cytologic evaluation of the sputum is a relatively simple method of detecting malignant disease of the lung. It is futile to perform this test on saliva. It is necessary to obtain a proper sputum specimen and to process it promptly.

Various sputum production techniques may be used by the inhalation therapist to promote a deep and productive cough. In rare instances one may resort to transtracheal aspiration to obtain a satisfactory sputum specimen.

Pulmonary function tests

Pulmonary function tests are useful in documenting the presence and degree of functional impairment in various disease states. Also, applied serially in time, they help to evaluate the response to therapy and progression of disease.

The main types of pulmonary function tests include spirometry, lung volumes, diffusing capacity, and lung compliance.

Spirometry

In this test the flow of air is measured in volume/unit time. Most commonly, the expiratory phase of the respiratory cycle is studied. Commonly obtained measurements include vital capacity, residual volume, and total lung capacity.

Vital capacity (VC) is the total volume of air exhaled after a full inspiration and forced expiration. Normally, 80% of this volume is exhaled in 1 second and is called the forced expiratory volume (FEV_1). In obstructive lung disease the patient is unable to breathe out fully and, therefore, the vital capacity and the FEV_1 are both reduced, as is the $FEV_1/VC\%$. In restrictive lung disease the chest cannot expand fully and therefore the vital capacity is low. There is decrease in lung compliance. However, airway resistance is normal and the FEV_1 is therefore not reduced proportionately, which causes the $FEV_1/VC\%$ to be normal or high (Fig. 5-6).

Residual volume represents the air that cannot be removed from the lungs, even by forceful expiration. One technique for measuring the residual volume is through the use of a body plethysmograph; another is a helium dilution test in which the patient is connected to a spirometer circuit containing helium. After several minutes of rebreathing, the degree of dilution of helium is measured.

Total lung capacity represents the volume to which the lungs can be expanded with the greatest inspiratory effort. Normal values for pulmonary function tests are displayed in Table 5-1.

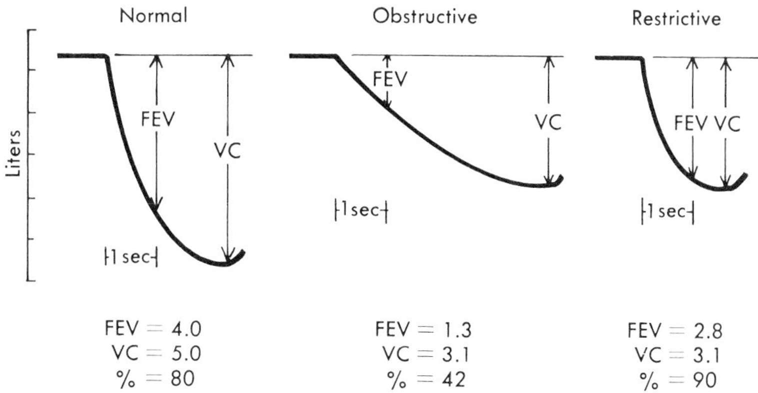

FIG. 5-6
Measurement of the forced expiratory volume, FEV_1, and vital capacity, VC. The patient makes a full inspiration and then exhales as hard and as fast as possible. As the patient exhales, the pen moves down. The FEV_1 is the volume exhaled in one sec; the VC is the total volume exhaled. Note the differences among the normal, obstructive, and restrictive patterns. (From West, J. B.: Disturbances of respiratory function. In Harrison's Principles of internal medicine, ed. 7, New York, 1974, McGraw-Hill Book Co.)

TABLE 5-1
Normal pulmonary function tests

Test	Age 20-39	Age 40-59	Age 60+
VC (liters)			
Men	3.35-5.90	2.72-5.30	2.42-4.70
Women	2.45-4.38	2.09-4.02	1.91-3.66
FEV_1 (liters)			
Men	3.11-4.64	2.45-3.98	2.09-3.32
Women	2.16-3.65	1.60-3.09	1.30-2.53
FEV% (FEV_1/VC%)			
Men	77	70	60
Women	82	77	74
Residual volume (liters)			
Men	1.13-2.32	1.45-2.62	1.77-2.77
Women	1.00-2.00	1.16-2.20	1.32-2.40
Total lung capacity (liters)			
Men	4.80-7.92	4.50-7.62	4.35-7.32
Women	3.61-6.18	3.41-6.02	3.31-5.86

Maximal mid-expiratory flow (MMEF) is a more sensitive measurement of expired air flow and is obtained from the mid portion of the spirogram.

Maximal breathing capacity or *maximal voluntary ventilation (MVV)* is another useful test of overall lung mechanics. Here the subject breathes as deeply and rapidly as possible for 15 seconds. The volume of exhaled air is multiplied by 4.

Blood gases

Analysis of *arterial blood gases* (ABGs) has become one of the most useful tests in pulmonary medicine. Determination of Po_2 in a sample of arterial blood gives a reliable estimate of the pulmonary O_2 transport function. Of course, this must be interpreted with a knowledge of the inspired O_2 tension.

The adequacy of *alveolar ventilation* is judged by Pco_2, while the *net* acid base status of the blood is reflected in the pH.

Blood gases may also be determined on venous blood. For cardiopulmonary evaluation, the best "venous" sample is the one obtained from the pulmonary artery, where there is complete mixing of blood, thus the term *mixed venous sample*.

NORMAL BLOOD GAS VALUES

	Arterial blood	*Mixed venous blood*
pH	7.40 (7.35-7.45)	7.36 (7.3-7.41)
Po_2	80-100 mm Hg	35-40 mm Hg
O_2 Sat	95%	70%-75%
Pco_2	35-45 mm Hg	41-51 mm Hg
HCO_3	22-26 mEq/l	22-26 mEq/l
Base excess (BE)	−2 to +2	−2 to +2

The pH measures the acidity or alkalinity of the blood. A low pH indicates acidemia. A high pH indicates alkalemia. The source of excess acid in acidemia (low pH) can be either respiratory, metabolic, or both. In *respiratory* acidemia an increased PCO_2 (hypoventilation) causes an increase in carbonic acid. In *metabolic* acidemia there is an accumulation of various metabolic acids.

The PO_2 measures the tension or the pressure of oxygen in the blood. A [illegible]

(acids or alkalis), an elevated PCO_2 leads to respiratory acidosis, whereas a low PCO_2 leads to respiratory alkalosis. Frequently, metabolic forces and the body's buffer systems are also active and, therefore, rapid changes in the pH are held in control.

HCO_3 (bicarbonate) and base excess are influenced by metabolic changes. Bicarbonate is an alkaline substance, and the term "excess base" refers to bicarbonates as well as other bases in the blood. An elevation in this parameter indicates metabolic alkalosis; a depression indicates metabolic acidosis.

Sometimes in order to evaluate the exact metabolic state of the patient, one must determine arterial blood gases, pH, and serum electrolytes. For example, a mild case of hypokalemic alkalosis along with respiratory acidosis may give normal arterial blood gases and pH. Unless one is aware of this interrelationship and measures the electrolytes along with the blood gases, one may never be able to detect the mild hypokalemic alkalosis and thus the presence of respiratory acidosis, the balance of which gives the false normal acid-base status.

Blood gases may fail to show major abnormalities at rest. In selected cases, a graded multistage exercise can be performed while O_2 consumption is either measured or estimated. Blood gases (at least arterial and ideally arterial and mixed venous) are obtained at various points during the exercise, at the peak and during recovery. Such a test is of great value in evaluating patients with symptoms of dyspnea and weakness.

Pleural fluid examination

Pleural fluid is easily accessible for examination by means of a diagnostic thoracentesis. When present, it may be secondary to and confirm the diagnosis of cancer, tuberculosis or other infections, pancreatitis, or rheumatoid arthritis.

Normally the pleural cavity is a potential space with moist membranes but no fluid present. However, in certain disease conditions fluid may accumulate in the pleural cavity creating a real space.

Pleural fluid consists of either transudates or exudates. *Transudates* pass through a membrane or are extruded from tissue, such as would occur in congestive heart failure, cirrhosis of the liver, and nephrotic syndrome. The protein content of transudates is less than 2.5 gm/100 ml. *Exudates* are composed of thicker cellular fluid that has escaped from blood vessels, such as would occur with inflammation and infection of the pleura. Accordingly, the protein content of exudates is higher, usually above 2.5 gm/100 ml.

The most common cause of transudates is congestive heart failure. Exudates are seen in various infections, inflammations, and malignancies. Bloody exudates raise the possibility of malignancy or pulmonary infarction.

For proper diagnosis a sample of the pleural fluid is obtained by thoracentesis, and then analyzed for its cell count and chemical and protein content. Complete bacteriologic studies are done including those for tuberculosis and fungi. Cytologic evaluation is necessary for malignant effusions. If suspicion of tuberculosis or carcinoma is high, a pleural biopsy may be obtained at the time of thoracentesis, increasing the diagnostic yield of the procedure.

Acute pancreatitis can cause pleural effusion. In this case the elevated amylase level in the pleural fluid will be diagnostic of the condition. Other subdiaphragmatic inflammatory processes can also cause effusions, which in the early stages are usually sterile transudates.

Another example of pleural effusion is *Meigs' syndrome,* which is usually transudate and is associated with carcinoma of the ovaries.

If the effusion has a milky appearance the presence of chyle is indicated and obstruction or rupture of the thoracic duct is implicated.

Following a thoracentesis a chest x-ray should be obtained to check for the possibility of pneumothorax induced by the pleural tap. Obtaining informed consent for this test is advisable.

Pulmonary perfusion scan

The pulmonary perfusion scan is obtained by injecting macroaggregates of radioiodinated albumin into a peripheral vein. These are trapped in the pulmonary capillaries and provide an indirect measure of blood flow to the lungs. The test is used in suspected cases of pulmonary embolism. Many disorders are reflected by a perfusion defect; therefore, this test is not specific for pulmonary embolism. When the pulmonary perfusion scan is normal, then the presence of a clinically significant pulmonary embolus is unlikely.

If, during pulmonary perfusion scanning, other organs are visualized (i.e., kidney, spleen, etc.), this should lead to a search for pulmonary arteriovenous fistula, which has allowed the passage of the macroaggregates to the arterial side.

Ventilation scan

A ventilation scan is made following the inhalation of a radioactive gas. If a perfusion defect is the result of embolism, ventilation will be intact and alveolar dead space visualized. If the perfusion abnormality is the result of obstructive lung disease, defective ventilation will also be present.

The combined use of ventilation and perfusion lung scanning has somewhat improved the diagnostic value of lung scanning.

[illegible]

[illegible]

[illegible] venous circulation. As part of the study, pressures should be measured in the pulmonary artery, right ventricle, and right atrium. These should then be correlated with the rest of the findings.

The patient is prepared for pulmonary angiography as for any cardiac catheterization procedure (p. 98). Informed consent is necessary.

Bronchoscopy and endobronchial biopsy

In this test a tube with a light source and a biopsy forceps is introduced into the tracheobronchial tree. Indications for and the value of this test have recently expanded because of the introduction of the flexible fiberoptic bronchoscope, which has a greater range and is safer and technically easier to use than other scopes.

Bronchoscopy is valuable in the evaluation of suspected neoplasm as well as in the work-up of hemoptysis of unknown cause. In carefully selected cases, this technique can be used to remove tenacious secretions from the tracheobronchial tree as a therapeutic measure.

Patient preparation and care. Premedication is usually necessary and informed consent is frequently obtained before bronchoscopy.

Hypoxia and cardiac arrhythmias number among the risks. The patient's vital signs should therefore be monitored until they are stable. Some hemoptysis is expected after a biopsy.

Bronchography

Bronchography involves the use of radiopaque material that is instilled into the tracheobronchial tree through a catheter. All of the tracheobronchial tree can then be seen on x-ray films. Diagnoses possible with the use of bronchography include bronchiectasis, obstruction in distal bronchi, and tracheobronchial malformation.

Patient preparation and care. Postural drainage may be instituted several days before the procedure if secretions are found to be excessive. The patient will be premedicated and will have nothing by mouth several hours before the procedure and until cough and gag reflexes are restored after the procedure.

A complication of this procedure is atelectasis or pneumonitis caused by the contrast medium blocking the distal bronchioles. The patient's temperature should therefore be monitored for 24 hours, and coughing should be encouraged.

Mediastinoscopy and open lung biopsy

These are surgical procedures performed in the operating room, usually under general anesthesia. In *mediastinoscopy* the scope is introduced from the suprasternal notch down to the anterior surface of the trachea in the superior mediastinum. The technique permits visualization and biopsy of paratracheal and subcarinal lymph nodes. It is a valuable test in the diagnosis of pulmonary malignancies and other mediastinal pathology, such as sarcoidosis.

Open lung biopsy is performed when all other lesser diagnostic tests have not yielded a diagnosis and when a definitive diagnosis is important to the care of the patient.

A limited thoracotomy is performed and the diseased tissue is resected for culture and pathologic evaluation. In general, the earlier the biopsy is performed, the more useful is the information obtained.

LABORATORY TESTS IN THE CLINICAL SETTING

Chronic obstructive pulmonary disease (COPD)

Chronic obstructive pulmonary disease is not one homogenous disease entity, but includes a heterogenous group of diseases of various etiologies, having in common a decreased flow of air in and out of the lungs. Three major subgroups are recognized: chronic bronchitis, emphysema, and asthma.

Laboratory tests

Pulmonary function tests, spirometry, lung volumes, and flow rates, are the cornerstone of the laboratory diagnosis of COPD. Not only do these tests document the presence of obstruction to the flow of air, but they also give an estimate of the severity of obstruction.

Chest roentgenograms are helpful in detecting severe emphysema, large bullae, or associated pneumonitis. The roentgenogram is a very insensitive test for the detection of COPD; there may be no radiologic evidence of disease even though severe degrees of disease and disability exist.

Arterial blood gases at rest may be normal in mild or moderate cases, but frequently will reveal some degree of hypoxemia (P_{CO_2} less than 70 mm Hg). In far advanced cases, severe hypoxemia and hypoventilation with respiratory acidosis may ensue.

Differential diagnosis

Functionally, the differences between pure emphysema and pure bronchitis are as follows. In pure emphysema, total lung capacity and the residual volume are increased much more than they are in pure bronchitis, in which the total lung capacity is often normal.

In the early stages of pure emphysema the arterial P_{CO_2} is normal because of an increase in ventilation that compensates for the decreased P_{CO_2}. There [illegible]

tacks," pulmonary function tests are relatively normal, the condition may well be classified as asthma. Of course, the patient's clinical history, age, and a multitude of other factors are to be considered before a definitive diagnosis is obtained.

Diffuse interstitial and alveolar lung disease (restrictive lung disease)

Under this heading are included numerous pulmonary disorders that have a similar clinical and laboratory presentation. The most frequent presenting complaint in these cases is dyspnea, initially exertional and ultimately present at rest.

Laboratory tests

A *chest roentgenogram* is very valuable in detecting the early abnormalities and in separating the interstitial from the alveolar varieties.

Pulmonary function tests are abnormal and have a fairly characteristic pattern, which is quite different from those observed in COPD. Here there is no obstruction to air flow, and FEV_1 and the total breathing capacity are normal or even increased. There is a decrease in vital capacity and total lung capacity. The major abnormality is a decrease in the diffusing capacity; thus this is the best test in estimating the severity of the disease process.

Arterial blood gases may be normal at rest. As the disease progresses, or if the patient is exercised, there will be a decrease in arterial O_2 saturation, while ventilation remains adequate.

Differential diagnosis

The diseases in the restrictive lung disease category are mostly diffuse and infiltrative. Because the clinical manifestations and physiologic abnormalities involved are very similar, a specific diagnosis may not be possible in many cases and a lung biopsy may be necessary. In cases in which a specific diagnosis would alter the treatment plan a lung biopsy is usually performed.

The causes of restrictive lung diseases are as follows:

1. Infections such as those caused by bacteria, fungi, and parasites, and the viruses of influenza, chickenpox, and measles.
2. Neoplasm
3. Metabolic disorders (uremic pneumonitis)
4. Physical agents such as blast or heat injury, oxygen toxicity, or postirradiation fibrosis
5. Hereditary infiltrative diseases, such as cystic fibrosis, familial idiopathic pulmonary fibrosis, and neurofibromatosis
6. Circulatory disorders, such as multiple pulmonary emboli, fat embolism, sickle cell anemia, foreign body vasculitis from parasites or drug addiction, pulmonary edema, and chronic passive congestion with fibrosis
7. Immunologic disorders, such as occur with hypersensitivity pneumonias, collagen diseases, and Goodpasture's syndrome
8. Occupational causes, such as mineral dusts and chemical fumes
9. Sarcoidosis
10. Histiocytosis X
11. Idiopathic pulmonary hemosiderosis
12. Pulmonary alveolar proteinosis
13. Desquamative interstitial pneumonia

Bronchiectasis

Bronchiectasis involves weakening of the bronchial wall structures, with subsequent dilation and secondary infections.

Laboratory tests

Chest roentgenogram is frequently abnormal, but in a nonspecific manner.

Bronchography is the usual diagnostic tool since the diagnosis of bronchiectasis depends on demonstrating the abnormal anatomy of the bronchial system.

The most common causative organisms are *Diplococcus pneumoniae*, *Hemophilus influenzae*, and *Bacteroides*. If the patient has had prior antibacterial therapy, superimposed *Staphylococcus* or *Pseudomonas* organisms may be involved.

Pneumonias

Pneumonias are discussed on p. 226.

Pulmonary embolism

Pulmonary embolism may mimic various acute and chronic lung diseases and is frequently misdiagnosed. Complete occlusion of the pulmonary artery may cause sudden death. Partial occlusion of a pulmonary artery or its branch may cause unexplained dyspnea or may mimic a pneumonia. If there is associated pulmonary infarction, there could be hemoptysis.

Laboratory tests

Chest roentgenogram could be perfectly normal in the presence of a significant pulmonary embolus. More frequently, there are nonspecific abnormalities, such as areas of atelectasis, infiltrate, or pleural effusion.

[illegible]

monary embolism, can produce an abnormal or "positive" lung scan.

Ventilation lung scan may help exclude some of these other causes.

Pulmonary angiography is the most specific diagnostic test for pulmonary embolism. It is used when the less specific tests have not yielded a clear picture, or when surgical intervention (inferior vena cava ligation, possible pulmonary embolectomy) is being considered. Heart pressures may be obtained during angiography and provide a hemodynamic assessment. In major vascular occlusion there is increased pulmonary artery pressure and possibly secondary tricuspid regurgitation.

The *electrocardiogram* is frequently abnormal but rarely helpful in a specific diagnosis. Changes include sinus tachycardia, right axis deviation, right heart strain, or right bundle branch block.

Carcinoma of the lung

Laboratory tests

X-ray examination of the chest is the most important initial diagnostic tool in carcinoma of the lung. Frequently the patient is completely asymptomatic while the routine x-ray film reveals a nodule. After identification of the nodule, serial laminograms are obtained to visualize possible calcification, which helps in the diagnosis of granuloma versus carcinoma but does not necessarily rule out either.

Bronchoscopy with bronchoscopic biopsy and, if possible, bronchoscopic aspiration for cytology, is of help, particularly in medially located lesions. Bronchial brushings are used for more distal lesions.

Scalene node biopsy is helpful when the lung cancer is inaccessible by bronchoscopy. The scalene fat pad contains lymph nodes that receive lymphatic drainage from the lungs. Therefore, a biopsy from this area often discloses carcinoma of the lungs, granulomatous infections, or sarcoidosis.

Sputum cytology can be helpful but the yield is low in peripheral lesions. The positive yield in cases of lung carcinoma ranges between 30% and 70%, depending on the eagerness and expertise of the pathologist and the adequacy of the specimen.

Needle biopsy is useful when the lesion is peripheral and nonresectable. The biopsy provides a tissue diagnosis before the institution of radiation and/or chemotherapy.

Thoracentesis and *needle biopsy of the pleura* should be performed in the presence of pleural fluid. The pleural fluid exudate is usually bloody. Fluid cytology may yield the diagnosis.

Mediastinoscopy is a very good method for visualizing the lymph nodes and obtaining a biopsy of the accessible ones.

Pulmonary function tests are frequently performed before thoracotomy. These tests are valuable in evaluating the feasibility of pulmonary resection, either lobectomy or pneumonectomy.

Alveolar hypoventilation

By definition elevated P_{CO_2} is equated with alveolar hypoventilation. When acute, this may be accompanied by respiratory acidosis, but when chronic the pH is frequently normal.

Differential diagnosis

Central nervous system diseases, various neurogenic and myogenic disorders, and severe musculoskeletal deformities, as well as COPD may all present with alveolar hypoventilation.

An interesting disorder is the sleep apnea syndrome in which alveolar hypoventilation is present *only* during sleep. Nocturnal sleep studies are necessary for a specific diagnosis. When the periods of apnea and hypoventilation extend into the day and are present during wakefulness, the clinical picture may be one of the "pickwickian syndrome."

Hyperventilation

The term hyperventilation implies decreased P_{CO_2}. When acute, this is accompanied by respiratory alkalosis. When chronic, the pH may be normal. Hyperventilation may be voluntary or involuntary, and when secondary to anxiety or present on a psychogenic basis, it is recognized as the "hyperventilation syndrome." A second common cause of hyperventilation is metabolic acidosis, in which hyperventilation is present as a compensatory mechanism.

6

DIAGNOSTIC TESTS FOR [illegible]

ANATOMY AND PHYSIOLOGY

Each kidney contains over 1 million nephrons, which are the functioning units of the kidney. Each is capable of forming urine. Each nephron is composed of two major units, the *glomerulus*, through which the blood is filtered, and a long *tubule* where the filtered blood is modified by the processes of reabsorption and secretion and converted into urine. The nephron and its blood supply are illustrated in Fig. 6-2. The tubule has a blind end that begins in the cortex of the kidney (Fig. 6-1). From there its path is tortuous, bending back on itself, in a section called the *first* or *proximal convoluted tubule*. The tubule then plunges down into the medulla, where its course is smooth, and then bends back to return to the cortex. The loop thus formed is called the *loop of Henle*. Within the cortex again, the tubule twists and turns in a section known as the *second* or *distal convoluted tubule* (Fig. 6-2). It finally joins the *collecting tubule*, which ends in the pelvis of the kidney.

The glomerulus is a tuft of up to 50 capillaries that begin with an afferent arteriole and end with an efferent arteriole (Fig. 6-2). The glomerulus is invaginated into the blind upper end of the tubule. The little sac thus formed is *Bowman's capsule*. The pressure of the blood within the glomerular capillaries causes the blood to be filtered into Bowman's capsule, where it begins to pass down the tubule. As the blood filtrate passes through the tubules, all substances useful to the body are reabsorbed while the end products of metabolism are cleared.

Because of their size, red blood cells and protein do not normally pass through the glomerular filter. Thus the fluid in Bowman's capsule is a protein-free filtrate of blood plasma. Capillary permeability is increased in many renal diseases, permitting plasma proteins to pass into the urine. Also, the glomerular membrane may be so injured by disease that it fails to function as a filter, permitting blood cells and plasma protein to leak through the injured capillary to be excreted in the urine.

The glomerulus is not the only capillary bed supplying the nephron. The efferent arteriole leaving Bowman's capsule goes on to form another capillary bed, this time a low pressure bed that supplies the tubules (Fig. 6-2). This low pressure in the peritubular capillary system causes it to function in much the same way as the venous ends of the tissue capillaries, with fluid being absorbed continually into the capillaries.

Laboratory tests for renal function are related chiefly to the two main functions of the nephron, that of glomerular filtration and tubular reabsorption. It is through these two mechanisms that the kidney clears the blood of unwanted substances.

The fluid that filters through the glomerular membrane into Bowman's capsule is called glomerular filtrate. The quantity of glomerular filtrate formed each minute in all nephrons is called the *glomerular filtration rate.* Normally, this averages about 125 ml/min. However, the normal rate may be as high as

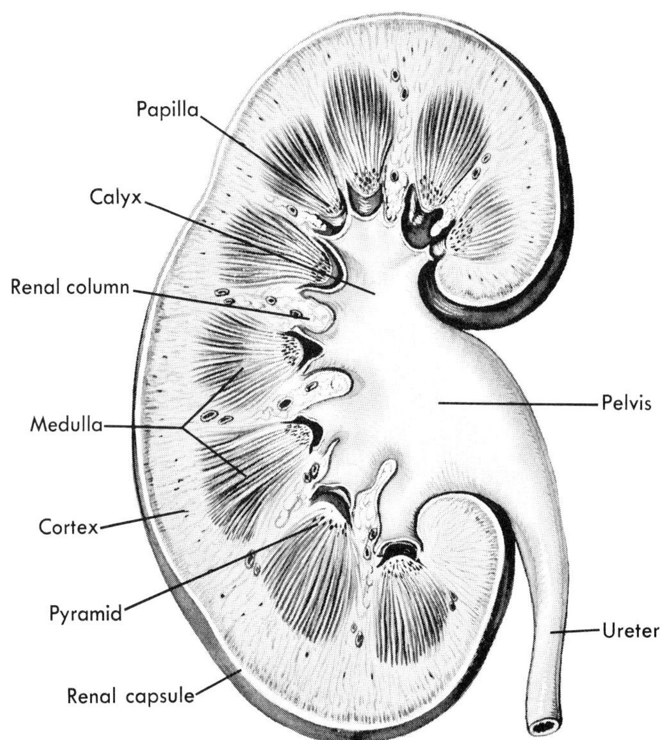

FIG. 6-1
Coronal section through the right kidney. (From Anthony, C. P., and Kolthoff, N. J.: Textbook of anatomy and physiology, ed. 9, St. Louis, 1975, The C. V. Mosby Co.)

200 ml/min. Usually over 99% of the glomerular filtrate is reabsorbed in the tubules. The remainder passes into the urinary bladder. The glomerular filtration rate will be determined by the filtration pressure and the filtration rate per unit of filtration pressure.

Tubular reabsorption is accomplished by active and passive transport

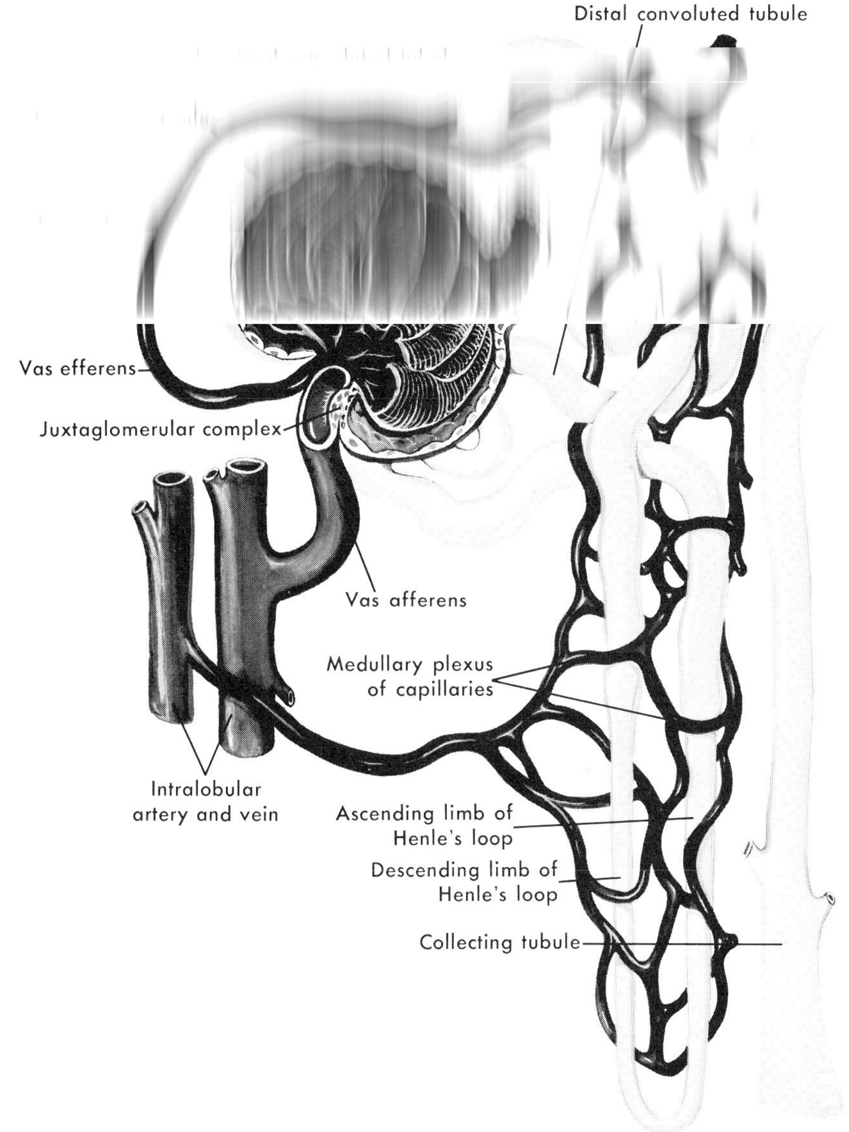

FIG. 6-2
The nephron and its blood supply. The wall of Bowman's capsule has been cut away to reveal the detail of the glomerulus. (From Schottelius, B. A., and Schottelius, D. D.: Textbook of physiology, ed. 17, St. Louis, 1973, The C. V. Mosby Co.)

across the membranes of the tubular system into the peritubular capillaries and interstitial tissue. Substances actively reabsorbed through the tubular epithelial cells include sodium ions, glucose, amino acids, calcium ions, potassium ions, phosphate ions, urate ions, and others.

Some solutes, such as urea, are *passively* diffused from the tubular fluid into the peritubular fluid in response to the concentration difference across the membrane and the permeability of the tubular membrane for the solute. Some substances, especially hydrogen, potassium, and urate ions, are *actively* secreted into the tubules.

Aldosterone

The adrenal cortex secretes a group of hormones called corticosteroids of which there are two major types: mineralocorticoids and glucocorticoids. Mineralocorticoids are so called because of their effect on electrolytes. Glucocorticoids are so named because they increase blood glucose concentration, although they also have an effect on protein and fat metabolism. Of the 30 different steroids isolated from the adrenal cortex, two have major importance in endocrine and renal function. They are *aldosterone,* the principal mineralocorticoid, and *cortisol,* the principal glucocorticoid.

Aldosterone is secreted by a very thin layer of cells located on the adrenal cortex just beneath the capsule. The major basic effect of aldosterone is to increase the rate of tubular reabsorption of sodium with a concomitant loss of potassium.

Large amounts of aldosterone may cause only a few milligrams per day of sodium to be lost in the urine. In such a case, although significant hypernatremia is present, the sodium concentration is not abnormal because the individual will become thirsty and dilute the sodium with water.

Conversely, a lack of aldosterone causes loss of as much as 20 gm of sodium per day into the urine.

Extracellular potassium concentration is one of the main factors regulating the rate of aldosterone secretion. When the potassium concentration increases, so does the aldosterone concentration, which in turn produces an increase in potassium excretion and sodium retention by the kidneys.

Another factor controlling the rate of aldosterone secretion is the *renin-angiotensin* system. This system is one of the main intermediaries by which sodium depletion exerts its effect upon aldosterone. Renin is an enzyme secreted by the juxtaglomerular cells in the walls of the renal afferent arterioles in response to decreased intravascular volume secondary to sodium depletion or to a change from the supine to the upright position. Renin then acts as a catalyst on one of the plasma proteins to produce angiotensin I and angiotensin II, which are potent stimulators of aldosterone. Water and salt retention is thus promoted in an effort to return the arterial pressure back to normal.

PATHOPHYSIOLOGY

The functioning nephron is made of glomerular, tubular, and interstitial tissue. Therefore, although a disease state may begin in a local spot, if it progresses it ultimately involves the whole kidney because the processes in the tubular system are dependent upon the production of a filtrate by the glomerulus. If the glomerulus is involved initially in a disease and becomes grossly abnormal with decreased perfusion and filtration, the tubules ulti- [illegible]

LABORATORY TESTS FOR RENAL FUNCTION

Glomerular filtration tests

Glomerular filtration is evaluated through clearance tests that measure the rate at which certain substances are cleared from the plasma. The testing substance must be freely filtered and neither reabsorbed nor secreted by the tubules for a true picture of glomerular filtration rate (GFR), which is usually 105 to 135 ml/min.

The clinical value of estimating the glomerular filtration rate (usually by creatinine clearance) rests in (1) the detection of impaired kidney function before symptomatic renal disease is manifest, (2) the estimation of the severity of the pathologic process, (3) the follow-up of the course of a disease (quantitating improvement or deterioration), and (4) the monitoring of the effects of treatment. The GFR also serves as a guide to prognosis.

Inulin clearance test

Inulin is a polysaccharide that is neither reabsorbed nor secreted by the renal tubular cells. It is completely cleared by the kidney and is, therefore, the best indicator of glomerular function. However, the inulin clearance test is cumbersome and not suitable for routine clinical work. It involves the intravenous injection of a priming dose of inulin followed by continuous infusion in an attempt to keep a uniform blood level. Urine flow during the test must be accurately measured. Plasma and urine inulin concentrations are measured and the glomerular filtration rate is estimated by the formula:

$$\text{GFR} = \frac{\text{Urine inulin concentration} \times \text{urine volume}}{\text{Plasma inulin concentration}}$$

NORMAL INULIN CLEARANCE
(Corrected to 1.73 sq m of body surface)

Males: 124 ± 25.8 ml/min
Females: 119 ± 12.8 ml/min

Serum creatinine and creatinine clearance test

Creatinine is an endogenous waste product originating from creatine and phosphocreatine of skeletal muscle. Creatinine clearance is a reliable estimate of glomerular filtration rate, since it is excreted by glomerular filtration and is not appreciably reabsorbed or secreted by the tubule cells. The serum creatinine level, therefore, rises when the glomerular filtration rate falls. At the same time the creatinine clearance rate, determined on a 24-hour urine specimen, is low.

This test is similar to inulin clearance except that instead of infusing inulin, the body's own sustained production of creatinine is used as the test agent. Urine and plasma concentrations of creatinine are measured and a timed urine is collected and measured for volume (at 2, 12, or 24 hours). Thus:

$$\text{Creatinine clearance} = \frac{U_{creat} \times \text{Urine volume}}{P_{creat}}$$

NORMAL CREATININE CLEARANCE

115 ± 20 ml/min

NORMAL SERUM CREATININE

0.6-1.2 mg%

Blood urea nitrogen (BUN) and urea clearance test (see also p. 18)

Urea is the end product of protein metabolism and similar to creatinine in that nitrogen is an endogenous waste product, cleared by the kidneys. An elevated BUN reflects a decreased glomerular filtration rate. Two factors make the BUN and urea clearance test less reliable than the creatinine clearance test: (1) urea, after being filtered, tends to diffuse back into the renal tubular cells and thus its clearance is dependent on the *rate* of urine formation, and (2) urea production varies according to the state of liver function and protein intake and breakdown. Thus urea clearance is infrequently used and BUN, although routinely used, must be interpreted with these limitations in mind.

NORMAL CREATININE CLEARANCE

115 ± 20 ml/min

Tubular function tests

Clinically, tubular function is best measured by tests that determine the ability of the tubules to concentrate and dilute the urine. Tests of urinary dilution are not as sensitive in the detection of renal disease as are tests of urinary concentration. This is especially valuable since the first function to be lost in renal disease is the ability of the kidney to concentrate urine.

Since the concentration of urine occurs in the renal medulla (interstitial fluids, loops of Henle, capillaries of the medulla, and collecting tubules), the disease processes that disturb the function or structure of the medulla produce early impairment of the concentrating ability of the kidney. Such diseases are acute tubular necrosis, obstructive uropathy, pyelonephritis, papillary

[illegible]

centration of all solids in the urine (p. 40). As routinely performed it is not an accurate test and would reflect only major deviations from the normal. This test is being replaced by the more accurate test of urine osmolality.

Urine and serum osmolality

The measurement of urine osmolality is a more refined and accurate test than specific gravity for determining the diluting and concentrating ability of the kidneys. Osmolality is an expression of the total number of particles in a solution. Plasma osmolality is the main regulator of the release of antidiuretic hormone (ADH). When sufficient water is not being taken in, the osmolality of the plasma rises, ADH is released from the pituitary gland, and the kidneys respond by reabsorbing water from the distal tubules and producing a more concentrated urine. The converse occurs with excessive water ingestion. With the decrease in plasma osmolality, ADH is not released and the urine becomes more dilute. The normal urine osmolality depends upon the clinical setting since normally, with maximal ADH stimulation, it can be as much as 1200 mOsm/kg of body weight and with maximum ADH suppression as little as 50 mOsm/kg. Thus urine osmolality should be interpreted in the light of what is known about the patient's hydration status and plasma osmolality.

Simultaneous determination of serum and urine osmolality is often valuable in assessing the distal tubular response to circulating ADH. For example, if the patient's serum is hyperosmolar or in the upper limits of normal ranges and the patient's urine osmolality measured at the same time is much lower, a decreased responsiveness of the distal tubules to circulating ADH is indicated.

In advanced renal medullary disease ability to concentrate urine is lost and, irrespective of the state of hydration or fluid intake, a dilute urine of *fixed* specific gravity or osmolality is excreted (hyposthenuria).

NORMAL URINE OSMOLALITY

50-1400	mOsm/L (range)
500-800	mOsm/L (random specimen)

NORMAL SERUM OSMOLALITY

280-295	mOsm/L (range)

Phenolsulfonphthalein (PSP) excretion test

Intravenously injected PSP is excreted by active transport at the proximal tubules at a rate proportional to renal blood flow. If renal blood flow and proximal tubular function are normal, 28% to 35% of the PSP will be excreted in the first 15 minutes after the IV injection.

Many factors can interfere with the accurate estimation of PSP excretion; incomplete emptying of the bladder, low urine volume, liver disease, congestive heart failure, low serum albumin levels, and various drugs can invalidate the test. Recent modifications of this test have tried to overcome these limitations by correlating the PSP dose injected to body size and limiting the collection time to 15 minutes. Since even kidneys with markedly diminished renal blood flow will excrete a relatively normal amount of PSP in 1 or 2 hours, the first 15 minutes of the test is the most sensitive measure of renal blood flow.

General evaluative tests for kidney function

X-ray film of the abdomen

KUB (kidney, ureter, bladder). This simple radiographic test gives an estimate of kidney position, size, and calcifications. This test should be reviewed before more extensive radiologic studies are performed.

Tomography. This test provides improved resolution at a desired level of the body and thus builds on the information available from simple plain films. It is helpful when the gastrointestinal tract or other organs blur the renal outlines.

Intravenous pyelogram (IVP). The intravenous pyelogram is obtained by injecting intravenously a contrast medium that, because it is cleared from the blood by glomerular filtration, can visualize the renal parenchyma and collecting system (calyses, renal pelvis, ureters, and urinary bladder) on multiple x-ray films.

This is a very valuable test and provides visualization of the entire urinary tract. The test is helpful in the diagnosis of renal masses and cysts, ureteral obstruction, retroperitoneal tumors, renal trauma, bladder abnormalities, etc. It also gives an estimate of renal function based on the appearance time and concentration of the contrast medium in each kidney. In the presence of moderate to severe renal disease with a compromised glomerular filtration rate visualization may be poor. If improved images are needed, a drip infusion IVP may be performed in which a larger volume of contrast medium is injected rapidly.

In this test there is a slight risk of an allergic reaction to the contrast material. The most severe reaction is anaphylaxis, which can be lethal.

Patient preparation and care. The patient remains fasting from midnight prior to the IVP in order to produce the moderate dehydration necessary for better concentration of the contrast medium. When a drip infusion IVP is to be performed, this fast is not necessary. In order that the films not be obscured by intestinal contents, a strong cathartic is administered the afternoon prior to the [illegible]

[illegible]

[illegible] indicates unilateral kidney disease. In such a case, the normal kidney shows some concentration of the dye before the abnormal one does.

It should be noted, however, that although this test is the best screening test for hypertension secondary to unilateral kidney disease, it does not differentiate between renal artery stenosis and chronic pyelonephritis or nephrosclerosis. If the patient has hypertension, the test does not differentiate between hypertension resulting from renal parenchymal disease or diffuse small vessel disease and that caused by obstruction of a major renal artery.

Retrograde pyelography. Retrograde pyelography is performed by passing a catheter from the urethra to the urinary bladder, then to the right or left ureter, and injecting a contrast medium. This test is more involved than the regular IVP, but provides detailed visualization of the urinary collecting system, independent of the status of renal function. It is very helpful in the diagnosis of ureteral obstruction.

Risks include the trauma of manipulation and the attendant risk of infection.

Patient preparation and care. The contents of the bowel should be cleared in order to avoid obscuring shadows on the x-ray films. Whether or not the patient remains fasting depends upon the type of anesthesia to be used.

Following the procedure the urine of the patient should be observed for amount, hematuria, and signs of urinary sepsis. Drainage from a ureteral catheter should be noted separately from that of the urethral catheter. Failure of the ureteral catheter to drain should be reported immediately.

Renal angiography. Renal angiography provides visualization of the entire renal arterial, capillary, and venous systems. This test is performed by introducing a catheter into the renal artery (selective angiography), or the aorta proximal to the origin of the renal arteries (aortorenal angiography), and injecting contrast material while rapid x-ray filming is performed.

This test is most helpful in the diagnosis of renal artery stenosis (renal vascular hypertension), renal masses, trauma, venous thrombosis, or obstructive uropathy.

Risks of the test are the same as in any selective angiographic study and include the possibilities of bleeding, thrombosis, damage to the vessel, and allergic reactions.

Informed written consent is necessary before the test is performed.

Patient preparation and care. Patient preparation may include administration of vitamin K or protamine sulfate, hematologic evaluation, administration of cathartics, and a skin prep. The contrast medium is an osmotic diuretic. Therefore, in order to avoid an overdistended bladder during the procedure, the patient should void immediately prior to the test.

The patient will be on bed rest 12 to 24 hours after the procedure. The puncture site should be checked for hematoma formation (manifest by swelling and bleeding). If this occurs pressure should be applied cephalad to the puncture and the physician should be notified.

Vital signs and the presence of peripheral pulses should be frequently evaluated. A base line of these physical assessments should have been established prior to the procedure.

Renal biopsy

Percutaneous biopsy of the kidney yields histologic information about both the glomeruli and the tubules, and thus may permit a precise diagnosis. The tissue is processed for light and electron microscopy as well as immunofluorescent studies and cultures when indicated. The precise histologic diagnosis thus made may be useful in the treatment of the patient and may also prove of prognostic value.

Risks include uncontrolled bleeding and hematuria and loss of the kidney. Informed consent is necessary.

Patient preparation and care. Since uncontrolled bleeding is a major risk, a complete hematologic evaluation is necessary. Preventive care consists in bed rest for 24 hours following the procedure and increased intake of fluids. Vital signs are monitored and hematocrit is determined frequently.

Ultrasound

Ultrasonic examination of the kidney is part of the abdominal ultrasonic examination. This test is most valuable in detecting renal or perirenal masses and is most helpful in the diagnosis of renal cysts.

Urine culture

Urine culture and sensitivity of the organism detected should be ordered in suspected genitourinary infection. In this test the colony count is important. Fewer than 10,000 viable bacterial units per milliliter of urine is probably of no significance. If 10,000 to 100,000 colonies are cultured, no positive conclusion can be drawn. There should be over 100,000 colonies before the infection is considered significant. However, samples of urine from the ureters and renal pelvis might contain fewer bacteria and still indicate infection, because bacteria multiply while the urine is being held in the bladder.

In the absence of symptoms, a positive urine culture should elicit an inquiry into how the specimen was collected. Unless it is a catheterized or midstream voided specimen with proper cleansing of the genitalia, contamination will occur.

[illegible]

the present time, the timed sequence IVP is the preferred screening test.

LABORATORY TESTS IN THE CLINICAL SETTING

Diseases primarily affecting glomerular structure and function

Acute glomerulonephritis

Acute glomerulonephritis is an acute inflammation that primarily involves the glomerulus, although some minor changes are noted in the tubules.

Diagnostic laboratory tests. Creatinine clearance studies are helpful in initially evaluating the extent of glomerular damage and following the progression of the disease. Further laboratory tests are usually needed to arrive at a definite diagnosis.

Characteristic urine findings are mild to moderate proteinuria, hematuria, RBC casts, granular casts, and, depending on the diffuseness and extent of involvement, blood urea nitrogen and creatinine retention indicating significant diminution of glomerular function.

Differential diagnosis. Previously, glomerulonephritis was immediately equated with poststreptococcal nephritis. However, many other diseases are known to have renal involvement with the typical picture of glomerulonephritis. Thus in the following discussion the other diseases will be mentioned and a differential diagnosis discussed.

Acute poststreptococcal glomerulonephritis. This is seen more frequently in children but also occurs in adults. It is an inflammatory reaction of the kidney glomerulus to deposition of immune complexes composed of antigen from the streptococcal organism and the body's own antibodies—thus the name "immune complex disease." For an etiologic diagnosis, necessary tests include a throat culture for group A beta hemolytic strep, and determination of the serum antistreptolysin-O titer to confirm the presence of the infecting organism.

Systemic lupus erythematosus nephritis. Kidney involvement in this systemic disease may present as acute glomerulonephritis. Diagnosis is suspected by the multiple organs involved in the disease process and confirmed by characteristic serologic tests including fluorescent antinuclear antibody, anti-DNA antibodies, and serum complement measurement. (See Chapter 11.)

Other diseases. The list of other diseases that may present as acute glomerulonephritis is long. Among the important ones are bacterial endocarditis, which is diagnosed by the clinical picture and blood cultures (see p. 85); viral hepatitis, diagnosed by the presence of the Australia antigen and by antibody tests; and malaria or syphilis, which are suggested by the clinical picture and blood smears or serologic tests.

In many other cases renal biopsy is needed for a specific diagnosis, (e.g., membranous glomerulonephritis, focal glomerulonephritis, Goodpasture's syndrome, etc.). Here light and electron microscopy as well as immunofluorescent studies may be necessary.

Chronic glomerulonephritis

Many of the disease processes presenting as acute glomerulonephritis may not heal completely and progress into a subacute or chronic phase with progressive destruction of glomerular function, the end-stage of which is called chronic renal failure.

Diagnostic laboratory tests. Persistent hematuria or proteinuria should lead the examiner to suspect latent chronic glomerulonephritis. As the disease progresses there will be a decrease in creatinine clearance and, after destruction of approximately 50% of glomerular function, serum creatinine and blood urea nitrogen levels may start rising. Urinary specific gravity is usually low (around 1.010) and fixed. A low serum complement level may be seen in active immunologic processes. In the early stages of chronic glomerulonephritis renal biopsy may be of help in diagnosis.

As the disease progresses and end-stage renal failure is present, even kidney biopsy may not yield a definite diagnosis. Hypertension frequently accompanies this stage. Anemia may appear in the far-advanced cases, and there would be serum elevation of potassium, decrease in serum sodium, and onset of metabolic acidosis.

Differential diagnosis. When chronic glomerulonephritis progresses to end-stage kidney disease with persistent azotemia and elevated creatinine levels, it is sometimes impossible to differentiate among the following conditions: the chronic stage of acute glomerulonephritis, end-stage pyelonephritis, and end-stage nephrosclerosis.

Nephrotic syndrome

The hallmark of the nephrotic syndrome is massive proteinuria (over 3.5 gm per day) resulting from increased permeability of the glomerular membranes to protein.

Different disease processes may lead to this syndrome, such as various types of glomerulonephritis, diabetes mellitus, amyloidosis, renal vein thrombosis, allergic reactions, drugs, and tumors. Edema, ascites, and pleural effusion are commonly present.

Diagnostic laboratory tests. The diagnosis of nephrotic syndrome is made when a 24-hour urine specimen contains 3.5 gm or more of protein; the protein is usually the albumin fraction of the serum proteins.

[illegible]

[illegible] acterized by the nephrotic syndrome in one stage of the disease. The more common ones include the following:

1. Nephrotic syndrome stage of acute glomerulonephritis, usually acute post-streptococcal, or any of the other acute glomerulonephritides
2. Metabolic causes such as diabetic nephropathy or amyloid kidney disease
3. Systemic disease such as systemic lupus erythematosus and certain malignancies (multiple myeloma)
4. Circulatory disease such as renal vein thrombosis or right-sided congestive heart failure
5. Nephrotoxins such as heavy metals and lead poisoning
6. Certain allergens, drugs, and infections

Diseases affecting tubular structure and function

Acute tubular necrosis

This disease, also known as lower nephron nephrosis, may follow renal circulatory impairment (shock of various types), or be the result of toxic damage to the kidney. There is also involvement of the glomeruli. However, the main pathology is at the tubular level.

Since acute tubular necrosis is reversible if properly managed and treated, it is important to make the correct diagnosis. The condition usually follows a state of shock, be it cardiogenic, toxic, or bacteremic, and it is usually the result of impaired circulation to the tubules.

The disease presents with a sudden onset of oliguria (urine volume less than 300 ml per day) associated with signs and symptoms of uremia.

Laboratory tests. The urine volume and specific gravity are low. Blood urea nitrogen and serum creatinine are elevated. Urinalysis may reveal proteinuria and hematuria. Serum potassium, phosphate, and sulfate levels may be elevated while sodium calcium and CO_2 will be decreased. Metabolic acidosis may be present.

Spontaneous recovery is frequent and usually occurs in a few days but may be delayed for 5 to 6 weeks. During the recovery stage a polyuric phase may occur with urine volumes of 5 to 20 liters per day. This state dictates careful management of fluid and electrolytes. When a diagnosis is not clear one may need to exclude obstructive uropathy by intravenous pyelography or retrograde pyelography or renal arteriography. Renal biopsy is not generally indicated.

Polyuric states

Differential diagnosis. When polyuria exists, the following possibilities should be considered. (The polyuric phase of acute tubular necrosis has already been mentioned.)

Diabetes insipidus. This is not a renal disease, but because of the absence of ADH, which is responsible for the reabsorption of water from the distal tubules, there is a massive polyuria sometimes approaching 15 to 20 liters a day. Although ADH is absent, the renal response to ADH is normal. An injection of ADH corrects the polyuria of diabetes insipidus, whereas polyuria secondary to renal tubular disease (nephrogenic diabetes insipidus) does not respond to ADH.

Recently, it has been found that chlorpropamide (Diabinese) has an action similar to ADH on the distal tubular cells and partially corrects the polyuria of diabetes insipidus. This is helpful in the differential diagnosis of diabetes insipidus versus renal tubular disease.

Renal tubular diseases. This group of diseases is also associated with polyuria because of the impairment of the reabsorption of water and electrolytes. Polyuric states can, therefore, be seen in hypercalcemic nephropathy, hypokalemic nephropathy, and in certain kinds of renal tubular acidosis of hereditary conditions.

Renal tubular disease also is usually associated with abnormal excretion of amino acids, such as cystinuria and the Fanconi syndrome.

Analgesic nephropathy. This disease simulates renal tubular acidosis and is characterized by polyuria and azotemia with a more or less fixed specific gravity. This is because of the tubular involvement secondary to the analgesics, which impair absorption. The most common of the analgesic nephropathies is the phenacetin nephropathy.

Congenital anomalies

Recognition of the congenital anomalies is important because of the predisposition of patients with these conditions to repeated urinary tract infection.

Diagnostic laboratory tests. The patient should be checked frequently with urinalysis and urine culture, which will identify the infecting organism. Intravenous pyelogram defines the anatomic or structural anomaly.

Differential diagnosis. Horseshoe kidney, ectopic kidney, or unusually mobile kidney may all be associated with ureteral obstruction and infection. Polycystic kidney may also predispose to infections. In addition, this may cause hematuria and may ultimately lead to chronic renal failure.

Renal vascular hypertension

[illegible]

of the renal artery. Significant narrowing of these arteries can result from either fibromuscular hyperplasia, which is common in females between 35 and 45 years of age, or an atherosclerotic plaque that narrows the renal artery to such a degree that an appreciable pressure gradient is created on either side of the obstruction. This situation triggers a hormone system called the renin-angiotensin system, which causes hypertension by the mechanism described on p. 120. The hypertension thus produced eventually affects the kidneys further by causing more nephrosclerotic changes in the renal arteries thus establishing a self-perpetuating cycle. It is imperative that patients with this disease be identified, particularly those in the younger age group for whom surgical correction is possible.

Laboratory tests. Renal vascular hypertension may manifest with minor, nonspecific urinary findings such as a few red blood cells with some RBC casts and a slight diminution of glomerular filtration rate (creatinine clearance).

Differential diagnosis. The tests employed for differentiating renal vascular hypertension from other hypertensions, as well as for presurgical evaluation, are listed below in the order of their importance and yield.

1. Timed (rapid) sequence IVP should be done in the absence of significant BUN elevation. Renal artery stenosis is suspected if the dye appears in one kidney 5 or 10 minutes after it appears in the other kidney. The IVP is also helpful in evaluating the kidney size, which is another parameter of renal vascular hypertension, the small kidney having the compromised vascular supply.
2. Peripheral blood renin levels should be assessed, and, if possible, independent measurement of the renin secretory rate from each renal vein should be accomplished by selectively catheterizing the renal veins.
3. Renal arteriography ultimately establishes the diagnosis. However, this

test should not be done until the patient has been screened with rapid sequence IVP.

Diseases associated with pure hematuria

Pure hematuria usually indicates a disease process below the nephron, which can be anywhere from the collecting ducts to the bladder. In this situation there are usually no RBC casts, and the microscopic examination of the urine shows gross RBCs.

Painless hematuria

If there is no pain associated with the hematuria the examiner should suspect renal tumors, renal tuberculosis, or inflammatory or malignant disease involving the structures below the nephron, that is, the collecting ducts, kidney pelvis, ureters, or bladder. Intravenous pyelography, retrograde pyelography, or renal arteriography are the diagnostic tests frequently used.

Painful hematuria

Nephrolithiasis is usually painful, particularly when calculi obstruct the urinary tract or move in the ureters. However, a big staghorn calculus located in the pelvis of the kidney may be asymptomatic and a cause of intermittent pure hematuria.

Pure pyuria and bacteruria

In an acute case of fever, chills, and pyuria the diagnosis is acute pyelonephritis. This usually affects the renal parenchyma as well as the tubules and the collecting ducts in the renal pelvis, and eventually the bladder. Under such circumstances it is imperative that a urine culture be obtained to identify the organism. The most common organism in an otherwise uncomplicated case is *E. coli.*

When there are repeated episodes of acute pyelonephritis, the examiner should investigate the kidney for any possible correctable structural conditions that may predispose to repeated episodes of pyelonephritis. Unless this is done and the condition is corrected, the patient may develop chronic pyelonephritis. Under such circumstances an IV pyelogram and an excretory cystourogram are usually done to rule out reflux at the cystourethral junction. Any indication of chronicity warrants a thorough investigation of the genitourinary tract for partial obstructive uropathy.

7

DIAGNOSTIC TESTS FOR
[illegible]
[illegible]

ANATOMY AND PHYSIOLOGY

The gastrointestinal (GI) system is unique both anatomically and functionally. Anatomically it begins in the oral cavity and ends in the anal orifice. Accessory organs, either located in the main digestive tract or opening into it, include the salivary glands, liver, gallbladder, pancreas, and appendix as illustrated in Fig. 7-1.

The digestive system forms a tube all the way through the ventral cavities of the body. It is, therefore, possible with fiberoptic scopes to directly visualize a good portion of the GI tract. In addition to this, the laboratory studies can be directed toward the GI functions: propelling the nutritional items from the oral cavity to the different parts of the digestive tract and breaking down these nutritional items into absorbable units by secreting digestive enzymes.

The anatomy and physiology of the accessory organs will be discussed separately.

LABORATORY TESTS FOR GASTROINTESTINAL DISEASES (GENERAL OBSERVATIONS)

Since a study of the gastrointestinal tract involves not only the main digestive tract, but the accessory organs as well, the diagnostic laboratory tests are covered under each division of the digestive tract and each accessory organ. A few general observations follow.

Direct visualization (endoscopy)

The fiberoptic scope allows direct visualization of previously inaccessible structures, and the usual endoscopic procedures can be performed more easily with less hazard and discomfort to the patient.

The fiberoptic scope consists of bundles of thin, flexible, transparent fibers through which light can be transmitted to different regions of the GI tract. The

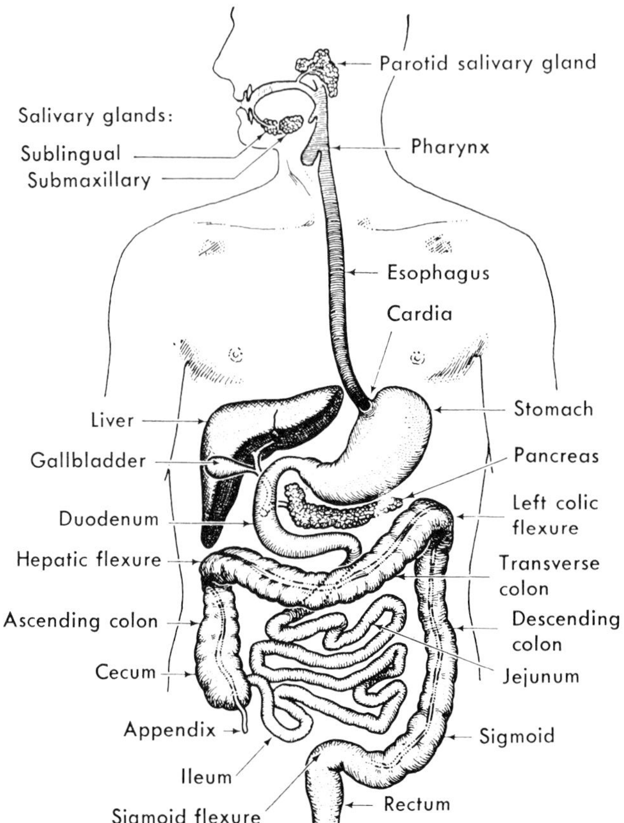

FIG. 7-1
The gastrointestinal system and accessory organs. (From Schottelius, B. A., and Schottelius, D. D.: Textbook of physiology, ed. 17, St. Louis, 1973, The C. V. Mosby Co.)

light from a light source is transmitted down some of the fibers; from the illuminated area the light is then reflected back up the remaining fibers to produce an image. The modern endoscope has a tip deflection of 180 degrees and is equipped with channels to permit the passage of biopsy forceps, cytology brushes, irrigating or injecting cannulas, snares, and/or cauteries.

Upper GI endoscopy permits visualization of all portions of the esophagus, stomach, and duodenum. The test is performed when it is necessary to confirm the x-ray evaluation and when upper GI bleeding is an emergency. A rare complication of upper GI endoscopy is perforation. Therefore, the patient should be observed for complaints of sharp pain in the stomach or chest.

Proctosigmoidoscopy and colonoscopy are discussed on pp. 150 and 151.

Elective procedures with endoscopy

With any of the endoscopic procedures one can combine other features such as obtaining biopsies and specimens for cytology. Photographs may also be taken through the endoscope. The following can also be performed:

1. Polypectomy. This procedure consists of the removal of polyps by snaring and electrocauterization.
2. Cannulation of the ampulla of Vater for retrograde cholangiography to visualize the bile duct, or pancreatography, which consists of injecting contrast material to visualize the pancreatic ducts.
3. Retrieval of ingested foreign objects.

film.

If a thorough study of the GI tract is necessary the most convenient procedure would be to perform the oral cholecystogram (p. 153) first, followed by the barium enema (p. 150) and then the upper GI series.

The upper GI series is performed for the purpose of visualizing the esophagus, stomach, and duodenum. A small bowel examination may be performed at the same session by requiring the patient to drink additional barium. The barium swallow is specific for visualization of the esophagus and involves various techniques to study the cardioesophageal junction and the mucosal pattern of the esophagus, and to demonstrate foreign bodies, hiatal hernia, or gastroesophageal reflux.

Before any radiologic studies are performed the dangers of introducing barium into the GI tract should be considered as well as the risks involved in preparing the patient for the procedure. The use of strong cathartics in the presence of obstructing lesions of the colon or small intestine or in the presence of active ulcerative colitis may be hazardous or life-threatening. The preparation of the patient or the introduction of the barium may aggravate acute ulcerative colitis or cause a partial obstruction to become complete.

A major disadvantage of contrast barium studies in the presence of gastrointestinal bleeding is the inability to associate an observed lesion with the bleeding site. If lesions are multiple, then the bleeding site should be established by panendoscopy.

Motility and pressure studies

Manometric studies are particularly valuable in evaluating esophageal function. An esophageal manometer is an instrument used to measure the pressure gradients generated by peristalsis as it progresses from the hypopharynx to the stomach. Abnormal pressure determinations can be helpful in diagnosing a number of disease entities, such as achalasia, esophageal spasm, or collagen vascular diseases (scleroderma or dermatomyositis), which also involve the esophagus.

Colonic motility studies are still in the experimental stages.

THE ESOPHAGUS

Anatomy and physiology

The esophagus (Fig. 7-1) extends from the pharynx to the stomach and has no secretory function. It is a collapsible tube about 10 inches long through which the bolus of food is propelled after having been swallowed. An initial peristaltic wave originates in the pharynx and secondary peristaltic waves originate in the esophagus if food still remains there. The lower end of the esophagus acts as a physiologic sphincter to prevent the reflux of food from the stomach.

Pathophysiology

Evidence indicates that the basic cause of esophageal pain is acid reflux resulting in irritation of the lower esophagus and secondary to a weak cardioesophageal sphincter. Recently, the hormone gastrin has been found to play a role in the maintenance of this sphincter integrity. Persistent reflux produces an irritated, swollen, and friable esophagus. Bleeding, esophagitis, and ulceration may result. Often, hiatal hernia coexists with the reflux.

Laboratory tests for esophageal disease

The barium swallow, motility tests, and upper GI endoscopy have already been described on p. 135. Cytologic examination is a helpful diagnostic adjunct provided it is done skillfully, with proper collection of specimens, and by an experienced examiner.

Bernstein test (acid perfusion test)

The Bernstein test demonstrates reflux esophagitis. Hydrochloric acid (HCl) 0.1% is started as a drip into the esophagus after normal saline has first been used. Spontaneous symptoms produced in the patient within one half hour after the HCl drip starts are indicative of esophagitis.

In order to verify whether or not the HCl is causing the esophageal symptoms, the drip should be switched to saline without the patient's knowledge as soon as pain develops. The distress should disappear after a few minutes and reappear again when the HCl drip is reinstated (again, without the patient's knowledge).

Test for esophageal acidity

A pH electrode attached to a manometric catheter and placed in the esophagus is the most accurate way of measuring esophageal acidity.

When the lower esophageal sphincter is located manometrically, the pH catheter and manometer are withdrawn to a level 2 cm above the sphincter. The patient is then asked to perform a Valsalva maneuver, to lift his legs, or to sniff vigorously. If no reflux is demonstrated, then the manometric catheter and the pH probe are reintroduced into the stomach for the purpose of instilling 300 ml of 0.1N HCl. The catheter is again withdrawn to the esophagus. The maneuvers described above for the production of reflux are repeated. If [illegible]

[illegible]

[illegible] agnosis of reflux esophagitis are radiologic studies demonstrating reflux of a contrast material, the Bernstein acid perfusion test, and the demonstration of esophageal acidity.

Differential diagnosis. Coronary heart disease is important in the differential diagnosis of reflux esophagitis with the clinical history being the most helpful. In reflux esophagitis a radiologic diagnosis of hiatal hernia is frequently made. However, the mere demonstration of hiatal hernia is not necessarily an indication that reflux exists; nor does it necessarily indicate that the symptoms produced are a result of the hiatal hernia causing the reflux. Many hiatal hernias are found in asymptomatic patients, and though an associated reflux has been shown to cause symptoms of esophagitis, hiatal hernia as a cause of esophagitis should be questioned. Esophagoscopy and biopsy are important in studying chronic esophagitis since this condition is not always the result of chronic acid reflux and may at times be caused by a fungal or viral disease, or even a neoplastic process. Therefore, esophageal biopsy is mandatory.

Diffuse esophageal spasm

Diffuse esophageal spasm is probably the second most common of the esophageal diseases. It is a disorder of esophageal motility and has various causes including reflux esophagitis.

Laboratory tests. The diagnosis is usually made radiologically with a cine-esophagogram that shows the disturbed segmental contractions without a peristaltic wave in the distal esophagus. The disorder can also be confirmed with manometric pressure studies of the different parts of the esophagus.

Differential diagnosis. Diffuse esophageal spasm is commonly associated with aging (presbyesophagus), ganglion degeneration (seen in the early stages of achalasia), mucosal irritation (most likely secondary to gastroesophageal reflux), obstruction of the cardia, and neuromuscular disorders (diabetic neuropathy and amyotrophic lateral sclerosis). Sometimes it may simply be idiopathic.

Achalasia

Achalasia is a motor disorder, the symptoms of which appear to reflect impaired cholinergic innervation of the esophagus.

Laboratory tests. The diagnosis is made with radiologic contrast studies showing the abnormal esophageal motor function with a characteristic beak-like narrowing of the distal esophageal segment, and by esophageal manometry showing a markedly increased lower esophageal sphincter pressure.

Differential diagnosis. Carcinoma of the lower esophagus and adenocarcinoma of the stomach with extension to the esophagus are sometimes radiologically difficult to differentiate from achalasia. Endoscopic study with biopsy is most helpful in the differential diagnosis.

Scleroderma (progressive systemic sclerosis)

Scleroderma involves the esophagus in approximately 80% of cases and is characterized by decreased esophageal peristalsis, mainly in the lower one-third of the esophagus.

Dermatomyositis

This is characterized by oropharyngeal dyphagia with difficulty in propelling the bolus from the mouth to the esophagus and decreased pressures of the upper esophageal sphincter on manometry.

Neurologic conditions

Neurologic conditions may possibly affect deglutition. One must be aware of the possibility of myasthenia gravis in deglutition problems. Edrophonium chloride (Tensilon) can be used for diagnostic testing. If the muscular weakness is caused by myasthenia gravis, the edrophonium injection will produce prompt relief.

Other conditions

The esophagus may rupture spontaneously, sometimes in previously healthy individuals. Usually x-ray films will show free air in the mediastinum with resultant mediastinal crunch and subcutaneous emphysema. Severe hemorrhage associated with vertical laceration of the gastroesophageal junction (Mallory-Weiss syndrome) occasionally occurs.

Plummer-Vinson syndrome consists of dysphagia associated with iron deficiency anemia and usually is found in elderly females.

THE STOMACH

Anatomy and physiology

The stomach in relationship to the rest of the digestive tract, the liver, and the pancreas is illustrated in Fig. 7-1. After the food enters the stomach it is stored, mixed with gastric juice, and then slowly emptied into the small intestine through the pyloric sphincter.

Gastric secretion

[illegible]

Cephalic stimulation results from the sight, smell, taste, or thought of food. Vagal impulses will then directly stimulate the parietal cells to secrete HCl and the mucosa of the antrum to secrete the hormone gastrin.

In the gastric phase partially digested protein and the distention of the antrum stimulate the release of gastrin. Gastrin is absorbed into the blood and carried back to the stomach to potently stimulate gastric acid secretion. It also moderately stimulates pepsinogen secretion and gastric and intestinal motility, as well as enhances sphincter mechanisms of the esophagus. When the pH of the gastric juice reaches 2.0, gastrin secretion usually stops.

The intestinal phase appears to be a more complex mechanism involving the release of intestinal gastrin and the inhibition of gastric secretion by various other hormones when fats and carbohydrates are in the small intestine.

Pathophysiology

The total gastric HCl secretion is determined by the parietal cell mass—by the number of parietal cells present and functioning. It has been shown that patients with duodenal ulcer have a secretion of HCl that is almost twice normal. Gastric ulcer patients secrete less acid than normal and gastric cancer patients secrete less still.

Laboratory tests for gastric acid analysis

Gastric acid studies are done for the following indications:

1. To determine whether the patient is able to secrete acid. This is done to establish the differential diagnosis of pernicious anemia and gastric ulcer.
2. To determine how much acid the patient secretes. This is indicated in rare conditions in which the clinical diagnosis strongly suggests peptic ulcer disease with an equivocal upper GI series. A high basal secretion (10 mEq

or more) is suggestive of active peptic ulcer disease. Very high secretory rates of acid are seen in tumors that secrete gastrin (i.e., Zollinger-Ellison syndrome).

3. To determine the type of surgery necessary. In hypersecretors, there is increased risk of stomal ulcer following ordinary gastric resection without vagotomy. If the patient is still having symptoms after a vagotomy for peptic ulcer, the completeness of the vagotomy should be ascertained by a Hollander test, which is explained below.

Basal secretion

The basal secretion rate is determined to ascertain how much acid the patient secretes without stimulation to do so. The patient is intubated under fluoroscopic visualization. The gastric contents are then aspirated continuously for 2 hours, with the aspirate titrated at half-hour intervals. A secretion of 6 mEq or more per hour is indicative of hypersecretion. A secretion of 15 mEq or more should lead one to suspect a hormonal abnormality affecting the parietal cells.

NORMAL BASAL ACID OUTPUT (BAO)

0-6 mEq/hr

Augmented histamine or Histalog test

This gastric secretion stimulation test should immediately follow the basal secretion test, since the capacity of the gastric cells to secrete, on a particular occasion, may not be significant in the basal state. With this stimulus (i.e., histamine or Histalog injection), a secretion of 50 mEq/hr or more indicates hypersecretion. The specimens are collected as in the basal state. This is a useful test to confirm the achlorhydria of pernicious anemia and in the diagnosis of the Zollinger-Ellison syndrome.

Diagnex blue test

With this test the presence or absence of acid can be determined without intubation. It involves the ingestion of a tablet of caffeine followed by a dye and an exchange resin. If the gastric contents have a pH of 3.0 or less, dye is released from the resin and excreted in the urine. If the results of this test are negative or inconclusive, a Histalog stimulation test is indicated.

Saline load test

This is a test to evaluate gastric outlet obstruction. A nasogastric Levin tube is inserted in the stomach. The gastric residue is aspirated and measured. Then, 750 ml of 0.9% (normal) saline is instilled. After 30 minutes the gastric contents are again aspirated and measured. If more than 400 ml of fluid is still present in the stomach, gastric outlet obstruction is suspected.

Hollander insulin test

This test is performed in order to determine whether a vagotomy has been complete or not. A 2-hour basal gastric analysis is performed as described above. The patient is then given an injection of insulin to produce hypoglycemia. The hypoglycemia should be 50% of fasting blood sugar. If the gastric secretion in any postinsulin hour (2 hours) exceeds that of the higher of the 2 basal hours, (pre-insulin fasting stage, two determinations) the va- [illegible]

[illegible]

rum gastrin levels are measured in the basal state and then again during calcium infusion. If the secretion of gastric acid approaches maximal levels and the serum gastrin levels rise appreciably with the calcium infusion, ectopic gastin production, such as is seen in Zollinger-Ellison syndrome, is suspected.

Gastric analysis using secretin

This is another test performed to differentiate the Zollinger-Ellison syndrome from hypersecretory states without inappropriate secretion of gastrin. Secretin is given intravenously and should cause a decrease in acid secretion. However, with Zollinger-Ellison syndrome the acid secretion is increased to maximal Histalog levels and the serum gastrin rises.

Serum gastrin level

Hypergastrinemia is one of the main characteristics of the Zollinger-Ellison syndrome, which is always accompanied by significant increase in gastric acid secretion. A marked elevation of gastrin is present also in pernicious anemia. This probably reflects the characteristic failure of patients with this disorder to secrete gastric hydrochloric acid, which is a potent, normal inhibitor of gastrin release.

Gastrin release is slightly elevated in the fasting serum of patients with gastric ulcer disease. Also, there is a slight elevation of gastrin levels in duodenal ulcer. However, it rarely reaches the levels found in the Zollinger-Ellison syndrome.

There is significant diminution of gastric acid in gastric carcinoma. Thus by the same mechanism of reciprocity, there will be increased gastrin secretion. In the Zollinger-Ellison syndrome, although there is high gastric acidity, which would normally suppress the gastrin secretion, there is an extremely high gastrin level, which indicates an autonomous tumor producing the excess gastrin.

Stimulation of serum gastrin can be accomplished by infusion of calcium and secretin. With calcium infusion intravenously, the response is a markedly elevated serum gastrin level. The response to secretin in normal situations is a diminution of the serum gastrin level, but in Zollinger-Ellison syndrome there is a paradoxical rise in serum gastrin.

NORMAL SERUM GASTRIN

40-150 pg/ml

Laboratory tests in the clinical setting

Gastritis

The most common disorder of the stomach is probably superficial gastritis secondary to ingestion of irritants such as aspirin and/or alcohol.

Laboratory tests. The diagnosis of gastritis is usually made by gastroscopy, since superficial gastritis may not be visualized by barium studies. However, the acute inflammatory edematous mucosa can easily be seen with a gastroscope and confirmed by gastric biopsy.

Gastric ulcer disease

Gastric ulcer disease is probably less common than gastritis.

Laboratory tests. The diagnosis depends on radiologic and gastroscopic examination. The combination of these two tests brings the diagnostic accuracy up to approximately 90% or 95%.

Differential diagnosis. In differentiating between benign and malignant gastric ulcer, radiologic examination of the stomach is an important diagnostic aid. However, during a gastroscopic procedure, a mucosal biopsy can be performed in suspected cases of carcinoma, and the diagnosis definitively made.

Cytologic examination of the gastric juice depends on the expertise of the pathologist. Accuracy varies from 30% to 80%. The yield is greater when the specimen is obtained during endoscopy.

Gastric acid examination is of some help. If true histamine-fast achlorhydria is present, then there is no good, reassuring way of ruling out the diagnosis of carcinoma. However, the presence of acid does not necessarily rule out carcinoma either.

If malignancy is not established with the above tests, strict medical therapy should be initiated. The radiologic examination should then be repeated between the second and third week of intensive medical therapy. If there is a reduction of the ulcer size by 50% or more, the lesion is probably benign and the medical regime should be continued for 2 or 3 more weeks until there is complete healing. The gastric studies and endoscopy should then be repeated.

Duodenal peptic ulcer

Laboratory tests. X-ray contrast barium study is very helpful in diagnosing duodenal ulcer. The demonstration of a crater on the films is the main characteristic of peptic ulcer disease. Endoscopy, however, is the most definitive way of making the diagnosis.

Differential diagnosis. Gastric juice analysis is usually not important in ordinary ulcer disease, with two possible exceptions: Histamine-fast achlor- [illegible]

[illegible]

[illegible] be visualized radiographically. However, the stoma and the ulceration can be visualized quite easily with the aid of a gastroscope.

Zollinger-Ellison syndrome

The Zollinger-Ellison syndrome is caused by non-beta islet cell tumors of the pancreas (a gastrin producing adenoma) and is characterized by profound gastric hypersecretion that causes a typical and severe malignant peptic ulceration.

Laboratory tests. As previously mentioned, an inappropriately high output of gastric acid, both in the basal and in the Histalog-stimulated states, is seen in this condition. If equivocal rises are seen, gastric acid measurements and serum gastrin determinations should be performed following calcium or secretin stimulation.

Complications of peptic ulcer

Hemorrhage. In upper GI hemorrhage it is essential to document the site of bleeding. Thus a vigorous, aggressive diagnostic approach is recommended. It is negligent to assume that the bleeding is from esophageal varices when the patient has cirrhosis of the liver. The bleeding might be a result of a gastric ulcer or a duodenal ulcer.

Laboratory tests. Intubation of the stomach should be performed on every patient with GI bleeding. This will help document whether or not the bleeding is from the upper part of the intestinal tract. If blood or "coffee ground" material is noted on aspiration, the stomach should be lavaged with iced saline. Following this, an attempt should be made to document the source of the bleeding, preferably by endoscopy. If this mode is not possible, an emergency GI series should be performed.

Perforation. Of patients with perforated ulcers, 85% have free air under the diaphragm that can be detected by x-ray examination of the abdomen with the patient in a reclining and an upright position. It should be noted, however, that the absence of free air under the diaphragm does not necessarily rule out perforation.

An elevated serum amylase level correlating with the clinical picture is extremely suggestive of perforation.

Occasionally, in equivocal cases, the perforation may be identified through the use of water-soluble contrast material (Gastrografin).

Gastric outlet obstruction. Obstruction of the gastric outlet may result from a number of causes. Ulceration and edema near the pylorus, scarring of the pyloric channel, and tumors are the most usual.

Symptoms commonly seen are vomiting, abdominal distension and occasionally pain. On physical examination a succussion splash and visible peristalsis are helpful diagnostic clues.

Laboratory test. Diagnosis is made by nasogastric aspiration and measurement of gastric residue. If, 4 hours after eating, the gastric residue is greater than 300 ml, or if the overnight gastric residue is greater than 200 ml, then a saline load test is performed.

Radiologically, a large distended stomach is frequently seen. Endoscopic and/or barium contrast studies are then considered. However, before any of these diagnostic studies are performed, it is always advisable to decompress and cleanse the stomach.

THE SMALL INTESTINE

Anatomy and physiology

The small intestine is a tube approximately 1 inch in diameter and 20 feet in length. It begins at the pyloric end of the stomach (duodenum), which can be seen in Fig. 7-1 in the shape of a C around the pancreas. The jejunum and ileum comprise the rest of the small bowel.

The chyme is propelled through the small bowel by segmentation contractions and peristalsis, and digestion is completed by the action of the intestinal juices.

Digestion and absorption

Through the process of digestion nutrients are reduced to simple components for transport across the intestinal mucosa to the portal blood system. Finger-like projections called villi and microvilli on the surface of the intestine increase the absorbing surface about 600 times that of an ordinary tube of equal length and circumference.

Only the salient features of fat, protein, and carbohydrate digestion and absorption are presented below.

The principal lipid, triglyceride, is digested in the duodenum and jejunum in the presence of bile salts and lipase (a pancreatic enzyme).

Protein digestion and absorption require a pH of about 6.5. In the duodenum, protein stimulates the release of secretin and pancreozymin, which in turn causes the release of bicarbonate and the pancreatic proteases. The latter require the enzyme from the mucosal surface, enterokinase, for activation.

Carbohydrate digestion takes place (1) in the duodenum by reaction with amylase from the pancreas and (2) on the surface brush border of the intestinal mucosa by the action of disaccharidase.

[illegible]

[illegible]

[illegible] may result from inadequate secretion of pancreatic enzymes. Carbohydrate malabsorption can be the result of a deficiency of brush border disaccharidase.

Laboratory tests for malabsorption syndromes

Stool examination

Stool examination for ova, parasites, and occult blood is very helpful. Cultures will determine the presence of bacterial infection or overgrowth, and microscopic examination for meat fibers and fat aids in the diagnosis of malabsorption.

Fecal fat content

This is the best screening test for determining overall malabsorption syndrome. The total 24-hour fecal fat should be less than 6 gm, given a daily intake of 75 to 100 gm of fat. If it is more than 6 gm, malabsorption is indicated. However, this does not differentiate between true malabsorption and maldigestion.

Inadequate specimen collection is suspected with a 3-day stool weight of less 300 gm.

Serum carotenes and prothrombin time

Since absorption of the fat-soluble vitamins is impaired in fat malabsorptive states, serum carotene levels and prothrombin time are diminished. The abnormal bleeding time results from vitamin K deficiency.

D-xylose absorption

This is a useful test, and a positive result usually indicates intrinsic intestinal disease. D-xylose is normally not metabolized and is absorbed intact.

Intrinsic intestinal disease, particularly in the proximal intestine, is reflected by diminished absorption of D-xylose.

Lactose tolerance test

This test will identify patients who are unable to digest lactose because of insufficient levels of intestinal lactase. Normally, after fasting and then ingesting 100 gm of lactose within 2 hours there will be a rise in blood glucose of at least 20 mg/100 ml. An abnormally low rise usually correlates with low levels of intestinal lactase.

Gastrointestinal x-ray films

Barium studies of the small bowel are extremely helpful in providing clues to the diagnosis of celiac disease, regional enterities, lymphomas, fistulas, etc.

Biopsy of the small intestine

Biopsy of the small intestine is of diagnostic value in the following conditions: celiac sprue, Whipple's disease, hypogammaglobulinemia, and abetalipoproteinemia. Biopsy may also be of value in the diagnosis of intestinal lymphoma, amyloidosis, eosinophilic enteritis, regional enteritis, intestinal lymphangiectasia, systemic mastocytosis, and parasitic infestations.

This test is not diagnostic although results may be abnormal in systemic scleroderma, acute radiation enteritis, tropical sprue, vitamin B_{12} deficiency, bacterial overgrowth syndromes, and folate deficiency.

Biopsy is performed by having the patient swallow a small metallic capsule attached to a polyethylene catheter. Suction is then applied to the mucosal wall. The biopsy specimen is obtained by triggering a small cutting blade.

In addition to tissue examination of the biopsied specimens, the intestinal cells can also be assayed for disaccharidase activity. This would help determine if there are enzymatic deficiencies of lactase, sucrase, or isomaltase. These deficiencies may be congenital or acquired and secondary to intrinsic small bowel disease.

Secretin test

The secretin test can be helpful in differentiating between malabsorption secondary to pancreatic disease and intrinsic intestinal disease. Secretin is a hormone that stimulates the production of pancreatic fluid high in bicarbonate content but low in enzyme content. After the passage of a double-lumen tube for separate gastric and duodenal aspiration, secretin is given intravenously. The gastric and duodenal contents are collected separately with the latter being measured for volume, bicarbonate content, and amylase activity. A volume of less than 1.5 ml/kg body weight per 30 minutes, or a bicarbonate concentration less than 70 mEq/L after stimulation indicates subnormal pancreatic function. Cytologic examination of the aspirate may be helpful in the diagnosis of carcinoma.

Flat film of the abdomen

In addition to the secretin test, a flat film of the abdomen that permits visualization of pancreatic calcification is extremely helpful in differentiating chronic pancreatitis from intrinsic intestinal disease as a possible cause of steatorrhea and malabsorption. Pancreatic pseudocysts can also sometimes be demonstrated on a flat film of the abdomen.

Celiac angiogram

[illegible]

There are two factors necessary for the formation of red blood cells: the extrinsic factor (vitamin B_{12}), which is found in meat, eggs, milk, and the like, and the intrinsic factor, which is produced by the gastric mucosa. The function of the intrinsic factor is to assure the absorption of vitamin B_{12}.

The Schilling test is performed by first giving the patient radioactive vitamin B_{12} orally. Two hours later a massive nonradioactive parenteral dose is given. About one third of the absorbed vitamin should appear in the urine; therefore, the presence of little or no radioactivity in the urine indicates gastrointestinal malabsorption. If there is absorption, ilial disease is ruled out as a cause of malabsorption; and since the vitamin was given without the intrinsic factor, pernicious anemia is also ruled out.

The same procedure is again followed with the addition of the intrinsic factor to the oral vitamin B_{12}. Nonabsorption of the vitamin B_{12} without the intrinsic factor, but absorption of it when the intrinsic factor is added, is diagnostic of pernicious anemia.

Occasionally, a patient may not absorb vitamin B_{12} with or without the intrinsic factor because of excessive bacterial invasion such as would occur in the blind loop syndrome. In this case, the results of the Schilling test return to normal after a course of antibiotic therapy.

Bile acid breath test

This is a relatively new, sensitive method of testing for malabsorption and/or small bowel bacterial overgrowth.

Most of the bile acids secreted in bile are reabsorbed in the distal small bowel and recirculated. Bile acids not absorbed enter the colon where bacteria deconjugate and metabolize different portions of the molecule, eventually producing CO_2.

If a small tracer amount of radioactive (^{14}C) bile salt is given by mouth it should, under normal circumstances, be absorbed from the small bowel and enter the bile salt pool. If small bowel disease exists or bacterial overgrowth of the small bowel is present, then the radioactive (^{14}C) bile salt is metabolized by the bacteria and $^{14}CO_2$ is produced. Eventually, this is extracted by the lungs. Thus by assaying the breath for radioactivity one can determine whether or not small bowel disease or bacterial overgrowth is present.

Under normal conditions practically no $^{14}CO_2$ should be present in the breath.

Tissue typing

A large portion of patients who have inflammatory bowel disease, particularly when associated with joint disorders such as arthralgias and arthritis, have tissue type HLA-B27. Thus tissue typing may identify certain genetic subgroups who are susceptible to inflammatory bowel disease.

Laboratory tests in the clinical setting

Malabsorption syndrome

The motility of the small intestine and its total surface area are factors in its absorptive capabilities, as are adequate pancreatic and biliary secretions. Thus, malabsorption syndromes are divided into two major categories: (1) those resulting from intrinsic disease of the wall of the small intestine with normal digestion but abnormal absorption because of the lesions of the bowel wall and (2) those caused by digestive problems related to pancreatic insufficiency or bile acid secretory problems causing delayed or inadequate absorption.

The initial screening test is a peripheral blood film to evaluate early folate deficiency. Low serum levels of iron, vitamin B_{12}, and folate will confirm the deficiency. Vitamin D and calcium absorption may be evaluated by an estimation of serum calcium, phosphorus, and alkaline phosphatase levels. Vitamin K absorption is evaluated by determination of the prothrombin time. A low level of serum albumin may reflect malabsorption of protein or protein-losing enteropathy. A low serum carotene level may indicate malabsorption of fat if dietary intake of carotene is adequate.

All of the more specific tests of malabsorption have been previously described.

Inflammatory intestinal disease (regional enteritis)

Initial suspicion of this disease comes from chronic intermittent diarrhea, fever, crampy abdominal pain, joint pains, and abdominal masses revealed by the physical examination. Perianal ulceration and stricture are quite common.

Laboratory tests. Nonspecific laboratory findings are leukocytosis, blood loss, anemia, undernutrition, hypoalbuminemia, hypocalcemia, hypokalemia, elevated sedimentation rate, elevated serum alkaline phosphatase level, hypoprothrombinemia, and macrocytic anemia.

The radiologic picture along with the clinical suspicion usually establishes the diagnosis. It is definitely established histologically. Fistulous tracts are common, particularly in the ileocecal region, and are virtually pathognomonic.

In the operating room, biopsies of the small intestine and lymph nodes provide adequate bases for microscopic diagnosis and rule out tuberculosis, various lymphomas, sarcoidosis, and fungous diseases. When the disease process involves the colon along with the small bowel, biopsies can also be [illegible]

or intussusception.

3. Extrinsic bowel lesions, such as adhesions, volvulus, or hernias.

Laboratory tests. Flat films of the abdomen are the single most important examination in suspected cases of intestinal obstruction. From the type of lumen pattern, the level of obstruction can more or less be determined: air-fluid levels are a hallmark of obstruction. If the symptoms are acute and the obstruction is suspected to be low in the intestine, barium should not be given orally. However, if the obstruction is thought to be in the colon, then a carefully administered barium enema may demonstrate the obstructive lesion.

The other laboratory findings of intestinal obstruction are nonspecific inflammatory findings such as leukocytosis, lactic dehydrogenase elevation, mild amylase elevation, and electrolyte abnormalities.

Differential diagnosis. The differential diagnosis would include paralytic ileus, and intestinal pseudo-obstruction. Laboratory tests are usually not helpful in differentiating these conditions from mechanical obstruction. One helpful clue can be found, however, on physical examination. In both of these conditions bowel sounds are significantly diminished, whereas in mechanical obstruction one can hear high pitched bowel sounds that come in rushes.

Mesenteric arterial insufficiency

The mesenteric arteries supply the splanchnic area. Atherosclerotic or other degenerative changes in these arteries or the celiac axis can produce pain that is steady and agonizing. Mucosal changes and mural deterioration lead to malabsorption, causing weight loss and symptoms of malabsorption.

Vascular insufficiency in elderly patients may contribute significantly to malabsorption. The syndrome in these patients may be at the subclinical level and be undetected if not looked for particularly.

To evaluate the vascular integrity of the GI tract, celiac angiogram and superior and inferior mesenteric angiograms are quite helpful in individual cases.

THE COLON

Anatomy and physiology

The large intestine is 5 to 6 feet in length and 2½ inches in diameter. It begins at the cecum and proceeds in turn as the ascending colon, transverse colon, descending colon, sigmoid colon, rectum, and anal canal (Fig. 7-1). The functions of the colon are the absorption of water and electrolytes from the chyme and the storage and elimination of waste products of digestion.

Laboratory tests for diseases of the large intestine

Radiologic examination—barium enema

Radiologic examination of the colon is a most important diagnostic tool. It should be noted, however, that acutely ill patients do not tolerate well the necessary preparation for barium enema. If the patient is not acutely ill a diagnosis can be determined by a simple barium enema or by air contrast barium enema, which is even more diagnostic. The barium enema is employed for the possible diagnosis of malignancies, benign growths, diverticular disease, and inflammatory disease of the GI tract, such as ulcerative colitis. Also included in this list are the bacterial granulomatous diseases such as tuberculous enteritis and colitis and amebic colitis.

In some of the conditions mentioned above the specific diagnosis can be made fairly well by the barium enema alone. However, often more direct visual examination and biopsy are necessary. Therefore, the second most important test in the examination of the colon is sigmoidoscopy and/or colonoscopy.

Patient preparation and care. The colon is thoroughly cleansed by means of diet, cathartics and/or enemas. If gas or feces are still present in the large intestine at the time of the examination the procedure may have to be repeated. Hence all care should be taken to adequately prepare the patient.

Because of the danger of an impaction caused by the barium in the large bowel, cleansing enemas or laxatives may be ordered to evacuate the residual barium.

The extensive preparation may have produced dehydration. Therefore, the patient should be encouraged to take fluids, unless medically contraindicated.

Sigmoidoscopy

Proctosigmoidoscopy can be performed for inspection of the rectum and sigmoid colon either by the conventional rigid tube sigmoidoscope or with the new fiberoptic proctosigmoidoscope. This test is used for two major reasons: (1) The lower 15 to 18 cm of the colon is difficult to visualize radiologically, particularly the sigmoid region, but is easily seen through a sigmoidoscope. (2)

The definitive diagnosis in certain conditions can be achieved through biopsy under direct visualization, which is possible with sigmoidoscopy. Ulceration is seen easily, and a biopsy is the determining factor in the differential diagnosis of many bowel disorders, particularly the different types of inflammatory bowel diseases.

Colonoscopy

schistosomiasis). This can be done by punch biopsy at the time of sigmoidoscopy or by suction biopsy via capsule.

Carcinoembryonic antigen (CEA) test

Initially, the carcinoembryonic antigen was thought to be relatively specific for carcinoma of the GI tract, including the liver and pancreas. However, later it was found that this antigen is relatively nonspecific. In clinical practice at the present time, the role of carcinoembryonic antigen is restricted mainly to follow-up studies. If a patient with known carcinoma has an elevated carcinoembryonic antigen level preoperatively or prior to therapy, and if this level rises on subsequent follow-up, it is a good indication of recurrence or growth of the carcinoma. However, in itself, since so many factors will cause an elevation, it is considered a nonspecific test and is not used for a definitive diagnosis of carcinoma of the GI tract. Highest titers of this antigen are found in carcinoma of the colon and pancreas.

THE GALLBLADDER

Anatomy and physiology

The gallbladder is a pear-shaped sac lying on the underside of the liver. Bile is produced by the liver and enters the gallbladder via the hepatic and cystic ducts to be concentrated and stored until needed.

During digestion, the gallbladder contracts and rapidly supplies bile to the small intestine through the common bile duct (Fig. 7-2). This contraction of the gallbladder and also the relaxation of the sphincter muscle is in response to a hormone (cholecystokinin) that is secreted by the intestine mainly in the presence of fats.

The most common disorders of the gallbladder are gallstone disease and cholecystitis.

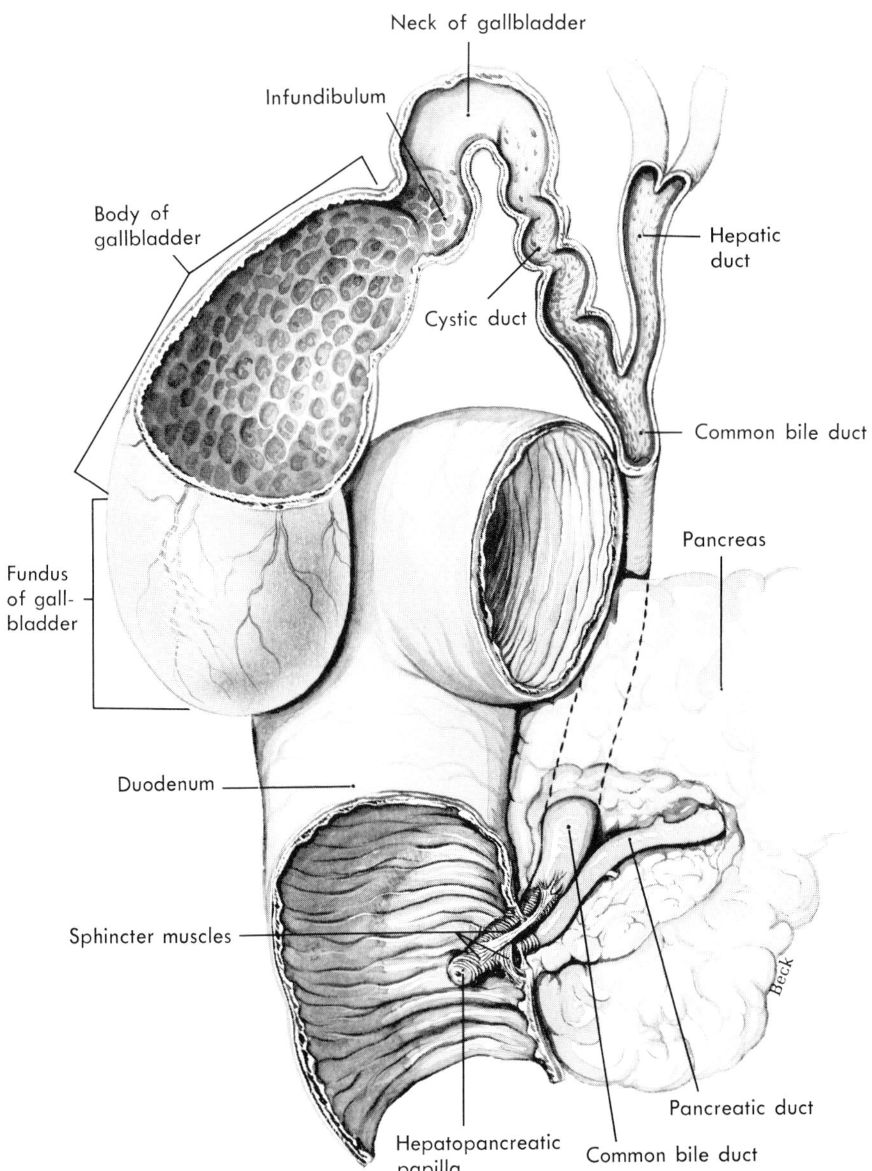

FIG. 7-2
The gallbladder and its divisions: fundus, body, infundibulum, and neck. Obstruction of either the hepatic or common bile duct by stone or spasm blocks the exit of bile from the liver, where it is formed, and prevents bile from ejecting into the duodenum. (From Anthony, C. P., and Kolthoff, N. J.: Textbook of anatomy and physiology, ed. 9, St. Louis, 1975, The C. V. Mosby Co.)

Laboratory tests for biliary tract disease

Flat film of the abdomen

If gallstones are calcified they are easily seen in flat films of the abdomen. Unfortunately, most gallbladder stones are cholesterol with less than 50% being calcified; therefore, contrast studies of the gallbladder are necessary.

Oral cholecystography

[illegible]

Intravenous cholangiography (IVC)

When an iodine contrast medium is given intravenously, both the biliary tree and the gallbladder can be visualized. However, since the visualization is much poorer than with oral cholecystography, tomography must frequently be used as well.

This study cannot be performed if hepatocellular disease or high grade obstruction of the biliary tree is present. In general, visualization is extremely poor if the serum bilirubin level is over 3 mg/100 ml.

Percutaneous transhepatic cholangiography

The visualization of the biliary tree achieved with this test helps to differentiate major obstructive jaundice from hepatocellular jaundice.

The liver is entered percutaneously with a plastic-sheathed needle. The needle is removed and the plastic sheath remains through which bile is aspirated and dye injected. Recently, a very thin, flexible needle known as the "Chiba" or "skinny" needle has been used with greater safety and success. Not only are there fewer complications such as peritonitis, bleeding, or sepsis, but also over 95% of obstructed biliary tracts and approximately 60% of normal biliary tracts are visualized.

Operative cholangiography

Cholangiography may also be performed during surgery. Dye is injected into the common bile duct or gallbladder. If a T-tube is left in, it can be utilized postoperatively for the injection of dye and thus cholangiography.

Endoscopic retrograde cholangiography

Fiberoptic endoscopy permits cannulation of the ampulla of Vater and retrograde injection of contrast material. Approximately 85% of obstructive lesions of the biliary tree can be visualized by this method by skilled endoscopists.

Retrograde cholangiography and percutaneous cholangiography have become two very helpful tools in delineating the biliary tree in obstructive jaundice.

Angiography

Selective hepatic arteriography can result in visualization of the cystic artery and gallbladder walls. However, this cannot consistently be accomplished in all cases; therefore, the diagnostic value of the procedure at this time is restricted to very select situations.

Abdominal ultrasonography

This is a noninvasive method of imaging the abdomen with the use of sound waves. Cystic lesions are well delineated and this method is particularly helpful in demonstrating a large, distended, obstructed gallbladder and stones within the gallbladder.

Computerized axial tomography

Tomography is described in more detail on p. 206. Briefly, this radiologic technique, applied to the right upper quadrant, permits visualization of the liver, biliary tree, and gallbladder. Thus obstruction with a distended gallbladder may be documented, as well as dilated bile ducts and gallstones in the gallbladder or biliary tree.

THE LIVER

Anatomy and physiology

The liver is the largest gland and the major metabolic factory in the human body. It lies immediately under the diaphragm, occupying most of the right upper quadrant (Fig. 7-1). The liver is involved in protein synthesis and other metabolic functions, regulation of blood volume, immune mechanisms, formation and excretion of bile, and the detoxification and excretion of toxic elements. The function of the liver is also important in the synthesis, esterification, and excretion of cholesterol.

Liver function tests and their physiologic basis

The routine screening tests for liver disorders has already been discussed in Chapter 1.

Bilirubin

This is the chief bile pigment in man. It is derived principally from the breakdown of hemoglobin, and is normally bound to albumin in the circulation. Bilirubin is then carried to the liver where it is conjugated with glucuronic acid. This *conjugated* bilirubin is more water soluble than the *free* bilirubin, and therefore is secreted more easily into the bile. Once within the intestine, the bilirubin is reduced to *urobilinogen* by the action of intestinal bacteria. Some of this urobilinogen is absorbed into the circulation and is either excreted in the urine or reexcreted in the bile. The rest of the intestinal urobilinogen is excreted in the stool as *fecal urobilinogen*.

Jaundice. Excessive bilirubin in the blood escapes into the tissues, which [illegible]

the excretion of bilirubin.

Bilirubin accumulates in the blood in all of these conditions and diffuses into the tissues to cause jaundice.

NORMAL SERUM BILIRUBIN

Direct or conjugated:	up to 0.3 mg/dl
Indirect or unconjugated:	0.1-1.0 mg/dl
Total:	0.1-1.2 mg/dl

NORMAL URINE UROBILINOGEN

2 hr:	0.3-1.0 Ehrlich units
24 hr:	0.05-2.5 mg/24 hr or
	0.5-4.0 Ehrlich units/24 hr

NORMAL FECAL UROBILINOGEN

75-350 mg/100 gm of stool

Since bilirubin is liberated when erythrocytes are destroyed, any condition that increases erythrocyte destruction results in hemolytic jaundice. In such a case, the serum enzymes (SGOT and SGPT) are normal. There is an increase in unconjugated (indirect) bilirubin in the serum and a mild to moderate increase in urobilinogen in the urine. There is frequently a significantly increased level of fecal urobilinogen. With this, other evidence of hemolysis should be looked for, such as reticulocytosis and dropping hematocrit.

Unconjugated hyperbilirubinemia may also be seen in conditions other than hemolysis. Two such conditions,which result from hepatic causes, are the Crigler-Najjar syndrome and Gilbert's disease. The only abnormality seen in these situations is an increased level of unconjugated (indirect) bilirubin with essentially normal liver function.

Conjugated (direct) bilirubin is elevated significantly in the blood in hepatic jaundice. This condition can be caused by viruses, or by toxins such as drugs, alcohol, etc., all causing a hepatitis. In these cases there is extreme elevation of the liver enzymes (SGOT and SGPT), a moderate increase in alkaline phosphatase levels, and the urine urobilinogen may or may not be increased. The fecal urobilinogen is normal. The cholesterol level is somewhat diminished, particularly the esterified fraction.

A marked elevation of alkaline phosphatase, particularly in primary biliary cirrhosis, is manifested in obstructive jaundice (or so-called cholestatic jaundice). Bilirubin is present in the urine and the urobilinogen level is normal, elevated, or decreased. SGOT and SGPT levels are slightly elevated, but much less so than in acute viral or hepatocellular jaundice.

In the case of posthepatic obstruction, such as a tumor of the ampulla of Vater, a carcinoma of the head of the pancreas, or a stone in the major common bile duct, there is complete absence of fecal urobilinogen. This gives the clay color to the stools. The cholesterol is increased. The alkaline phosphatase is markedly increased. The enzyme levels (SGOT and SGPT) are mildly to moderately elevated.

In summary, in the differential diagnosis of jaundice, besides evaluating the total bilirubin, one must:

1. Fractionate the bilirubin and look for evidence of indirect hyperbilirubinemia, which suggests hemolysis.
2. Look for evidence of elevated enzymes, particularly SGOT and SGPT, which suggests hepatocellular disease.
3. Look for evidence of alkaline phosphatase and cholesterol elevation, which points more toward obstructive jaundice.

Serum enzyme assays

Serum alkaline phosphatase is one of the most important determinations in the differential diagnosis of obstructive jaundice. For all practical purposes, a normal alkaline phosphatase strongly suggests liver pathology other than obstruction. Normal values are listed in Chapter 1 and Appendix A.

5′-Nucleotidase and serum leucine aminopeptidase are measured in conjunction with alkaline phosphatase because they are not related to bone destruction, as is alkaline phosphatase, and are not elevated in bone disease. However, they are not as sensitive as alkaline phosphatase in diagnosing obstructive jaundice.

NORMAL SERUM 5-NUCLEOTIDASE

0-1.6 units

NORMAL SERUM LEUCINE AMINOPEPTIDASE

50-220 units

The transaminases, serum glutamic oxaloacetic transaminase (SGOT) and serum glutamic pyruvic transaminase (SGPT), are liberated from destroyed cells. SGOT is found particularly in skeletal muscles, cardiac muscle, and liver while SGPT is found mainly in liver tissue. In the absence of cardiac or other muscle injury, the elevations of SGOT and SGPT are suggestive of hepatocellular damage.

NORMAL SERUM SGPT

1-36 U/ml

Serum protein determination is important because albumin is synthesized in the liver, and because serum globulins are produced by Kupffer cells. Therefore, in typical chronic liver disease, the albumin/globulin ratio is reversed with diminution of albumin and elevation of globulin, which is a broad gamma type of elevation.

Neoplastic and inflammatory diseases of the liver produce elevation of the alpha 2 globulin fraction, and sometimes biliary obstruction shows elevation in the beta globulin levels. Gamma globulin elevation is noted frequently with chronic active liver disease. See p. 13 or Appendix A for normal values.

Although this is a good screening test for overall extensive liver disease, the influence of nonhepatic factors on protein metabolism should be remembered.

Prothrombin time and vitamin K administration test

The increase of prothrombin time in liver disease may be the result of either malabsorption of the fat-soluble vitamin K or a deficiency in the formation of one of the clotting factors (I, II, V, VII or X, all of which are produced in the liver). The prolongation of prothrombin time would be manifested by bleeding tendencies.

The differential diagnosis of obstructive versus hepatocellular damage is made by giving an intramuscular injection of vitamin K. If the prothrombin time returns to a normal level or rises at least 30%, the implication is that the patient has obstructive problems rather than hepatocellular damage. However, continued prolongation of prothrombin time indicates severe hepatocellular damage.

NORMAL PROTHROMBIN TIME

12-14 sec

Blood lipid and cholesterol

Blood lipid and cholesterol levels are usually elevated in obstructive jaundice and particularly in Zieve's syndrome (fatty liver), in which case there is extreme elevation of cholesterol and triglycerides. In chronic liver disease cholesterol levels are diminished. In both obstructive and chronic liver disease the percentage of esterified cholesterol is diminished. See p. 12 or Appendix A for normal values.

Other tests helpful in evaluating liver function

Blood ammonia levels. Blood ammonia levels are elevated in severe liver cirrhosis, especially following GI bleeding. This occurs because ammonia is usually metabolized to urea in the liver and is then excreted by the kidney. However, in the presence of marked liver disease, ammonia levels would be elevated. It has been suspected that some of the hepatic encephalopathy is probably a result of a high ammonia level in the cerebrospinal fluid, which interferes with the normal function of the central nervous system. In association with elevated ammonia, blood urea nitrogen will also be diminished.

NORMAL PLASMA AMMONIA

20-150	mcg/dl (diffusion)
40-80	mcg/dl (enzymatic method)
12-48	mcg/dl (resin method)

Sulfobromophthalein excretion test (Bromsulphalein, BSP). This is a general screening test for overall liver function. It is a relatively simple test that can be done mainly on patients who are not jaundiced and is an index to the extent of parenchymal disease in that it gives some indication of hepatocellular damage and cell loss. The results are, however, also elevated in obstructive disease and are therefore not helpful in differentiating the causes of jaundice.

BSP dye is administered intravenously and is almost completely cleared from the blood in approximately 45 minutes by the normal liver.

Hepatic scanning. This is a means of visualizing the liver by giving a tracer dose of radioactive technetium sulfur colloid and by imaging its uptake by the reticuloendothelial system of the liver.

Under normal conditions a homogenous uptake is seen. This test can be helpful in diagnosing masses, abscesses or cysts of the liver, which would appear as "cold" spots—that is, as areas of decreased isotope uptake.

Percutaneous needle liver biopsy. Percutaneous biopsy is a safe method of establishing the pathologic and microscopic picture of the liver cell. It is most useful in the diagnosis of diffuse parenchymal disorders of the liver. It is also helpful in differentiating disseminated granulomatous focal disease from tumors.

The major indications for needle biopsy are:

1. Unexplained hepatomegaly and hepatosplenomegaly
2. Persistently abnormal results of liver function tests
3. Suspected systemic or infiltrative disease
4. Sarcoidosis or miliary tuberculosis
5. Suspected primary or metastatic liver malignancy

Needle biopsy should not be performed if the prothrombin time is sig- [illegible]

[illegible] on his right side for 2 to 4 hours following the biopsy. In general, ambulation is not permitted for 24 hours.

Peritoneoscopy. This is a useful but not a routinely employed way of studying patients with liver disease. The procedure is performed by introducing the peritoneoscope into the peritoneal cavity and thus directly visualizing the gallbladder, liver, and serosal lining with a minimum of discomfort and hazard to the patient. It is additionally helpful in determining the site for the liver biopsy, which can be performed under peritoneoscopy.

Alpha fetoprotein ("fetal" $alpha_1$ globulin). This is a unique protein found in the blood of patients with carcinoma of the liver. If it is detected in the blood of a patient with chronic liver disease, and if it persists, it is suggestive of primary carcinoma of the liver. Normally, in the adult there are only trace amounts detected by radioimmunoassay.

Ultrasonography. This is a helpful means of identifying cystic lesions and abscesses of the liver.

Computerized axial tomography. This can be helpful in imaging masses or cysts of the liver (see pp. 154-160).

Selective hepatic angiography. Hepatic angiography permits visualization of the arterial supply of the liver and is helpful in delineating neoplastic lesions.

Hepatitis B surface antigen (HBsAg). This was previously known as the Australia antigen and is an antigenic marker for hepatitis B virus, which causes long incubation hepatitis (previously known as serum hepatitis).

The most sensitive way of assaying for HBsAg is by radioimmunoassay. When present, it is diagnostic of hepatitis B infection.

Hepatitis B surface antibody (anti-HBs). Anti-HBs can also be assayed and is indicative of previous infection with hepatitis B virus.

e antigen. This antigen is frequently found in sera of patients who have chronic active liver disease associated with hepatitis B surface antigenemia. Its presence alerts one to the possibility that persisting liver enzymes could be indicative of chronic active hepatitis, the diagnosis of which is made by liver biopsy.

THE PANCREAS

Anatomy and physiology

The pancreas is comprised of two major types of tissues: the acini, which secrete digestive juices into the duodenum, and the islets of Langerhans, which secrete insulin and glucagon into the bloodstream.

In response to the entry of food into the small intestine and to the hormones secretin and cholecystokinin, the pancreas secretes pancreatic juice into the intestinal tract.

Pancreatic juice contains bicarbonate and water to neutralize the acidic chyme and enzymes for digesting proteins, carbohydrates, and fats.

Laboratory tests for pancreatic function

Serum amylase and lipase

Amylase is the digestive enzyme for carbohydrate. In pancreatitis the serum amylase level is usually between 200 and 500 units and in biliary tract disease over 1000 units. Even though serum amylase levels are also elevated in mumps and in renal insufficiency, the test is indicated in patients with upper abdominal pain. Serum lipase parallels the amylase, though it rises slightly later and persists in the serum longer than the amylase.

NORMAL SERUM AMYLASE

4-25 U/ml

NORMAL SERUM LIPASE

0-1.5 Cherry-Crandall
2 U/ml or less

Urine amylase

This test is limited because of the wide range in the normal value. Normally, the urinary excretion of amylase ranges from 50 to 700 U/ml. In pancreatitis there is usually an elevated excretion.

A more useful modification is to measure a 2-hour urinary amylase and correlate this finding with the serum amylase and lipase levels.

Hypotonic duodenography

This is another barium study performed for the purpose of detecting pancreatic disease. Barium is introduced by nasal catheter into the duodenum, which has been rendered atonic through the injection of an anticholinergic drug, such as propantheline bromide (Pro-Banthine). Pancreatic masses may then be seen impinging upon the flaccid duodenal wall. Men with prostatism should void immediately prior to the procedure, restrict fluids for several hours following the procedure, and be checked for voiding, because transient urinary retention is a side effect sometimes experienced with anticholinergic drugs.

Endoscopic retrograde pancreatography

[illegible]

Abdominal angiography

Angiography can help visualize the arterial supply of the pancreas and thus helps to delineate mass lesions of this organ.

Computerized axial tomography

This technique is described on p. 206. It permits visualization of the pancreas, helps to delineate masses and cysts, and demonstrates calcification.

Other specific tests of pancreatic function

The secretin test, described on p. 146, is indicated when pancreatic insufficiency is a possibility. Intestinal malabsorption tests have already been described and should be used when pancreatic insufficiency is suspected.

Laboratory tests in the clinical setting

Acute and chronic pancreatitis and pancreatic carcinoma are usually accompanied by abdominal pain, whereas pancreatic insufficiency is usually manifest more by malabsorption and malnutrition than by abdominal pain.

Acute pancreatitis

In this disease of variable causes the locally released enzymes destroy the gland.

Laboratory tests. Amylase and lipase are released from the pancreas and these levels will rise in acute pancreatitis. The hematocrit, probably reflecting intravascular volume contraction, also rises. Serum triglyceride levels may also be elevated. Methemalbumin may be found in the serum if the pancreatitis is hemorrhagic. If the common bile duct has been obstructed by an edematous pancreas, the serum bilirubin level will be elevated.

Chronic pancreatitis

This condition is usually the result of repeated injury of the pancreas. The cause is frequently alcohol.

Laboratory tests. Amylase and lipase show variable elevations. Pancreatic calcification is common. Results of the secretin test are usually abnormal, and endoscopic retrograde pancreography shows diagnostic changes.

Cystic fibrosis

The clinical features of this genetic illness are chronic pulmonary disease, pancreatic dysfunction, and a high concentration of sodium and chloride in the sweat. Mucus plugs the pancreatic ducts, the intestinal mucous glands, and the bronchial tree. The pulmonary symptoms are usually more significant than the pancreatic.

Laboratory tests. The electrolyte concentration of the sweat will be elevated to 60 mEq/L or more. The normal concentration is less than 40 mEq/L.

There will also be evidence of malabsorption, mainly because of maldigestion, with resultant steatorrhea.

8

DIAGNOSTIC TESTS FOR ENDOCRINE DISORDERS

The endocrine system is a very complex system with one common denominator. The organs of the endocrine system all produce small amounts of very active chemical substances known as hormones, which alter body metabolism. Each of the hormones is manufactured by one particular organ and is secreted into the bloodstream to exert its influence on other organs or tissues ("target tissues").

The established endocrine system, illustrated in Fig. 8-1, is comprised of the following organs: hypothalamus, anterior and posterior pituitary, thyroid, parathyroids, adrenals, pancreatic islets of Langerhans, ovaries, testes, and placenta.

The endocrine system has inherent checks and balances so that most of the endocrine function tests depend not only on excess production or underproduction of a particular hormone, but also on the reciprocal effects such over- or underproduction has on other endocrine organs. For example, excess cortisone production from the adrenal glands suppresses production of ACTH by the pituitary gland. There is, therefore, a differential diagnosis as to the location of the main pathologic process.

THE THYROID GLAND

Anatomy and physiology

The thyroid gland (Fig. 8-2) consists of two lobes with a connecting portion (isthmus), giving the gland an H-shaped appearance. There is one lobe on each side of the trachea. This gland is unique among the endocrine glands because of its large amount of stored hormone and its slow rate of excretion.

The principle hormones secreted by the thyroid are *thyroxine* (T_4) and *triiodothyronine* (T_3). These hormones stimulate the oxidative reactions of most of the cells of the body, help to regulate lipid and carbohydrate metabolism, and are necessary for the normal growth and development of the

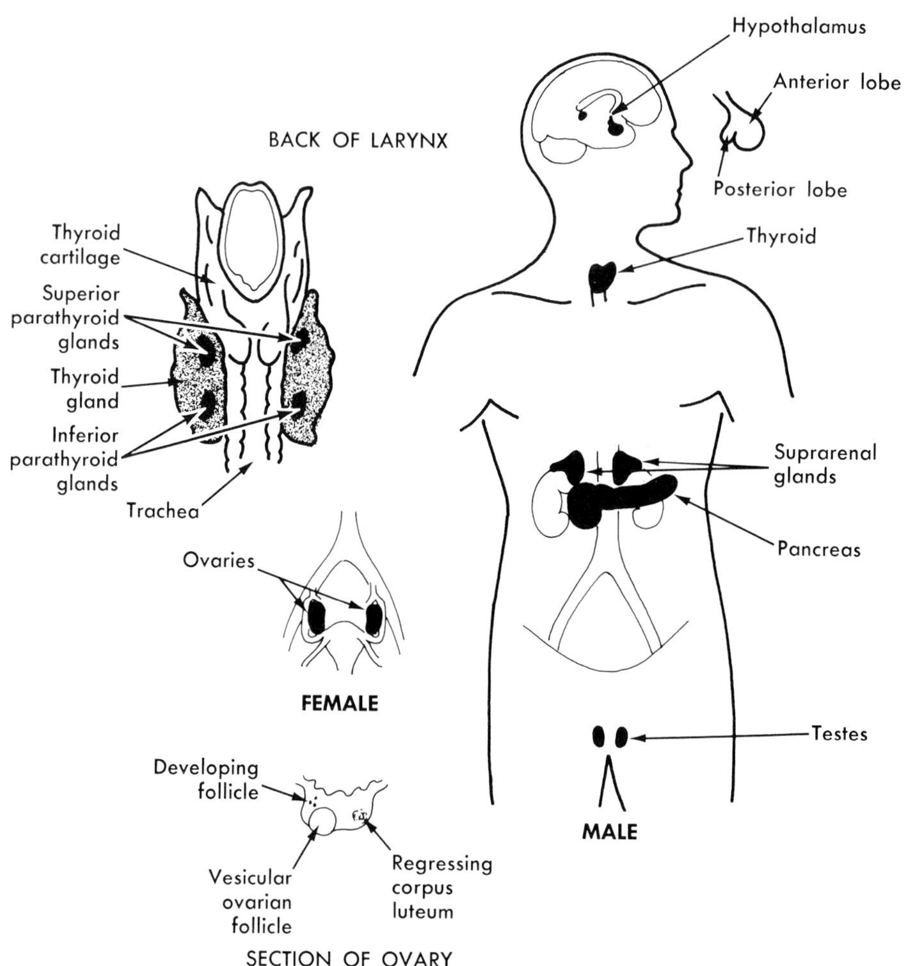

FIG. 8-1
The endocrine system.

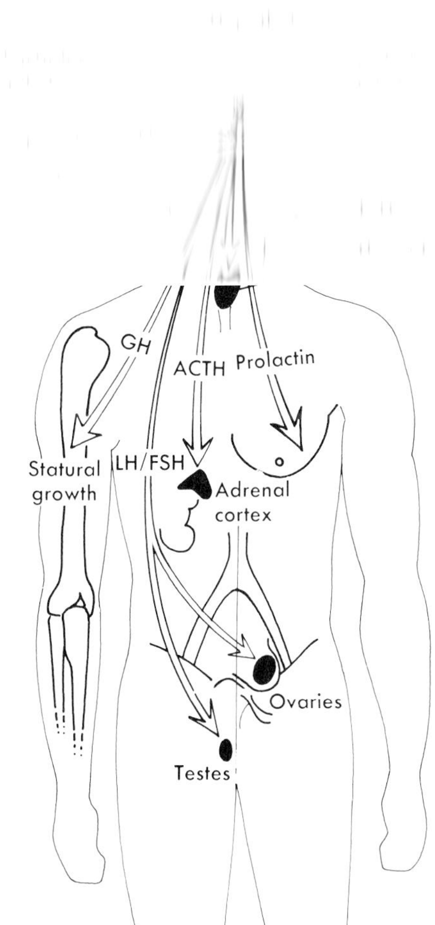

FIG. 8-2
The interrelationships between the pituitary gland, the hypothalamus, and the target organs.

organism. Most of the action of the thyroid hormone is mediated through the sympathetic nervous system. This is why beta adrenergic blockers are effective in controlling symptoms of hyperthyroidism.

The first step in the synthesis of the thyroid hormone is absorption of dietary iodide from the small intestine into the circulation. The circulating iodide that is not taken up by the thyroid gland is cleared by the kidneys through glomerular filtration. After entering the thyroid, iodide is oxidized and combines with the amino acid tyrosine within the protein molecule thyroglobulin, where the thyroid hormones triiodothyronine (T_3) and thyroxine (T_4) are formed and stored.

The next step is the release of T_3 and T_4 from the thyroid gland. Under the influence of the thyroid-stimulating hormone (TSH) from the anterior pituitary gland, thyroglobulin is hydrolyzed and T_3 and T_4 are released into the circulation. Of the circulating thyroid hormones, 99.95% of the T_4 and 99.5% of the T_3 are bound to serum proteins, particularly to thyroxine-binding globulin (TBG). These hormones are inactive when bound to serum proteins. Therefore, only very small amounts of unbound thyroid hormone circulate to provide biologic activity. Although the proportion of unbound T_3 in the serum is greater than that of unbound T_4, there is more total circulating T_4. The protein-bound hormones are, therefore, more likely to reflect T_4 levels. However,

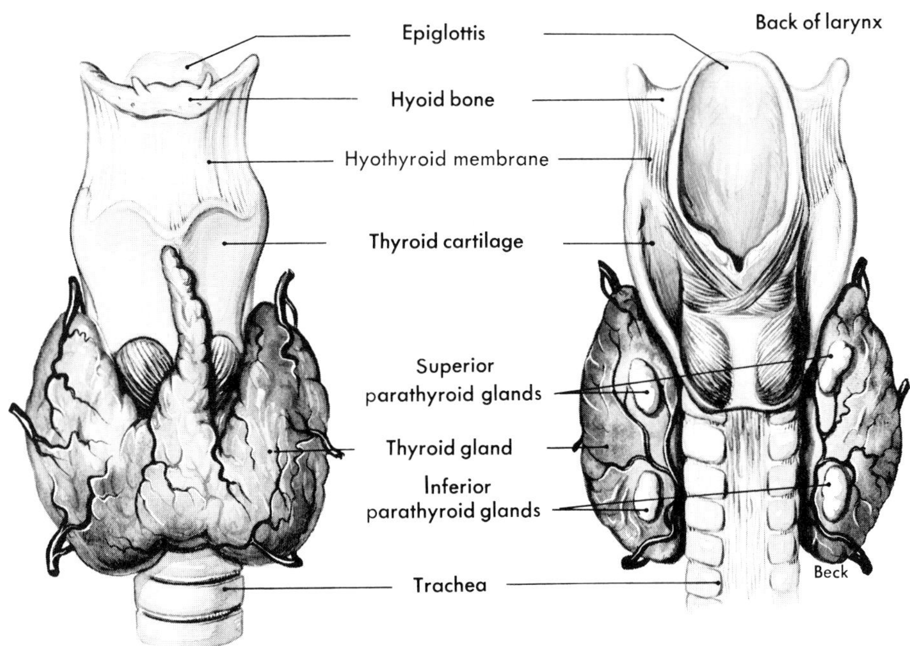

FIG. 8-3
The thyroid and parathyroid glands. (From Anthony, C. P., and Kolthoff, N. J.: Textbook of anatomy and physiology, ed. 9, St. Louis, 1975, The C. V. Mosby Co.)

T_3 is four times more potent than T_4 and only one sixth less plentiful in the unbound state.

The regulation of the thyoid gland occurs through a feedback system (Fig. 8-3) consisting of three main components: (1) the thyroid gland, which secretes T_3 and T_4, (2) the anterior pituitary gland, which secretes the thyroid-stimulating hormone (TSH), and (3) the hypothalamus, which secretes thyrotropin-releasing factor (TRF). TRF then stimulates the release of TSH and [illegible]

[illegible]

[illegible] rate (BMR) is no longer considered *the* test for thyroid disease; in its place is a whole complex of thyroid function tests. New techniques for the identification of the thyroid hormones have been developed, resulting in a more specific and accurate determination of the metabolically active thyroid hormone factors.

Basal metabolic rate (BMR)

In the past the most important thyroid function test was the basal metabolic rate. A low level BMR indicated hypothyroidism that was associated with hypercholesterolemia. These measurements plus the clinical picture were sufficient reason to initiate therapy.

Protein bound iodine (PBI)

With the discovery of protein bound iodine in 1950 and the introduction of radioactive iodine uptake of the thyroid gland, the BMR became obsolete. At that time there was widespread use of the PBI and the RAI uptake. However, the PBI as a thyroid function test is limited, particularly because any condition that increases or decreases the level of proteins that carry thyroxine also falsely increases or decreases the amount of PBI. In addition, exogenous iodine preparations interfere extensively with the test. Thus the value of the PBI test remains limited.

Radioactive iodine (RAI)

The radioactive iodine, or ^{131}I, test is still used. A small tracer dose of ^{131}I is given intravenously, and the amount that enters the gland provides an indirect measure of thyroid activity. The test has, however, become less specific, particularly in detecting hypothyroid states, because of the increased use of iodinized food, which suppresses the RAI uptake.

Butanol-extractable iodine (BEI)

As a slight improvement on the measurement of serum PBI, the measurement of butanol-extractable iodine was introduced during the early 1950s. This test eliminates exogenous contamination with iodine. However, it is a time-consuming and technically difficult test and does not solve the most common problems in testing thyroid function: interference from organic iodides and from factors that influence thyroxine-binding globulin (TBG).

Serum thyroxine (T_4) determination

The most dramatic improvement in thyroid function tests occurred between 1960 and 1966 with the development of a direct determination test of thyroxine, which effectively eliminates the problem of exogenous iodine contamination. The test is also known as the Murphy-Pattee and T_4(D) (T_4 by displacement) test. It is a radiochemical procedure that measures the ability of serum T_4 to displace radioactive thyroxine from thyroxine-binding globulin (TBG). The development of this test was motivated by the recognition of the specificity of thyroxine-binding protein. This method is absolutely specific for thyroxine and therefore free from all iodine interference. It is, however, affected by thyroxine-binding globulin (TBG), which, if elevated, will give elevated T_4 results.

T_4 can also be measured by the radioimmunoassay method, which may be even more accurate.

Serum triiodothyronine (T_3) determination

Soon after the introduction of the T_4 determination, a technique for the estimation of T_3 was developed. T_3 is much less stable than T_4 and occurs in very small quantities in the active form. Yet the ability to measure T_3 in the serum is clinically important when the patient has all of the symptoms of hyperthyroidism but a normal serum level of T_4. In such a patient, T_3 measurements may identify a T_3 thyrotoxicosis, a very rare clinical entity. There are two methods available for its measurement: (1) T_3 by displacement, which involves competitive protein binding, and (2) T_3 by radioimmunoassay (T_3[RiA]), an elaborate antigen-antibody reaction requiring special reagents.

Free thyroxine and free thyroxine index

It is the free, unbound thyroxine that enters the cell, is metabolically active, and is not affected by TBG abnormalities. This is, therefore, the measurement that would be of most diagnostic value. However, free thyroxine is cumbersome and difficult to measure clinically. Instead, T_4 and T_3 uptakes are measured, and the results of these in vitro determinations are multiplied. The resulting product not only correlates very well with the true level of free thyroxine but is also unaffected by TBG. This mathematical product is frequently referred to as the free thyroxine index. However, certain laboratories have been creating confusion by reporting it as T_7 or T_{12}.

Comparison of T_4, T_3, and free thyroxine

At the present time, the most useful and accurate tests for evaluating thyroid function are the T_4 determination (Murphy-Pattee) and the T_3 determination (either by displacement or radioimmunoassay method). The free throxine index can then be calculated. The result will reflect changes of free thyroxine and will not be influenced by TBG changes. Radioactive iodine uptake is also employed in situations in which the T_3 and T_4 results are [illegible]

[illegible]

[illegible]	[illegible]	[illegible]
Thyroxine-binding globulin (TBG)	10-26 μg/dl (expressed as T_4 uptake)	
Free thyroxine index	0.9-2.3 ng/dl	0.1-1.5 ng/dl

Thyroid scan

The thyroid scan is of greatest value in studying solitary thyroid nodules. Radioactive iodine is injected intravenously, after which the overall pattern of thyroid gland radioactivity can be visualized. Thus hyperactive and hypoactive areas can be localized, and the size of the gland can be determined. Hyperactive areas will indicate a hyperfunctioning nodule ("hot nodule"), and will thus differentiate between diffuse hyperplasia and toxic nodule as a cause of thyrotoxicosis. Hypoactive areas indicate a hypofunctioning nodule ("cold nodule") and thus increase the suspicion of carcinoma. The hot nodule is seldom malignant. Also, thyroid scanning provides some guidelines for therapy in hyperthyroidism when ^{131}I therapy is contemplated.

Measurement of serum thyroid-stimulating hormone

The most reliable and accurate test for primary hypothyroidism is the measurement of the thyroid-stimulating hormone, which is elevated in this condition. A normal serum level of TSH excludes primary hypothyroidism, because an absence of thyroid hormone in the serum stimulates the pituitary gland to produce more than the normal amount of TSH.

Thyroid-stimulating hormone suppression test

This test is used to rule out primary hyperthyroidism when the T_3 and T_4 values are borderline. It is, however, not of value in making the diagnosis of hypothyroidism. The test is based on suppressing the thyroid-stimulating hormone by giving the patient oral T_3, the most active form of thyroid hormone. If this is followed by suppression of TSH, hyperthyroidism is ruled out.

Thyrotropin-releasing hormone (TRH) stimulation test

The hypothalamus produces the thyrotropin-releasing hormone, which stimulates the release of TSH and causes the synthesis of new TSH in the pituitary gland. This test, therefore, measures diminished pituitary TSH reserve. The response to TRH stimulation is supranormal in patients with hypothyroidism of thyroid origin, whereas little or no response occurs in patients with thyrotoxicosis. This lack of response is an excellent test to confirm thyrotoxicosis. The test is also of value in the recognition and differential diagnosis of pituitary and hypothalamic hypothyroidism. In the former no response to TRH stimulation is expected.

TSH stimulation test

This test is performed by injecting TSH in patients who have low T_3 or T_4 for any reason. Usually the thyroid gland is suppressed because of exogenous thyroid intake. A positive response suggests that the patient does not need exogenous thyroid and that the thyroid gland is normal but temporarily suppressed because of the exogenous thyroid intake.

This test is also helpful in differentiating between primary and secondary hypothyroidism. If there is no response, primary hypothyroidism is suggested.

Tests for circulating antibodies

Antithyroglobulin antibody. Moderate to high titers of an antithyroglobulin antibody are found in the serum of patients with Hashimoto's thyroiditis, indicating that this condition is an autoimmune thyroid disease.

Long-acting thyroid stimulator (LATS). This antibody is an immunoglobulin directed against some component of the thyroid cell plasma membrane. This abnormal thyroid stimulator differs from TSH and is found in approximately 50% of patients in the active phase of Graves' disease.

Summary of thyroid tests

The most accurate and most commonly used tests for evaluating thyroid function at the present time are:

1. T_4 (Murphy-Pattee) method, which is also officially designated as T_4(D)
2. T_3 determination
3. Free thyroxine index
4. TSH

To further test the homeostatic controls and feedbacks, sophisticated tests employed are:

1. TSH stimulation
2. TSH suppression
3. TRH stimulation

Of historical value only is the determination of protein bound iodine (PBI), butanol-extractable iodine (BEI), and basal metabolic rate (BMR).

The thyroid scan is still the most valid test for detecting hot or cold nodules of the thyroid. For medullary carcinoma of the thyroid, increased concentration of calcitonin in the serum is diagnostic.

Thyroid function tests in the clinical setting

Simple diffuse nontoxic goiter

The patient with a simple goiter will have a normal metabolic state, which [illegible]

imoto's disease. The thyroid function tests (T_3, T_4, and free thyroxine index) may be variable, depending upon when these tests are performed during the course of the thyroiditis. Therefore, the patient may be metabolically normal, slightly hypothyroid, or hyperthyroid. In addition, in Hashimoto's thyroiditis the antithyroid antibody and microsomal antibody levels are usually elevated.

Hypothyroidism

In hypothyroidism the T_4 Murphy-Pattee, T_4 resin exchange or radioimmunoassay, and the free thyroxine index are all decreased.

An elevated TSH level in a patient with symptoms of hypothyroidism is nearly diagnostic of hypothyroidism. Because of the decrease of serum thyroxine level, the feedback suppression of TSH is not present; thus the TSH level is markedly increased.

The Achilles tendon reflex is another test used in the evaluation of thyroid function. In hypothyroidism, there is a delay in the relaxation phase of the reflex.

Diffuse toxic goiter (Graves' disease)

Along with the clinically unique hypermetabolic picture the following laboratory tests will show elevated levels: T_3 resin uptake or radioimmunoassay, T_4 Murphy-Pattee, and the free thyroxine index.

TSH is normal or low normal.

Differential diagnosis. Thyroid scan will distinguish diffuse goiter from a nodular goiter or a toxic nodular goiter. In diffuse toxic goiter there will be a uniform increase in the uptake of radioactive iodine, whereas in toxic nodule there will be one area of excessive uptake of radioactive iodine. In this case the surrounding tissue will show diminished uptake.

Neoplasms of the thyroid

Thyroid neoplasms may be either adenomas or carcinomas. Both usually present as a solitary nodule and the patient is usually euthyroid. If the neoplasm is functioning antonomously it will accumulate ^{131}I, and the thyroid scan will show a hot nodule. If this is associated with frank thyrotoxicosis it is called toxic adenoma.

Carcinoma of the thyroid is very similar in appearance and consistency to the nodular goiter. ^{131}I uptake will most frequently demonstrate a cold nodule. However, a hot nodule does not rule out the possibility of carcinoma. Microscopic examination of biopsied tissue is necessary to make a definitive diagnosis.

In medullary carcinoma of the thyroid, elevation of the calcitonin level is the hallmark of the diagnosis. In recent years thyroid ultrasound has been of some help in differentiating cystic benign tumors from solid thyroid tumors.

THE PARATHYROID GLANDS

Anatomy and physiology

There are four small parathyroid glands so closely associated with the thyroid that for some time they were often removed during thyroidectomy (Fig. 8-2). The parathyroid hormone is essential for life and is responsible for the maintenance of ionized calcium in the blood as well as for the renal reabsorption of calcium and excretion of phosphate.

Low serum calcium levels, by a feedback system, trigger an increase in the production of the parathyroid hormone. Magnesium is also important in the release of the parathyroid hormone, which acts on bone, kidney, and intestine to increase serum calcium levels. Osteoclasts, in response to the parathyroid hormone, release bone salts into the extracellular fluid, thereby raising both calcium and phosphate levels in the plasma. The renal tubular cells, in response to the parathyroid hormone, increase reabsorption of calcium and decrease reabsorption of phosphate from the glomerular filtrate.

Calcitonin, a potent hypocalcemic hormone, has effects opposing those of the parathyroid hormone because it increases renal calcium clearance.

Vitamin D also plays an important role in calcium homeostasis by increasing the efficiency of intestinal calcium absorption.

Laboratory tests for parathyroid function

Tests for hyperparathyroidism

Evaluation of parathyroid function was discussed in Unit One in the section on calcium and phosphate. Evidence of hypercalcemia is still essential for the diagnosis of hyperparathyroidism. However, additional tests that have also been advocated will be discussed.

Phosphate clearance. This is not a very accurate test and has many variables. Excessive parathyroid hormone accompanied by an increase in phosphate excretion provides the physiologic basis for the test.

Phosphate reabsorption test. The parathyroid hormone prevents renal tubular reabsorption of phosphorus. The phosphate reabsorption test is accomplished by comparing the creatinine clearance with the phosphate clearance. This comparison gives the amount of phosphate reabsorbed by the tubules per minute, and is therefore some indication of the level of parathyroid hormone [illegible]

[illegible]

hypercalcemias caused by other conditions.

It is also known that thiazide diuretics given to patients with hyperparathyroidism increase the serum calcium level.

Parathyroid hormone measurement by immunoassay is available and is being used more and more frequently. However, a uniform standardization is still not available for widespread clinical use. In addition to the determination of the parathyroid hormone level, in the differential diagnosis of hyperparathyroidism resulting from adenoma vs hyperplasia, the calcium infusion test is done. This test suppresses the parathyroid hormone level in hyperplasia but not in adenoma.

Tests for hypoparathyroidism

The parathyroid hormone assay is becoming more available but is still not uniformly standardized for practical clinical purposes.

Tests for pseudohypoparathyroidism

In pseudohypoparathyroidism, serum calcium, phosphate, and alkaline phosphatase levels are elevated. However, the parathyroid hormone level is normal or slightly elevated in contrast to hypoparathyroidism, in which the level is low. Also, in pseudohypoparathyroidism there is no response to parathyroid hormone administration in the serum and urinary values of calcium, phosphate, and alkaline phosphatase, indicating an end-organ resistance phenomenon.

Test for metastatic carcinoma to bone

Bone scanning. Bone scanning is used to detect carcinoma that has metastasized to bone. A radioactive isotope of elements that are involved in bone

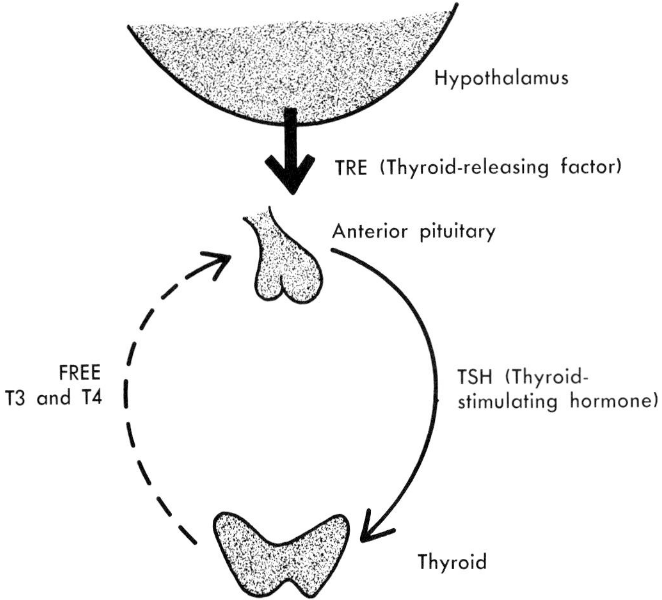

FIG. 8-4
The regulation of the thyroid gland through a feedback system.

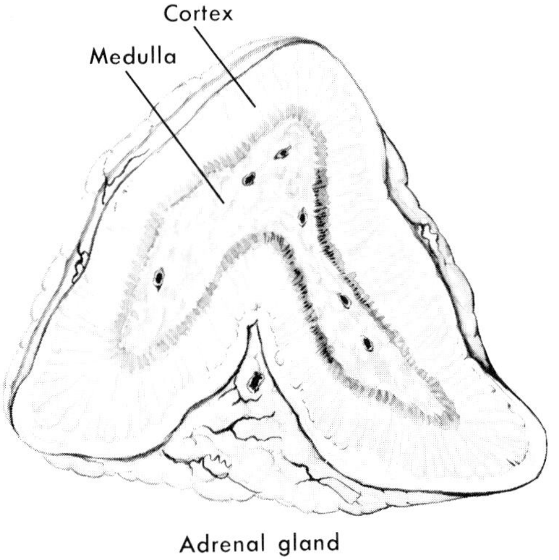

FIG. 8-5
The adrenal gland. (From Schottelius, B. A., and Schottelius, D. D.: Textbook of physiology, ed. 17, St. Louis, 1973, The C. V. Mosby Co.)

metabolism is used to detect the foci of metastatic tumors in advance of detection by x-ray films.

THE ADRENAL GLANDS

Anatomy and physiology

A right and a left adrenal gland overlap the upper ends of the kidneys. These glands are composed of two distinct parts, the medullary or inner [illegible]

of proteins, carbohydrates, and lipids

2. The mineralocorticoid, *aldosterone,* which predominantly affects sodium and potassium excretion
3. The sex steroids, *androgens* and *estrogens,* which primarily affect secondary sex characteristics

Terminology

An understanding of a portion of the biochemistry and physiology of steroids is helpful.

The carbon atoms on the basic steroid nucleus are numbered in sequence from 1 to 17. The steroids derived from this basic nucleus are of two structural types, the C-19 steroids and the C-21 steroids.

The C-19 steroids have predominantly androgenic activity and carry methyl groups at positions C-18 and C-10. If there is also a ketone group at the C-17 position, they are called *17-ketosteroids.*

The C-21 steroids have predominantly either glucocorticoid or mineralocorticoid properties and have 2-carbon side chains (C-20 and C-21) attached at position 17 of the molecule. There are also methyl groups at C-18 and C-19. The C-21 steroids that also possess a hydroxyl group at position 17 of the steroid nucleus are called *17-hydroxycorticosteroids (or 17-hydroxycorticoids).*

Adrenocorticotropic hormone (ACTH)

The role of the anterior pituitary gland in adrenal cortical secretion is displayed in Fig. 8-6. Adrenocorticotropic hormone is stored in and released from the anterior pituitary gland. The release of stored ACTH is governed by a corticotropin-releasing factor (CRF) in the hypothalamus, which in turn is governed by plasma cortisol levels, stress, and the sleep-wake cycle. The

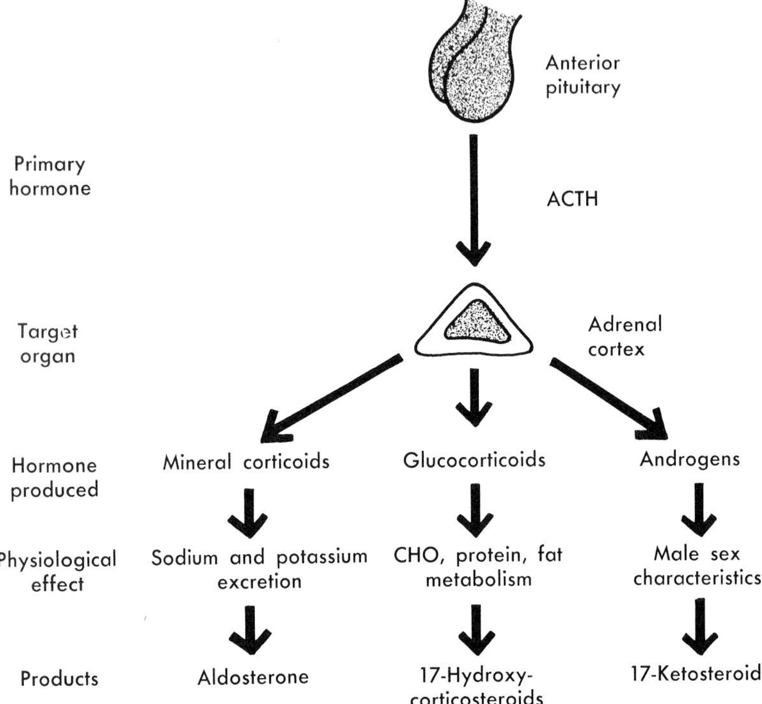

FIG. 8-6
The steroid hormones of the adrenal cortex, their physiological effects and products.

plasma ACTH level roughly follows a diurnal pattern, being highest just prior to waking and lowest just prior to retiring. In certain types of stress (emotional trauma, surgery, pyrogens) the ACTH levels rise. However, the circulating cortisol is the principal regulator of ACTH and CRF release. This is a negative feedback mechanism (Fig. 8-5) that, when plasma cortisol is low, causes a release of CRF. When plasma cortisol is high there is a decrease in the release of CRF. A low plasma cortisol level increases the responsiveness of the anterior pituitary adrenocorticotropic cells to CRF. Thus a smaller amount of CRF, in the absence of cortisol, will cause an inappropriate increase in ACTH.

Aldosterone (see also pp. 120 and 121)

Aldosterone, a mineralocorticoid secreted by the adrenal cortex, is the chief electrolyte-regulating hormone of the adrenal gland. The kidneys require aldosterone for the normal reabsorption of sodium, which leads to a secondary loss of potassium. Normally, an increase in total body sodium triggers a decrease in the rate of aldosterone secretion, causing the kidney to lose large quantities of sodium until the total body sodium level is back to normal. Conversely, if the total body sodium falls below normal or if serum potassium concentration rises, the rate of aldosterone secretion increases so that sodium is retained and potassium lost.

Aldosterone secretion is also under the control of the hormone renin, which is secreted by the kidney cells in hypovolemic or hyponatremic states. The renin-angiotensin-aldosterone system is described on p. 120.

Laboratory tests for adrenocortical function

Absolute determination of individual adrenal hormone values

Plasma cortisol levels. Cortisol, the most potent glucocorticoids, is also the most abundant of the major circulating adrenocorticosteroids.

Plasma cortisol levels are obtained in the morning and also in the evening, preferably at 8 A.M. and 8 P.M. In the healthy person the secretion rate is higher in the early morning hours and lower in the evening hours. This diurnal variation is interrupted if there is any disturbance of the hypthalamopituitary axis or if there is an autonomous lesion in the adrenals producing the excess cortisol levels. Extreme elevation of the plasma cortisol level without diurnal variation is very suggestive of autonomous carcinoma.

Although there is a definite tendency for serum cortisol levels to be high in the morning hours and low toward the evening hours, one determination may be misleading because cortisol secretion is spasmodic. For example, a low morning specimen may have been collected in the absence of such a spasmodic increase in secretion. A falsely low level would result. Several determinations taken every half-hour would be of more value than a single determination.

NORMAL PLASMA CORTISOL

8 A.M.: 5-25 μg/dl
8 P.M.: $<$ 10 μg/dl

24 hour urine steroids. The next best test for evaluating adrenal function is the 24-hour collection of urine for hydroxycorticosteroids and ketosteroids. The principal determinations with normal values appear below.

17-hydroxycorticosteroids (17-hydroxycorticoids). These steroids are measured in a 24-hour urine specimen as Porter-Silber chromogens. (The Porter-Silber reaction is a sensitive index of adrenocortical function.) The 17-hydroxycorticoids include the C-17, C-20, and C-21 hydroxysteroids, that is, those steroids with hydroxyl groups on C-17 (carbon number 17) and a ketone group on C-20 and C-21.

Elevated hydroxycorticosteroids in the urine usually indicate either primary or secondary hyperadrenalism, and elevated ketogenic steroids have more or less the same implication.

NORMAL 17-HYDROXYCORTICOSTEROIDS (24 HOUR URINE)

Male: 5.5-14.5 mg/24 hr
Female: 4.9-12.9 mg/24 hr
Lower in children
After 25 USP units ACTH, I.M.: a two- to four-fold increase

17-ketosteroids. The urine 17-ketosteroids are those C-19 steroids that also contain a ketone group at C-17 (carbon number 17) of the steroid nucleus. They are determined by the Zimmerman reaction.

Extreme elevation of the 17-ketosteroids suggests an autonomous tumor that is secreting mainly androgenic steroids. Ketosteroids are also elevated in virilizing syndromes, particularly in the adrenogenital syndrome. In such a situation, there is also an elevation of urinary pregnanetriol and pregnanediol.

NORMAL 17-KETOSTEROIDS (24 HOUR URINE)

Male: 8-15 mg/24 hr
Female: 6-11.5 mg/24 hr
Children (12-15 yr): 5-12 mg/24 hr
(<12 yr): <5 mg/24 hr
After 25 USP units ACTH, I.M.: 50%-100% increase

Ketogenic steroids. This term refers to the C-21 hydroxycorticoids that can be oxidixed to 17-ketosteroids in vitro and thus can be measured by the Zimmerman reaction.

NORMAL 24 HOUR URINE KETOGENIC STEROIDS

5-23 mg/24 hr

Aldosterone levels. Usually, aldosterone levels are ordered in hypertensive patients. At the present time hypertensive patients are being classified as high aldosterone, high renin producers or as high aldosterone producers without high renin production. The latter group is considered to have relatively benign hypertension, whereas the high renin, high aldosterone producers are thought to be vulnerable to the vascular catastrophes associated with hypertension and vascular disease. Aldosterone determination is, therefore, becoming very important. It should be performed under controlled situations in which the sodium and potassium intakes, as well as the supine and standing states, are closely monitored, because a potent stimulus to the release of renin is a low sodium diet for 4 to 5 days followed by a 4-hour period in the upright posture.

NORMAL PLASMA ALDOSTERONE

0.015 μg/100 ml

NORMAL 24 HOUR URINE ALDOSTERONE

2-26 μg/24 hr

Elevated aldosterone levels. Elevated aldosterone levels can be found in primary aldosteronism resulting from aldosterone-producing adenomas or [illegible] routinely in hypertensive patients. However, it seems reasonable that they will be performed routinely as a criterion in the selection of appropriate treatment, since renin suppression may be the treatment of choice in certain types of hypertension, whereas aldosterone suppression would be the treatment in other types.

Opinion is currently divided regarding the value of aldosterone and renin determinations in the overall management of essential hypertension. One group strongly advocates the "renin profiling" of hypertensive patients, thus categorizing them into a high renin and high aldosterone group, a normal renin group, and also a low renin and high aldosterone group. The patients are then treated accordingly. However, the opposing view is that renin profiling presently is neither standardized nor practical and therefore should not be performed in the evaluation of hypertensive patients.

Plasma ACTH levels. Adrenocorticotropic hormone (ACTH), also known as the adrenocortical-stimulating hormone, governs the secretion of glucocorticoids and the sympathetic response to stress from the adrenal glands.

ACTH levels are elevated when there is primary adrenal deficiency, particularly of the hydrocorticosteroid levels, causing the reciprocal elevation of plasma ACTH.

Extremely high levels of ACTH are found in ectopic ACTH-producing tumors or in pituitary adenomas in which there is increased secretion of ACTH.

NORMAL PLASMA ACTH AT 8 A.M.

<150 pg/ml

Feedback mechanisms and tests that reflect interdependency of hormones

These tests measure, by means of stimulation and suppression, the integrity of the functions of the hypothalamus and the pituitary and adrenal glands.

ACTH stimulation test. The ACTH stimulation test demonstrates the ability of the adrenal glands to produce steroids. Forty units of ACTH are infused within 8 hours. If the patient responds with an increase in plasma cortisol levels, any significant primary adrenal hypofunction is ruled out. However, this test is not of much clinical help.

Aldosterone stimulation test. One of the best stimulators of aldosterone secretion is the lowering of serum sodium level. This can be accomplished with a potent diuretic such as furosemide (Lasix), which will significantly stimulate aldosterone production, or with a low sodium diet.

Dexamethasone suppression test. Dexamethasone (Decadron) is a synthetic steroid with actions similar to, but much more potent than, cortisone. Therefore, very small doses suppress pituitary ACTH production, which is reflected in the urine by decreased corticosteroid levels.

The overnight dexamethasone suppression test is probably the most widely used, practical, and informative procedure available in the initial evaluation of Cushing's syndrome. The test is performed by giving a small amount of dexamethasone (2 mg) toward evening. Serum cortisone levels or the urinary excretion of 17-hydroxycorticosteroids is measured the following morning. This test can be performed on an outpatient basis. If suppression is normal (50% decrease in cortisone production), Cushing's disease or syndrome is effectively ruled out. However, nonsuppression necessitates hospitalization of the patient for a higher dose of dexamethasone with the suppression test.

Aldosterone suppression (desoxycorticosterone test). The administration of desoxycorticosterone (Doca) along with large amounts of salt will suppress aldosterone production. If the patient has primary aldosteronism there is little or no suppression, but a patient with essential hypertension has a suppression of greater than 50%, which is the normal suppression.

The Doca is administered intramuscularly, 10 mg every 12 hours for 3 days. Urinary aldosterone measurements are performed of 24 hour specimens collected before Doca administration and after the final injection on the third day.

Laboratory tests for adrenal medullary function

The adrenal medulla is a part of the sympathetic nervous system. It differs from other ganglia of the sympathetic nervous system because it secretes more epinephrine (adrenaline) than norepinephrine, and it secretes its hormones directly into the bloodstream; this classifies it as an endocrine organ.

The adrenal medullary function is not routinely tested except when there is a clinical picture of hypertension or pheochromocytoma, a tumor of the adrenal medulla.

Adrenal radiography

Radiographic visualization of the adrenal glands may reveal calcification caused either by tuberculosis associated with Addison's disease or by carcinoma of the adrenal.

An intravenous pyelogram and a tomogram may be of value in further delineating the size and shape of the adrenal gland and displacement of other organs resulting from adrenal gland pathology.

Adrenal venography and angiography may be helpful for further radiographic delineation.

Retroperitoneal air insufflation is no longer recommended, since it can be dangerous and there are better ways of delineating and visualizing the adrenal [illegible]

[illegible]

[illegible]

[illegible] gories, excess production of glucocorticoid (e.g., Cushing's syndrome) and excess production of mineralocorticoid (e.g., primary hyperaldosteronemia). However, these clinical syndromes may have overlapping features.

Cushing's syndrome. This syndrome may be produced by (1) adrenocortical hyperplasia, which is caused by some type of hypothalamic dysfunction, (2) adrenal adenoma or carcinoma, (3) ectopic ACTH production, or (4) a pituitary adenoma.

When Cushing's syndrome is clinically suspected, one should proceed as follows:

An *overnight dexamethasone suppression test* should be performed. If suppression is normal Cushing's syndrome is ruled out. If there is no suppression, the patient should be hospitalized and a higher dose of dexamethasone given, usually 2 mg every 6 hours for 3 days. If there is suppression of cortisol by more than 50% of the control, adrenal hyperplasia secondary to hypothalamic dysfunction is suggested. In this setting, the serum ACTH level may be slightly decreased, normal, or slightly elevated. If there is no suppression, one of the following is suggested: (1) ectopic ACTH-producing tumor causing adrenal hyperplasia, or (2) adrenal neoplasia, either adenoma or carcinoma.

At this point, a *plasma ACTH* determination is done. An extremely elevated plasma ACTH level suggests an ACTH-producing tumor causing adrenal hyperplasia. If the ACTH is low, an adrenal neoplasm is suggested.

A urinary 17-ketosteroid determination is called for at this point. If normal, adenoma is suggested; if high, adenocarcinoma.

Mineralocorticoid excess syndrome. This syndrome is usually caused by primary hyperaldosteronism resulting from adenoma (aldosteronemia) and is usually associated with clinical hypertension. Serum aldosterone levels are elevated with failure of the elevated aldosterone to be suppressed with the salt-loading test. Because of the elevated aldosterone levels there will be lowering of plasma renin activity, low potassium, low chloride, elevated CO_2 content, and alkalosis.

Hypofunction of the adrenal cortex

Hypocorticalism may be either primary, in which the adrenal is unable to produce sufficient quantities of hormone (Addison's disease), or secondary, the result of failure of the pituitary gland to secrete ACTH.

Addison's disease (primary hypoadrenalism). In this condition there are low serum cortisol levels and diminished hydroxy- and ketosteroids. However, there is marked elevation of ACTH in response to lowered serum cortisol levels. MSH (melanin-stimulating hormone) is elevated and there is no response to the ACTH stimulation test.

Secondary hypoaldosteronism resulting from pituitary failure. Isolated pituitary ACTH hyposecretion is rare and is usually associated with panhypopituitarism. The best test with which to measure the pituitary ACTH reserve in this situation is the *metyrapone test*, described on p. 185. A poor response to this test suggests secondary hypoadrenalism caused by failure of the pituitary to produce ACTH.

Hyperfunction of the adrenal medulla

Pheochromocytoma. Abnormally large amounts of catecholamines are released into the circulation in pheochromocytoma. A small percentage of these catecholamines is excreted unchanged in the urine. Some of the adrenal medullary hormones appear in the urine as metanephrine, and the major portion of the hormones will be excreted as vanillylmandelic acid (VMA), which is a metabolic by-product of catecholamine degradation. Therefore, a complete work-up of a patient with possible pheochromocytoma should include a 24-hour urine collection with determinations of VMA, catecholamines, and metanephrine, any one of which might be elevated in a given case of pheochromocytoma. Pheochromocytoma is characterized by hypertension with marked vasomotor changes and thus enters into the differential diagnosis of hypertensive patients.

THE PITUITARY GLAND

Anatomy and physiology

The pituitary gland is protected in the bony cavity of the sella turcica and is covered by the dura mater. The hypothalamus is attached to the pituitary gland by a stalk, and the two act together to control the functions of the target organs. The hypothalamus controls the pituitary by inhibiting and releasing factors. The pituitary, in turn, exerts its effect on various peripheral endocrine organs. The relationships of the pituitary gland and the hypothalamus to the target organs are shown in Fig. 8-7.

The seven known hormones secreted by the anterior lobe of the pituitary gland are:

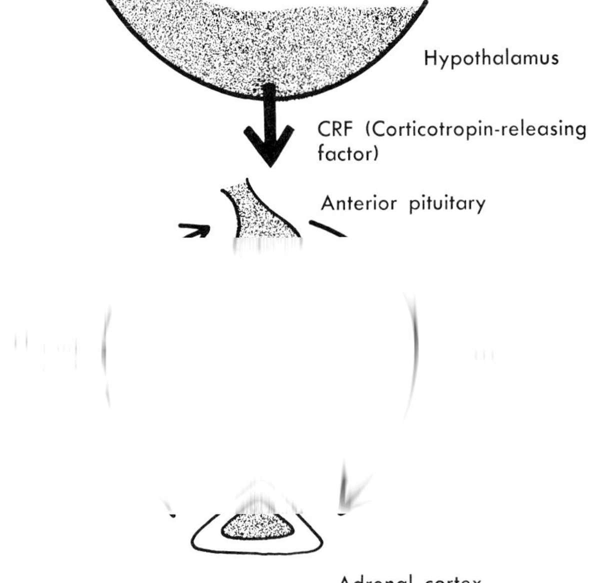

FIG. 8-7
The role of the hypothalamus and anterior pituitary gland in adrenal cortical secretion.

1. Growth hormone (GH), which has a general effect on growth
2. Prolactin, which controls the secretion of milk by the mammary glands
3. Thyroid-stimulating hormone (TSH), which stimulates the formation and release of thyroid hormones
4. Adrenocorticotropic hormone (ACTH), which controls the secretion of the adrenal cortex
5. Luteinizing hormone (LH), which initiates ovulation and luteinization in the ovary
6. Follicle-stimulating hormone (FSH), which stimulates estrogen secretion and the growth of the graafian follicle in women and spermatogenesis in men
7. Melanocyte-stimulating hormone, which affects pigment metabolism

The posterior pituitary hormones are vasopressin (antidiuretic hormone, ADH) and oxytocin, which are manufactured in the hypothalamus and stored in and released from the posterior pituitary gland.

The releasing factors secreted by the hypothalamus are as follows: corticotropin-releasing factor (CRF), gonadotropin-releasing factor (GRF), thyrotropin-releasing hormone (TRH), and growth hormone–releasing factor (GHRF). Additionally, there are three known inhibiting factors secreted by the hypothalamus. They are: prolactin-inhibiting factor, melanocyte-inhibiting factor, and a growth hormone–inhibiting factor (somatostatin).

The releasing factors stimulate the synthesis and release of the specific pituitary hormones. These factors reach the pituitary gland by the hypothalamic-pituitary venous plexus. The pituitary hormones, ACTH, FSH, LH, and TSH, are also controlled by a negative feedback loop in which the concentration of the circulating hormone secreted from the target gland suppresses the elaboration of the corresponding pituitary hormone.

Laboratory tests for pituitary function

Most of the tests performed for pituitary function have already been described under the different target organs, the thyroid and the adrenals. An adenoma of the pituitary gland initially increases secretion by the target organ. For example, there may be an increase of thyroxine and of the hydroxysteroids or ketosteroids initially because of stimulation of the thyroid and adrenal glands. Later on, as more pituitary tissue is destroyed, there is diminution of the pituitary secretions and secondary failure of the target organs.

Growth hormone measurement

The growth hormone (GH) is elevated in gigantism in children and in acromegaly in adults. This is usually the result of eosinophilic adenomas of the pituitary. Measurements of the GH are taken during the course of a glucose tolerance test. Normally, the release of serum growth hormone is suppressed by glucose administration. Therefore it is important to demonstrate a lack of suppressibility of elevated GH levels with glucose administration.

Because the growth hormone is usually the first of the pituitary hormones to become deficient, tests of growth hormone secretory capacity are diagnostic for hypopituitarism.

It is necessary to employ a stimulatory test when there is a question of hypopituitarism because the resting growth hormone values may normally be near zero. The most potent and reliable means of causing a marked increase in serum growth hormone are insulin-induced hypoglycemia, oral administration of L-dopa, and intravenous administration of arginine. The fasting state is required for the insulin tolerance and L-dopa tests. Only water is allowed prior to the arginine test.

Insulin tolerance test. Just as growth hormone secretion is suppressed by glucose administration, it will be stimulated by insulin-induced hypoglycemia.

Following the injection of insulin the blood glucose level will fall promptly, reaching its lowest point in about 30 minutes. The mild symptoms of hypoglycemia thus produced will resolve spontaneously in normal individuals. A 50% reduction of the basal value will be enough to increase the growth hormone concentration to 5 ng/ml or more within 45 to 60 minutes after administration of insulin.

Oral and intravenous glucose should be kept available since severe hypoglycemia may occur in patients with hypopituitarism and an increased sensitivity to insulin. This test is potentially dangerous; however, it is very specific and reliable and will substantiate the results of other tests.

The integrity of the pituitary-adrenal axis may also be confirmed with this test, since hypoglycemia will also cause a release of ACTH and cortisol.

L-Dopa test. L-Dopa, 0.5 gm, is given orally and blood samples for growth hormone determination are obtained every 30 minutes for 2 hours. Normally, [illegible]

[illegible]

and thus causes more compound S and less cortisol to be secreted. The diminshed values of cortisol stimulate the pituitary to produce ACTH in a negative feedback mechanism. In the normal individual, the administration of metyrapone should cause more ACTH production from the pituitary and result in an increase in urinary hydroxysteroids and ketosteroids.

X-ray films of the skull

It is usually advisable to take an x-ray film of the skull to evaluate the sella turcica, a depression in the sphenoid bone of the skull where the pituitary gland rests, for volume and erosion or enlargement.

A spinal fluid examination and a measurement of the visual fields should also be performed.

Vasopressin injection

In diabetes insipidus a vasopressin (antidiuretic hormone, ADH) deficiency is present, manifested by excessive urine output that may amount to up to 12 to 15 liters per day. The patient will respond to a vasopressin injection with a decrease in urine output, thus documenting the deficiency and the normal responsiveness of the renal tubules to the hormone.

Recall that ADH is secreted by the hypothalamus and posterior pituitary gland and promotes increased water reabsorption from the distal tubules and collecting ducts.

Posterior pituitary function tests

Specific gravity

After overnight fasting a morning specific gravity will give a rough measurement of the concentrating ability of the kidney as well as an indication of whether or not there is an adequate amount of vasopressin.

Water deprivation test

This test is used in suspected cases of diabetes insipidus.

After several hours of controlled water deprivation the urine should be concentrated. In diabetes insipidus the patient will not only be unable to concentrate the urine, but also, because of a continued loss of water, the serum osmolality will be relatively higher in spite of the lower urinary specific gravity or osmolality. Since the kidney tubules function normally in diabetes insipidus, an injection of vasopressin will correct the abnormal concentrating ability of the kidneys and bring the osmolality of both urine and serum back to normal.

Pituitary function tests in the clinical setting

Hypopituitarism

Hypopituitarism is manifested by the malfunction of the target organs. Since the capacity to secrete growth hormone is usually the first of the pituitary hormonal functions to become deficient, a normal L-dopa test will be sufficient to exclude pituitary insufficiency when the diagnosis is clinically unlikely. However, if the clinical picture presents a significant possibility of hypopituitarism, the other tests mentioned above should also be performed and correlated with the clinical state.

Hyperpituitarism

If excess production of growth hormone occurs before epiphyseal closure, the individual will be abnormally tall (gigantism). If this occurs after epiphyseal closure, acromegaly results.

The standard glucose tolerance test with blood samples being measured for growth hormone and glucose will confirm the diagnosis. Normally, the growth hormone level will decrease to below 5 ng/ml or become undetectable. In acromegaly the growth hormone levels will be greater than 5 ng/ml.

Inappropriate ADH secretion syndrome

Serum and urine osmolality are measured when inappropriate ADH secretion syndrome is suspected. These tests have already been described on p. 123 of Chapter 6.

Normally, hyperosmolar serum stimulates the osmoreceptors and the posterior pituitary produces ADH in an attempt to dilute the blood. The individual is also thirsty, a physiologic sign of hyperosmolar blood. Conversely, when there is hypoosmolarity ADH is not secreted and the individual excretes a diluted urine. In the so-called inappropriate ADH secretion syndrome there is hypoosmolarity of the blood in association with a relative hyperosmolarity of the urine, indicating a malfunction of the normal osmolar response of the osmoreceptors, an excess of exogenous vasopressin, or a production of a vasopressin-like hormone that is not under the regular control of serum osmolarity.

The inappropriate secretion of ADH has been described in multiple disease entities, such as bronchogenic carcinoma or other types of cancer, in congestive heart failure and inflammatory pulmonary lesions, in some metabolic diseases such as porphyria, and in some patients who use diuretics excessively.

The diagnosis is made by simultaneous measurement of the urine and [illegible]

[illegible]

[illegible]

Clinically the following four types of hypoglycemia are most frequently encountered.

Reactive hypoglycemia

This is the most common type of hypoglycemia and is usually seen in diabetic and some prediabetic patients. Reactive hypoglycemia is thought to be the result of inappropriate release of insulin when the blood sugar is low. It occurs because of a lag in insulin release when the blood sugar is high, causing a delayed release after the blood sugar has already started to lower.

Hypoglycemia caused by insulin-producing tumors

Insulinomas from the pancreas cause hypoglycemia. Occasionally, non-insulin secreting tumors cause hypoglycemia, particularly large retroperitoneal sarcomas.

Iatrogenic hypoglycemia

Both insulin injections and long-acting oral hypoglycemics cause this type of hypoglycemia.

Alcoholic hypoglycemia

Alcoholic hypoglycemia is common in chronic alcoholics who drink for a few days without eating.

9

DIAGNOSTIC TESTS FOR HEMATOLOGIC DISORDERS

The anatomy and physiology of blood formation is discussed in Chapter 2.

LABORATORY TESTS

Bone marrow examination

The bone marrow, which produces millions of blood cells daily (hematopoiesis), is the major site of the formation of blood. In the adult the red bone marrow is found in only a few locations, mainly in membranous bones, such as the vertebrae, the sternum, and the ribs. The most accessible region for bone marrow examination is the sternum, by means of sternal puncture, or the iliac crest. Since the bone marrow is the center of hematopoiesis, the system that actually produces the blood can be examined when a disorder in this production is suspected.

A bone marrow examination is diagnostic in the following diseases.

Leukemias

The examination is helpful especially if there is a differential diagnostic problem with the peripheral smear, such as leukemia versus leukemoid reaction, or in aleukemic leukemia in which the peripheral smear is not diagnostic of leukemia. In the bone marrow examination the ratio between myeloid cells and erythroid cells is decidedly increased in leukemia with an increase of early immature forms. In the differential diagnosis between chronic myelogenous leukemia and leukemoid reaction, in the former there is decreased leukocyte alkaline phosphatase and also the presence of Philadelphia chromosome.

Iron deficiency anemia

In the early stage of iron deficiency anemia a bone marrow examination reveals normoblastic hyperplasia, but the severe iron deficiency later restricts erythropoiesis (the formation of red blood cells) to the basal level. The normoblasts are small with frayed edges. Smears stained for iron reveal storage iron to be absent.

Megaloblastosis

Although at the present time the levels of vitamin B_{12} and folic acid in the blood are being relied on increasingly for the diagnosis of macrocytic anemia, a bone marrow aspiration reveals megaloblasts in both vitamin B_{12} and folic [illegible]

[illegible]

[illegible]

Hemolytic anemias

The bone marrow is important in documenting hemolysis as a possible cause of anemia, although the different causes of hemolytic anemias are not differentiated.

Hypoplastic or aplastic anemias

The diagnosis of these anemias can be made only through a bone marrow examination, which reveals hypocellularity.

Evaluation of bleeding disorders

Usually, bleeding results from either failure to clot normally or failure to prevent excessive clotting due to consumption of clotting factors. An example of the first condition is excess heparin intake or some clotting factor deficiency. An example of the second condition is disseminated intravascular coagulopathy.

Theory of blood coagulation

The theory of blood coagulation should be known in order to understand the various laboratory tests designed to demonstrate defects in the coagulation mechanism.

The process of blood coagulation is one of the most complicated in the body. At least thirty-five compounds take part in the formation of a firm clot, which is made up of an insoluble network of fibrous material called *fibrin*. The clotting process is divided into four stages, which are described below and illustrated in Table 9-1. The corresponding laboratory tests that reveal disorders in each stage and the various blood factors (Roman numbers) involved are also included in Table 9-1.

TABLE 9-1
Theory of blood coagulation and corresponding tests

Blood coagulation				Corresponding tests and excreted results
Stage I	*Platelets*			Platelet count (low)
	Contact factor			Clot retraction (deficient)
				Tourniquet test (positive)
				Prothrombin consumption time (abnormal)
Stage II	*Platelet factor*	Ca^{++} →	Thromboplastin ↓	Prothrombin time (normal)
	Thromboplastin generation factors	VIII		Partial thromboplastin time (abnormal)
		IX		
		X		Prothrombin consumption time (abnormal)
		XI		
		XII		
Stage III	*Prothrombin*	Ca^{++} →	Thrombin ↓	Prothrombin time (abnormal)
	Accelerator factors	V		Partial thromboplastin time (normal)
		VII		
		X		
Stage IV	*Fibrinogen*	→	Fibrin	Venous clotting time (abnormal)
			XIII	Plasma fibrinogen (abnormal)
				Protamine sulfate test (abnormal)
				Clot lysis (abnormal)

Stage I: Release of platelet factors. When blood comes in contact with a rough area on the blood vessel endothelium, such as that caused by a cut in the vessel or, very commonly, a patch of cholesterol-lipid substance, clumps of platelets begin to attach to the rough area within a matter of seconds. The platelet membranes then rupture and a substance is released that initiates the clotting mechanism.

Stage II: Thromboplastin generation. The platelet factors, in union with calcium ions and other coagulation factors present in normal blood, form a substance called thromboplastin.

Stage III: Conversion of prothrombin to thrombin. Thromboplastin then catalyzes the conversion of prothrombin, a circulating inactive protein, to thrombin. Calcium ions are also necessary for this conversion, along with other substances known as accelerator factors. Vitamin K is necessary for the synthesis of prothrombin, which takes place in the liver.

Stage IV: Formation of fibrin. Thrombin then catalyzes the conversion of fibrinogen, another circulating inactive protein, to fibrin, the final mesh that forms the clot.

Tests in hemorrhagic disorders

Stage I: A defect in the clotting mechanism at the platelet hemolysis stage, such as the thrombocytopenias, may be confirmed by the following tests.

Platelet count. Because stage I depends on platelet clumping and hemolysis with the release of the platelet factor, a decrease in platelets affects the clotting mechanism at its initiation.

Clot retraction. Normally, after about an hour the blood clot shrinks and becomes much firmer. Platelets play a major part in the mechanism of clot retraction; therefore, a deficiency in this mechanism indicates a platelet problem (thrombocytopenia).

[illegible] amount to be left in the serum, thus shortening the serum prothrombin time.

Stage II. Defects at this stage of the clotting mechanism, such as classical hemophilia, Christmas factor deficiency, or deficiency of factors VIII, IX, X, XI, and XII, may be indicated by the following tests.

Prothrombin time (PT time). A calcium-binding anticoagulant is added to the patient's serum in this test. The time between the addition of the calcium and the appearance of a fibrin clot is the prothrombin time. The prothrombin time primarily shows defects in stage III and is therefore normal when the defect is at stage II.

Partial thromboplastin time (PTT). This test is very sensitive to defects in stage II. Another name for this test is the kaolin-cephalin clotting time. It is a measurement of the clotting time of plasma, free of calcium ions and poor in platelets, performed under conditions that standardize the steps not wanted in the measurement. Thus it measures factors XII, XI, X, IX, VIII, V, II, and I. Deficiency of factor VIII is the cause of classical hemophilia, the most common hereditary coagulation factor deficiency.

The PTT is often used instead of the coagulation time for the control of anticoagulation with heparin.

Stage III. Defects of sufficient severity at this stage of the clotting mechanism, such as vitamin K deficiency, liver disease, and prothrombin suppression caused by Coumadin, will be manifest by an abnormal prothrombin time. The partial thromboplastin time is normal unless the defect is severe. These tests are described above.

Stage IV. A defect at this stage, such as consumptive coagulopathy (disseminated intravascular coagulopathy), results in an abnormal prothrombin time. Conditions associated with consumptive coagulopathy are: (1) obstetrical complications such as abruptio placentae and amniotic fluid embolism, (2) surgical complications, particularly from surgery following prostatic carcinoma, (3) conditions associated with shock and diminished flow, (4) excessive burns, and (5) excessive sepsis. Abnormalities are also seen in the following tests.

Venous clotting time (VCT). This procedure, initially described by Lee and White in 1913, is based on the principle that whole blood, when exposed to a foreign surface, forms a solid clot. The time required for the solid clot to form is the clotting time. Increases in clotting time and abnormality of the clot help to monitor treatment.

Plasma fibrinogen. Normally, fibrinogen is converted to fibrin, and the clot separates from the plasma. The fibrinogen is then measured indirectly.

Clot lysis test. This test is a measure of circulating fibrinolysins, which if present in sufficient quantities can dissolve the blood clot.

Protamine sulfate test. Normally, thrombin catalyzes the conversion of fibrinogen to fibrin, which then forms the scaffolding of the blood clot. Fibrinolysins may attack either fibrinogen or fibrin to prevent the formation of the fibrin scaffolding. This test depends on the presence of the fibrin before clots are formed. Protamine sulfate acts on the fibrin and allows it to clot even in the presence of secondary fibrinolysins. However, if the fibrinolysins are primary, a protamine sulfate reaction is not elicited because there is no fibrin on which the compound may act.

Summary

If the patient has platelet count abnormalities, defective clot retraction, a positive tourniquet test, and abnormal prothrombin consumption test, the defect is most likely at stage I.

If the patient has a normal prothrombin time and abnormal partial thromboplastin and prothrombin consumption times, the defect is at stage II.

If the patient has an abnormal prothrombin time and normal partial thromboplastin time, the defect is at stage III.

An abnormal venous clotting time, plasma fibrinogen level, clot lysis test, and protamine sulfate test indicate a defect at the stage IV.

After these tests, individual factor assays must be performed to define which particular factor is involved in the defect. These assays are rarely indicated, and are performed only in major centers.

Blood typing and cross-matching

Before a blood transfusion is given, the blood group of the recipient and of the donor must be determined to ensure the similarity of the antigenic and immune properties of the blood of the two individuals. If the necessary precautions are not taken, red blood cell agglutination (clumping) and hemolysis (release of hemoglobin) may result. This is called a transfusion reaction and can lead to the death of the recipient.

In an emergency in which there is not time to actually determine the type of antigens on the red blood cell membranes (blood type) of the donor and recipient, the bloods can be cross-matched. This procedure determines if agglutination will occur and requires mixing the cells of the donor with the defibrinated serum of the recipient. The reverse procedure is then performed: the cells of the recipient are cross-matched against the serum of the donor. The antigen is contained on the red blood cells and the antibody is contained in the serum.

[illegible]

[illegible] and can cause transfusion reactions if they are transfused into persons with incompatible blood types.

ABO blood groups. Individuals may have either A antigens, B antigens, both, or neither on their red cells. In the latter case, the blood type is usually type O.

If an individual *does not* have type A red blood cells, antibodies known as "anti-A" agglutins will be present in the serum. If this person is transfused with type A blood, these agglutinins will agglutinate the type A red blood cells of the donor. The same is true if an individual *does not* have type B red blood cells. The serum will contain antibodies known as "anti-B" agglutinins, which will agglutinate type B red blood cells. If the individual has both A and B (Ab group) antigens on the red cells, no agglutinins (antibodies) are present and the individual can receive any type of blood ("universal recipient"). If the individual is type O, with neither A nor B antigens on the red cells, the serum will contain both anti-A and anti-B agglutinins. Both A and B blood types will be agglutinated if given to the type O individual. However, since the red cells of the type O individual cannot be agglutinated by the serum of any other blood group, these persons are called universal donors.

Rh groups. Most individuals possess an antigen on their red cells called the Rh factor. These persons are said to be Rh positive, whereas those persons who do not possess the factor are said to be Rh negative. Antibodies (agglutinins) to the Rh factor do not occur spontaneously as in the ABO group. If an Rh negative individual is transfused with Rh positive blood, anti-Rh agglutinins develop slowly against the Rh positive blood. This causes no ill effects unless the person is subsequently again transfused with Rh positive blood. Then the anti-Rh agglutinins that formed in the serum as a result of the first transfusion will agglutinate the cells of the second Rh positive transfusion. Of course, Rh negative blood does no harm to an Rh positive person.

If an Rh negative mother is carrying an Rh positive fetus, the antigen from the blood cells of the fetus causes antibody production in the serum of the mother. The firstborn child usually shows no ill effects, but with subsequent pregnancies the antibodies in the mother's serum have increased and are sufficient to cause agglutination and hemolysis of the red cells of the fetus, unless the mother has been exposed to Rho Gam previously by transfusion with Rh positive blood.

Tests in hemolytic disorders

The term hemolysis refers to the destruction of red blood cells with the release of hemoglobin into the surrounding medium. Its presence and degree are usually measured indirectly through an evaluation of the compensatory erythropoiesis that follows hemolysis. Some of the indirect tests include (1) the reticulocyte count, (2) determination of the amount of unconjugated bilirubin in the serum, (3) bone marrow tests showing erythrocytic hyperplasia, and (4) determination of the amount of urobilinogen in the feces (a rarely used test because it requires complete fecal collection). Results of these indirect methods of measuring hemolysis are, however, invalid in the presence of anything that suppresses erythropoiesis, such as infection. Other tests, which are directly related to hemolysis are described below.

Haptoglobin determination

This test involves electrophoresis or radioimmunodiffusion. It is a sensitive and reliable test of hemolysis although it is not quantitative. When there is a release of hemoglobin, such as would occur with hemolysis, it will bind with a group of alpha globulins of plasma called haptoglobin. Thus in the presence of hemolysis the level of free haptoglobin will fall.

When megaloblastic anemia is the result of the hemolytic component haptoglobin levels are low. They may also be low after hemorrhage and may be congenitally absent in some normal individuals. Levels are increased by infection, inflammation, and malignancy.

NORMAL HAPTOGLOBIN LEVEL
(varies with method)

100 mg/100 ml

Osmotic fragility

This test is based on the principle that erythrocytes will hemolyze in hypertonic solution. Water will enter the cell, causing the cell to become more spherical until it finally ruptures. If the cell is already spherical, as in hereditary spherocytosis, it takes less water intake to cause a rupture (increased osmotic fragility). Conversely, if the cell is thin and flat, as in obstructive jaundice and thalassemia, more water intake is necessary before the cell will rupture (decreased osmotic fragility). The chief limitation of this test is its nonspecificity, since increased fragility will occur whenever there are spherical cells.

Autohemolysis

This test is nonspecific but will broadly group some of the congenital hemolytic anemias. It is based upon the principle that normal erythrocytes will resist incubation with usually less than 5% lysis for 48 hours at 37° C [illegible]

[illegible]

lins (Ig) on the surface of the red cells. The antiglobulin serum, known as Coombs serum, is secured from a rabbit that has been injected with human globulin.

In the direct Coombs test, the patient's washed red cells are mixed with Coombs serum. The mixture is then examined for agglutination. If the human red cells are coated with immunoglobulins, agglutination will occur. The test is called direct because only one step is needed—adding the Coombs serum directly to the washed cells. A positive direct Coombs test is found in hemolytic disease of the newborn, hemolytic transfusion reactions, and in idiopathic acquired hemolytic anemias.

The indirect Coombs test requires two steps. The first step may be done in one of two ways:

1. Red cells of known antigenic makeup are exposed to serum containing unknown antibodies. The second stage detects whether or not the antibody combines with the red cells. Agglutination at the second stage proves that a circulating antibody to one or more antigens on the red cells is present. The antibody may then be more specifically identified since the red cell antigens are known.
2. Red cells of unknown antigenic makeup are exposed to serum containing known antibodies. The second stage detects whether or not the antibody combines with the red cells, thus identifying the antigen on the red cells.

In the second stage of the indirect Coombs test, Coombs serum is added to the red cells, which have been washed to remove unattached antibodies. The Coombs serum then causes agglutination if a specific antibody has coated the red cells.

The indirect Coombs test is used to detect IgG antibodies (anti-Rh_0 [D]); demonstrate autoantibodies in the serum of patients with autoimmune hemolytic anemia; demonstrate other antigen-antibody reactions involving white cells, platelets, and tissue cells; and demonstrate hypogammaglobulinemia and agammaglobulinemia.

Erythrocyte enzyme assays

At least fourteen forms of hemolytic anemia are associated with a deficiency of erythrocyte enzymes. Although quantitative assays are necessary for the identification of most of these anemias, simple screening tests are available for two of the more common forms of hemolytic anemia: glucose-6-phosphate dehydrogenase deficiency (favism, G-6-PD) and pyruvate kinase deficiency. The screening test involves the use of long-wave ultraviolet light with which the erythrocytes are activated. Most oxidative compounds will precipitate a hemolytic crisis when these enzymes are deficient.

Tests for the gammopathies

Protein electrophoresis

The serum proteins, part of which are immunoglobulins in solution, will migrate and separate into distinct layers in response to an electrical current passed through the solution. This is because each immunoglobulin has its own specific electrical charge, rate at which it moves, size, and shape.

The solution to be charged is placed on paper or cellulose acetate strips. After the proteins separate they are stained. The normal pattern will be diffuse since no single protein is in excess, and the immunoglobulins will diffuse in the gamma band. However, if a single protein does dominate there will be a peak or a spike at the gamma band, or less frequently at the beta band of the electrophoresis. This peak is often called the M component. Serum protein electrophoresis will give a quantitative numerical value of the amount of protein in each electrophoretic band. This is sometimes expressed in percentage of the total proteins on each band.

Immunoelectrophoresis

The purpose of immunoelectrophoresis is to classify immunoglobulins found in the serum. Usually this test is performed after the simple serum protein electrophoresis shows a spike in the gamma band, thus identifying the type of the excess immunoglobulin. The different immunoglobulins are designated as immunoglobulin G (IgG), immunoglobulin M (IgM), immunoglobulin A (IgA), immunoglobulin D (IgD), and immunoglobulin E (IgE).

Immunodiffusion

After serum electrophoresis identifies a spike (M component) and immunoelectrophoresis identifies the type of immunoglobulin in the M component, immunodiffusion quantitates the amount of abnormal immunoglobulin. This test uses an antiserum to produce a reaction between antibody and antigen in a supporting medium.

Hemoglobin electrophoresis

Electrophoresis is useful for detecting hemoglobins A, S, C, E, and D. As with protein electrophoresis, described above, hemoglobin will migrate in solution in response to an electrical current. However, this migration is relative. Therefore, known reference hemoglobins are important to the test. In normal adult red blood cells, hemoglobins A_1, A_2, and F are present, with only a trace of the latter two.

The hemolytic anemias

In the hemolytic anemias the life span of the red blood cells is shortened as a result of the greatly accelerated destruction of the mature red blood cells.

Diagnostic laboratory tests

Hemolysis can be documented with the appearance of bilirubinemia, reticulocytosis, urobilinogenemia, or urobilinogenuria.

Differential diagnosis

Hemolytic disorders may be caused by a defect in the red blood cells, which may be either congenital or acquired (vitamin B_{12} or folic acid deficiency), or by factors extraneous to the red blood cells, such as transfusion incompatibility, chemical agents, and the like. The following list contains the more commonly encountered hemolytic anemias along with the laboratory tests most helpful in the differential diagnosis.

Hemolytic anemias caused by defective erythrocytes*

A. Congenital
   1. Membrane defects, such as occur in hereditary spherocytosis (spherocytosis on the peripheral smear and an increase of osmotic fragility and autohemolysis)
   2. Hereditary deficiencies in the Embden-Meyerhof pathway (anaerobic glycolysis), such as occur in pyruvate kinase deficiency (low levels of erythrocyte pyruvate kinase [PK] shown by specific assays of the red blood cell glycolytic enzymes)
   3. Abnormalities of the phosphoglucokinase oxidative pathway, such as glucose-6-phosphate dehydrogenase (G-6-PD) deficiency; more than

*The tests in parentheses are the diagnostic tests for each type of hemolytic anemia.

100 varieties have been described; hemolysis is precipitated sometimes by the ingestion of various drugs and fava beans (erythrocyte enzyme assays)

4. Qualitative abnormalities in globin peptides—hemoglobinopathies such as hemoglobin C disease and sickle cell disease (hemoglobin electrophoresis)
5. Quantitative abnormality in globin peptide synthesis—thalassemias (hemoglobin electrophoresis shows an increase of hemoglobin F in thalassemia major; a decrease of normal hemoglobin A_1 and a relative increase of hemoglobin A_2 in thalassemia minor)

B. Acquired
   1. Vitamin B_{12} deficiency (serum B_{12} levels, Schilling test)
   2. Folic acid deficiency (folic acid levels)
   3. Paroxysmal nocturnal hemoglobinuria (plasma hemoglobin)

Hemolytic anemias caused by extraerythrocytic factors*

A. Extracorporeal factors
   1. Isoantibodies caused by ABO or Rh incompatibility (blood-typing and cross-matching)
   2. Chemical agents and drugs such as phenylhydrazine, benzene, and lead (peripheral smear for lead)
   3. Infectious agents such as malaria (malaria parasites on thick smear)
   4. Physical agents such as aortic valve disease
   5. Certain animal poisons such as snake and brown recluse spider venoms
B. Conditions developing within the body
   1. Idiopathic acquired hemolytic anemias (Coombs positive)
   2. Secondary hemolytic anemias (Coombs negative) such as those associated with sarcoidosis (node biopsy and Kveim test), liver disease (liver function tests), Hodgkin's disease (node biopsy), disseminated lupus erythematosus (antinuclear antibodies), renal cortical necrosis (renal sediment and renal function tests), and thrombotic thrombocytopenic purpura (bone marrow and peripheral smear)

The gammopathies

Normal human serum contains proteins that can be separated into different types by serum protein electrophoresis. These different types are albumin, alpha I globulin, alpha II globulin, beta globulin, and gamma globulin.

The gamma globulins may be further separated into the following immunoglobulins: immunoglobulin G (IgG), immunoglobulin A (IgA), immunoglobulin M (IgM), immunoglobulin D (IgD), and immunoglobulin E (IgE).

All of the immunoglobulins have combinations of light and heavy polypeptide chains, classified according to molecular weight. The normal im-

*The tests in parentheses are the diagnostic tests for each type of hemolytic anemia.

munoglobulins in the body are involved in the antigen-antibody reactions that protect the human organism from infective agents and are of paramount importance in immunologic and allergic reactions.

The gammopathies are a group of disorders in which neoplastic cells produce an excess of a single immunoglobulin. The abnormal proteins produced by the cell tumors are called paraproteins or M components (M stands for myeloma or macroglobulinemia) and belong immunologically to the immu- [illegible]

4. Alkaline phosphatase: increased

Specific tests

In *multiple myeloma* bone marrow study reveals the presence of plasma cells in sheaths or isolated islands. Serum or urine protein electrophoresis reveals a homogeneous spike either in the gamma range or alpha I or II range. Immunoelectrophoresis usually yields abnormal quantities of immunoglobulin G. However, some multiple myelomas have been reported to be associated with abnormal production of immunoglobulin A, immunoglobulin D, and immunoglobulin E.

In the *macroglobulinemias* serum protein electrophoresis yields mainly immunoglobulin M. Bone marrow study reveals infiltration with lymphocytes rather than plasma cells.

In *benign monoclonal gammopathy,* so called because the tumor is thought to stem from a clone of cells, there will usually be a spike on serum protein electrophoresis although the patient is asymptomatic. This combination is thought to represent either a latent form of multiple myeloma, which may develop into an active form, or it may represent an extensive immunologic response to some unknown antigen and have a perfectly benign course.

Also classified under gammopathies are heavy chain disease, alpha heavy chain disease, gamma chain disease, and light chain disease. However, it is beyond the scope of this book to discuss these entities, since they are extremely rare.

10

DIAGNOSTIC TESTS FOR NEUROLOGIC DISORDERS

ANATOMY AND PHYSIOLOGY OF THE BRAIN

The brain consists of three major parts: the cerebrum, the cerebellum, and the brain stem. The cerebrum is the largest division and is divided into two hemispheres, each of which has five lobes. The *cerebrum* is the highest integrative center of the nervous system and is responsible for sensation, perception, memory, consciousness, judgment, and will. The *cerebellum* is located just below the posterior portion of the cerebrum and functions in the control of skeletal muscles. The *brain stem* is composed of the midbrain, pons, and medulla oblongata, which connects the brain with the spinal cord and controls breathing, heart rate, and blood pressure.

The three meninges or membranes that envelop the brain and spinal cord are the *dura mater, arachnoid mater*, and *pia mater* (Fig. 10-2). Their names imply their qualities: the dura is the strong, tough outer layer; the arachnoid is a delicate layer between the dura mater and the pia mater; and the pia adheres to the brain surface like a delicate skin and contains blood vessels.

A potential space called the *subdural space* lies between the dura mater and the arachnoid mater. Between the arachnoid mater and the pia mater lies an actual space, called the *subarachnoid space,* which is filled with cerebrospinal fluid.

The *skull* is rigid and unyielding, and has very little space for anything but the brain. The skull can expand to accommodate hemorrhage, tumors, or fluid until a person is 12 or 13 years of age, when the skull sutures close. After this age anything in the skull taking up space pushes the brain down into the foramen magnum, the largest bony foramen in the skull. The foramen magnum lies at the lowest part of the skull and encircles the brain stem. Pressure from above pushes the brain down, and the brain stem, with small cerebellar tonsils on each side, becomes impacted in the foramen magnum. This is a very critical anatomic area because the brain stem is involved with consciousness, control

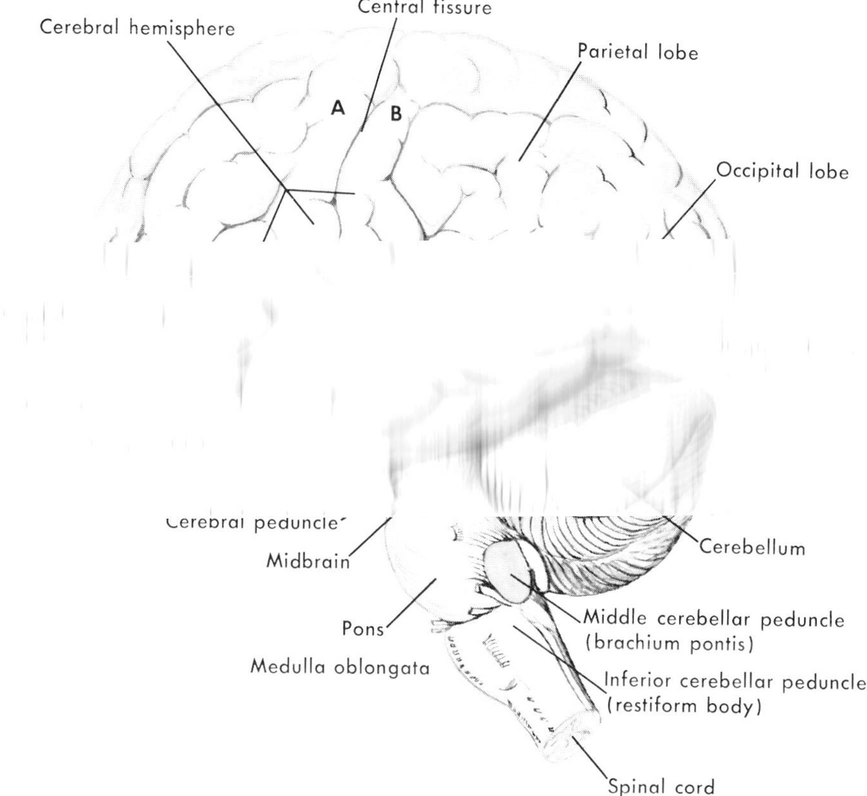

FIG. 10-1
The brain. (From Schottelius, B. A., and Schottelius, D. D.: Textbook of physiology, ed. 17, St. Louis, 1973, The C. V. Mosby Co.)

of blood pressure, heart rate, and respiration. If the brain stem does become impacted in the foramen magnum, it results in Cheyne-Stokes respirations, erratic breathing patterns, abnormal pupillary responses, and impairment of consciousness.

A second critical anatomic area is at the midbrain above the pons, where a sharp edge of dura separates the posterior fossa from the rest of the skull, dividing it into two compartments. This sharp edge of dura is positioned next to the midbrain on either side. If there is pressure on one side from a tumor, intracerebral hemorrhage, or the like, this uncus can be pushed down against the brain stem to the point where the brain stem is confined and held by the sharp edge of the dura. The third nerve comes out of the brain stem and travels in this area. The uncus can catch the third nerve, causing a dilated pupil on that side, or it can push the brain stem over to catch the third nerve on the other side, causing a dilated pupil on the other side.

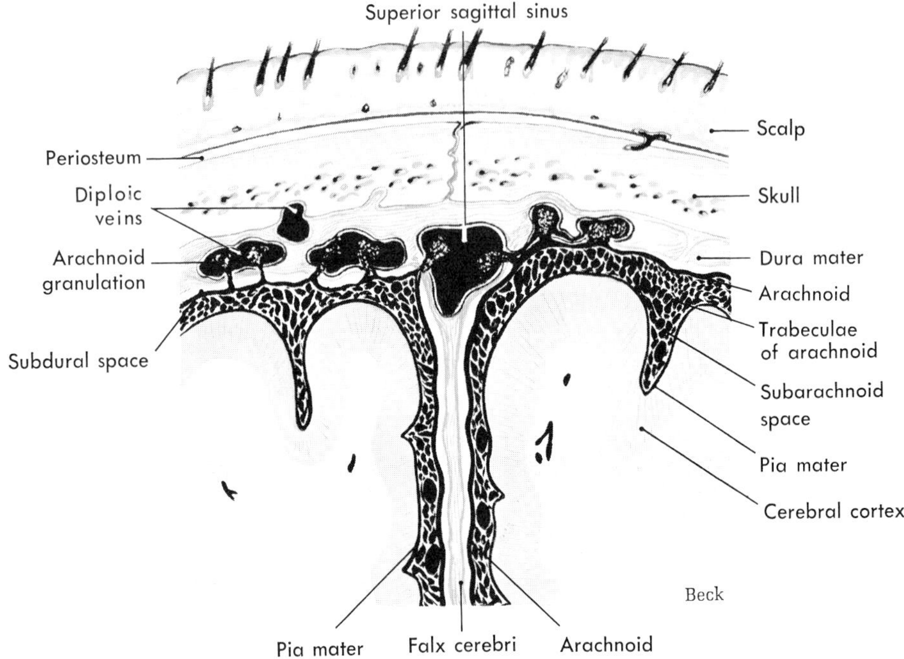

FIG. 10-2
The meninges of the brain as seen in coronal section through the skull. (From Anthony, C. P., and Kolthoff, N. J.: Textbook of anatomy and physiology, ed. 9, St. Louis, 1975, The C. V. Mosby Co.)

LABORATORY TESTS IN BRAIN DISORDERS

In neurology the diagnosis and evaluation of the patient are usually much more dependent on the history and physical examination and expertise of the examiner in the interview than on laboratory tests. However, there are some laboratory tests that are valuable in evaluating and diagnosing neurologic conditions.

The cerebrospinal fluid (CSF)

The cerebrospinal fluid (CSF) is the part of the central nervous system (CNS) that is most accessible to the clinician. The CSF is secreted by the cerebral vessels and the choroid plexuses, a cauliflower-like growth of blood vessels projecting into the lateral third and fourth ventricles of the brain. This fluid is continually secreted from the choroid plexus to pass into the fourth ventricle and from there into the subarachnoid cistern, where it diffuses over and around the brain and spinal cord. Although the spinal cord ends at the second lumbar vertebra, the subarachnoid space with its CSF extends to the second sacral vertebra.

The brain floats in CSF and is thus protected when the head receives a blow. Without the protection of the spinal fluid and meninges, the brain would

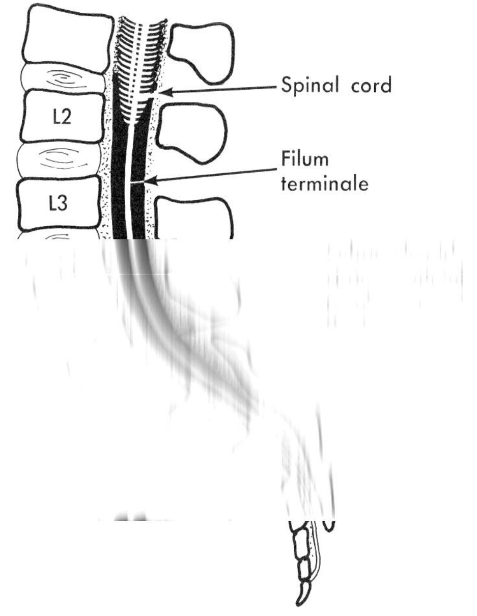

FIG. 10-3
The end of the spinal cord (lumbar vertebra 1-2).

probably be unable to withstand even the minor traumas of everyday living.

The spinal fluid is obtained through two sources: lumbar puncture and cisternal puncture. Cisternal puncture should not be performed by the inexperienced. However, lumbar puncture is a relatively harmless procedure and is easily done with some expertise.

Spinal tap and examination of CSF is done in many neurologic conditions for diagnostic purposes. It is performed in a few situations for therapeutic reasons. In bacterial meningitis it is absolutely indicated for diagnosis and management. It is also indicated in most cases of suspected cerebral hemorrhage, with a few exceptions.

Procedure for spinal tap

The spinal tap is usually performed with an 18 gauge needle introduced between the fourth and fifth lumbar vertebrae or between the fifth lumbar and first sacral vertebrae. The opening and closing pressures can then be measured and the Queckenstedt test can be performed at the same time. In this test, pressure is placed on the external jugular veins while the spinal needle is connected to a manometer. If the fluid level rises and falls promptly with pressure on the jugulars and release of that pressure, there is no blockage of the free flow of CSF in the spinal column.

The Queckenstedt test should be done when the pathology is suspected to be in the spinal canal and not in the cranium. If there is pressure in the cranium, it is increased with this maneuver, and the brain stem may be pushed into the foramen magnum.

Gross appearance of spinal fluid

Blood. Blood in the spinal fluid may mean one of two things: either the tap was a bloody tap or intracranial hemorrhage may be indicated. The tap may be bloody because the spinal puncture is a blind procedure and a small vein or a venous plexus covering the spinal cord can be hit easily.

There are a few things that will help in differentiating between the two. Crenated red cells (red blood cells that show a scalloped border) are an indication that the hemorrhage is longer-standing than would be expected from a bloody tap. Also, the accidental bloody tap usually clears up after the initial bloody fluid and the fluid becomes relatively clear. If the tap is atraumatic but the fluid is bloody, subarachnoid hemorrhage is certain. Clear fluid helps in eliminating the possibility of intracranial hemorrhage and is helpful in the diagnosis of infections. If there is purulent infection, the test is not valid for protein determinations because the results will be obviously elevated.

Color. The normal CSF is a water-clear fluid. A xanthochromic (somewhat gold) fluid usually indicates the presence of either old blood or extreme elevation of protein in the CSF.

Turbidity indicates increased white and red cells as well as increased protein, in which case some kind of infectious process should be suspected.

If the CSF is frankly purulent, it is an indication of purulent meningitis and meningoencephalitis.

Microscopic examination of the CSF

The microscopic examination should be performed immediately after the CSF specimen is obtained. The specimen should be stained for both gram and acid-fast bacilli, and an indirect india ink stain for some specific fungi should be done. Normal values are found in Appendix A.

The cell count and differential. In a clear fluid a slight elevation of lymphocytes with slight protein elevation and a normal blood sugar level usually indicates an aseptic type of meningitis that may be viral or caused by a collagen disease.

An elevation of cells in proportion to the protein elevation suggests poliomyelitis. On the other hand, normal cell count in the presence of elevated protein, the so-called albuminocellular dissociation, strongly suggests Guillain-Barré syndrome.

Protein elevation is also encountered in almost all serious pathologic conditions of the CNS. However, it should be noted that sometimes total protein may not be elevated in certain conditions (multiple sclerosis) when, qualitatively, immunoelectrophoresis may reveal abnormal proteins in 50% of the cases.

If the patient is having CNS symptoms but does not have an elevated protein, a metabolic abnormality affecting the central nervous system is very likely (for example, hepatic encephalopathy or diabetic encephalopathy).

Cultures of the CSF

When the CSF is purulent it is imperative to perform a culture. The patient's life may depend upon an accurate determination of the organism and its [illegible]

[illegible] meningitis, such as meningococcal meningitis, *Hemophilus influenzae* meningitis, or any bacterial meningitis. Viral meningitis is characterized by an elevated cell level and normal glucose level.

The glucose determination also becomes important when differentiating between viral meningitis and tubercular meningitis. Tubercular meningitis is characterized by decreased CSF glucose but viral meiningitis is not. Both diseases may be similar in protein level and cytologic picture, making the CSF glucose level the sole differentiating factor.

A simultaneous determination of serum blood glucose and CSF glucose should be obtained because, to be significant, the CSF glucose should be lower than two thirds of the blood glucose. There is a direct relationship between elevated blood glucose and elevated CSF glucose, since the composition of the CSF depends on filtration and diffusion from the blood.

Cytology

In suspected neoplasm (primary or metastatic), cytologic examination of the CSF may aid in the diagnosis of the malignancy.

VDRL (Venereal Disease Research Laboratories) test

The VDRL test should be performed on the CSF in cases of suspected syphilis of the central nervous system, particularly if a positive serologic examination is to be evaluated in view of a negative history and tertiary CNS syphilis is to be ruled out.

Radiologic examination of the skull and spinal column

Other accessible organs in evaluating the CNS are the skull and spinal column as seen on x-ray films.

X-ray film of the skull

This test requires the cooperation of the patient and is performed to verify fractures, abnormal calcification of a tumor, or unilateral tumors.

X-ray films will reveal fractures when there has been trauma. When a neoplasm is suspected, particularly a multiple myeloma, x-ray films may be diagnostic. Calcification of the pineal gland, which is located between the two halves of the thalamus, is normal. If there is enlargement of one of the hemispheres because of a brain tumor or infarction, the midline structures, including the pineal gland, will be pushed to the contralateral side. This is well visualized radiologically as a shift of the pineal gland from the midline and is an important diagnostic sign of intracranial disease. Intracranial calcification is also seen in toxoplasmosis.

X-ray films of the spinal column

Radiologic examination of the spinal column in the cervical region is important for evaluation of headaches and pain involving the upper extremities.

X-ray films of the lumbosacrum are frequently obtained for evaluation of lower extremity pain, particularly when it is of sciatic distribution, caused by rupture of an intervertebral disk, and narrowing of intervertebral foramina.

Brain scan

A brain scan requires a cooperative patient and is often performed as a diagnostic test because it is relatively atraumatic and therefore should precede more invasive methods.

This test depends on changes in the permeability of brain capillaries. Embryologically, brain tissue is skin and therefore, like skin, is a barrier tissue. There is, then, a blood-brain barrier that can be broken down by pathologic conditions such as a tumor, abscess, hemorrhage, focal injury, gunshot wound, and subdural hematoma. The radioisotopes that have been injected will concentrate in the involved area of the brain. The character and speed of isotope uptake will give a clue to the cause of the alteration of the blood-brain barrier, be it tumor, subdural hematoma, encephalitis, or vascular accident.

This test is very helpful in patients who have clear-cut lateralizing signs and symptoms, such as acute appearance of hemiparesis or speech deficit. A normal brain scan taken during the first few days following the appearance of symptoms strongly suggests cerebral thrombosis without development of hemorrhagic infarct, and rules out brain tumor or hemorrhage.

Computerized transaxial tomography (CAT scan; CTT)

Tomography is a special x-ray technique that allows visualization of a specific layer of tissue. The CAT scan literally shows the examiner a slice of the brain much as it would appear in the pathology lab. This technique is based on the principle that tissues of varying density, such as white matter, ventricular fluid, gray matter, and neoplasms, will absorb x-ray photons differently. On routine skull film this difference is not visible. However, a new EMI scanner developed in England uses a sensitive detector that permits 28,000 different density readings, in conjunction with a 180 degree x-ray scan of the head, and utilizing a computer storage and retrieval system. With this system it is possible to obtain on demand from the computer a three-dimen- [illegible]

[illegible] nature and the relative ease with which it is performed. At the present time the main problem is the cost factor, which is a major debate issue between health care providers and health care financial underwriters.

Electroencephalogram (EEG)

An electroencephalogram requires the cooperation of the patient and is performed to reveal focal abnormalities. The two halves of the brain are electrically identical in their function. Therefore, the left and right EEG patterns should be identical. Spike discharges in one area indicate a focal abnormality. Generalized slowing in the EEG waves indicates diffuse pathology in both hemispheres. This test is abnormal in 75% of patients with seizures, tumors, and subdural hematomas.

Electroencephalography is used to document focal epileptic lesions. However, there is a certain false negative in the EEG documentation of patients with chronic epilepsy.

In identifying a possible space-occupying lesion a normal EEG with a normal brain scan almost excludes a supratentorial brain tumor.

In brain injury concussions the EEG helps in differentiating diffuse lesions from focal lesions.

Lastly, the EEG is becoming more and more important in defining cerebral death, particularly for medicolegal reasons in organ transplantation programs.

Patient preparation and care. The patient should have clean hair free of any preparations or foreign objects. A meal is usually taken before the procedure since hypoglycemia may produce an abnormal EEG.

Sleeping electroencephalogram

This test is requested when the routine waking electroencephalogram is normal and yet a seizure or tumor is still suspected. The electrical rhythms of the brain are more unstable during sleep, when the pattern changes markedly. Abnormalities can sometimes be seen during sleep that cannot be seen when the patient is awake. A sleeping and waking EEG are always performed on patients who have seizures only during sleep. A sleeping EEG may occasionally show an abnormality in a situation in which a tumor is suspected and a diagnosis cannot be confirmed.

In addition to the sleeping EEG, sometimes the EEG is taken after injection of metrazol, which is a CNS stimulant and may cause abnormal electrical discharge from a focus that is latent otherwise.

Echoencephalogram

This test does not require the cooperation of the patient. It is, therefore, a useful test for agitated patients.

The echoencephalogram is obtained by placing a titanium dioxide crystal at the head of the patient. This crystal emits a very high frequency sound wave that is echoed back when it hits an interface. Because sound travels at different rates through different densities, a change in density is recorded as a blip on the oscilloscope.

The third ventricle of the brain is in the exact center of the brain and the echos arising from the two walls of the third ventricle are called the M spike. A shift of the M spike greater than 3 mm is considered abnormal. The M spike may be shifted away from the lesion in unilateral subdural hematoma or neoplasm, or it can be shifted toward the lesion when there is generalized atrophy. The echoencephalogram should be correlated with the EEG and the brain scan for accurate interpretation of echo shifts. In addition to a shift in the M spike, one can evaluate enlargement of the third ventricle by measuring the distance between the sides of the spike. In a patient with severe neurologic lateralizing signs, inability to obtain an echoencephalogram suggests marked destruction and displacement of the third ventricle because such displacement and destruction makes recording of the M spike impossible. Bilateral pathology would prevent any shift of midline structures; thus one might have a perfectly normal echoencephalogram in the presence of bilateral hemispheric pathology.

Electromyogram (EMG)

An electromyogram is a graph of the electrical potentials generated in individual muscles, which are usually tested at rest, with slight voluntary contraction, and with maximal contraction. This is accomplished by inserting a sterile needle electrode into the muscle to be tested. The electrical activity generated by the conduction mechanism of skeletal muscles is then amplified and displayed on a cathode-ray oscilloscope.

The electromyogram determines the following: (1) muscle denervation, (2) the level or area of nerve injury, (3) the presence of intrinsic muscle disease (dystrophies and myopathies), and (4) the occurrence of reinnervation.

The electromyogram is indicated as an aid in: (1) the diagnosis and the differential diagnosis of a large group of neuromuscular disorders involving the lower motor neuron, (2) determining the management of peripheral nerve injuries, (3) differentiating the apparent paralysis of the malingerer or the patient with hysteria, and (4) planning patient rehabilitation programs.

[illegible]

[illegible]

[illegible]

[illegible] direct injection of a dye in the carotid artery, either right or left, as indicated by the symptoms.

Angiography carries with it a small risk of about 1% from stroke, allergic reaction to the dye, or shock. It is important in detecting tumors, abscesses, hemorrhage, and thrombosis.

Patient preparation and care. The patient is kept fasting, but is given liquids, either orally or intravenously, before the procedure. Adequate hydration will prevent excessive concentration of the contrast medium in the cerebral vasculature.

Puncture sites are surgically prepared. Dentures are removed as well as all foreign objects in the hair. The hair should be clean, combed, and not braided. Before premedication is given, a base line record of neurologic status and vital signs is obtained for comparison after the procedure.

Following the procedure vital signs and neurologic status are monitored, and the puncture site observed for bleeding or swelling.

Pneumoencephalogram (PEG)

In this test air is injected into the spinal fluid space in the lumbar area. Since this spinal fluid space is connected to the fluid spaces in the cranium, some of the air bubbles up and fills these fluid spaces in the head. The ventricles of the brain can then be visualized on x-ray films. If the brain has been displaced by the ventricles it will be evident. This test is usually performed when there is suspicion of hydrocephalus, increase or decrease of ventricular size, or deformity or displacement of the cerebral ventricles.

Since the introduction of CAT scan, the use of pneumoencephalography has significantly diminished.

Patient preparation and care. The patient is kept fasting in the event that a craniotomy may be necessary and because of the nausea associated with the procedure.

Following the procedure the patient is evaluated frequently relative to the base line vital signs and neurologic status already established. Particular attention is paid to pupillary size and reactivity, and alertness. The patient will remain flat in bed for the first 24 to 48 hours. An elevated temperature, headache, nausea, and vomiting commonly are experienced.

Myelogram

This test is performed by injecting a contrast medium into the spinal fluid. An x-ray film is then taken in order to visualize lesions suspected of causing cord compression. These lesions may be secondary to discogenic disease or neoplastic disease of the spinal column.

Patient preparation and care. The patient is kept fasting before the procedure and a base line record of neurologic status and vital signs is obtained before premedication is given so that they may be closely monitored when the patient returns to the unit.

Following the procedure the patient is kept flat in bed for 24 hours and encouraged to drink. If the dye has not been completely removed then another x-ray film may be taken following the original procedure. In such a case, at no time should the patient's head be lower than the rest of his body lest the dye move into the head and be irretrievable.

On occasion the patient may develop a chemical meningitis, manifested by a stiff neck and mild fever. Smears and cultures will rule out infectious meningitis, although the clinical picture and the mildness of the symptoms will be helpful distinguishing features.

LABORATORY TESTS IN THE CLINICAL SETTING

Cerebrovascular diseases

Atherosclerotic thrombosis

In most circumstances the clinical picture is quite characteristic of atherosclerotic thrombosis of one of the cerebrovascular branches. However, if a differential diagnostic problem arises, then the following tests are usually performed.

CSF examination is usually done to exclude cerebral hemorrhage or other possibilities. Characteristically, the CSF is clear with perhaps a slight increase in leukocyte count. The protein level may be normal or slightly elevated.

Skull x-ray films are taken to rule out other diseases and are usually unremarkable. Rarely, they show a shift of the pineal body resulting from cerebral swelling.

EEG and radionuclide scan are of limited value. *CAT scan* is informative but not essential.

Cerebral angiography is a definitive diagnostic procedure if a problem concerning a differential diagnosis exists. However, because of its invasive nature it is not performed unless absolutely indicated.

Cerebral embolus

In the differential diagnosis between embolus and thrombosis the history and the clinical setting are most important. Usually, one looks for predisposing [illegible]

Hemorrhage

CSF examination is the most important diagnostic test for hemorrhage, which is usually revealed by gross blood except in rare conditions in which the hemorrhage is relatively small and/or remains intracerebral and does not communicate with the ventricles or subarachnoid space.

When there is gross blood there is a differential diagnosis between true hemorrhagic fluid and traumatic tap. In the latter the CSF pressure is usually normal or low, the first sample is bloody and later clears, and the fluid will clot. Additionally, after centrifugation the supernatant fluid in the traumatic tap is clear compared to the xanthochromic or pink discoloration characteristic of subarachnoid hemorrhage.

CAT scan is highly diagnostic of even a small amount of hemorrhage up to 1.5 cm. This procedure may obviate the need for lumbar puncture, which carries a small risk, especially if there is elevation of intracranial pressure and possible herniation of the cerebral tonsils.

The EEG is usually nondiagnostic in cerebrovascular disease.

The carotid or vertebral angiogram is the single most important diagnostic test for determining the cause of intracranial hemorrhage. It is performed as soon as possible after the patient is stabilized for possible surgical intervention.

CAT scan is helpful if there is a localized blood clot and/or concomitant hydrocephalus.

Transient ischemic attacks

Aortic arch angiography is the most important diagnostic test performed to evaluate and detect carotid artery obstructive lesions, which may be correctable surgically.

Trauma to the central nervous system

Acute trauma to the brain

The CSF is usually hemorrhagic with elevated pressure. These findings are directly related to prognosis.

X-ray films of the skull are taken to determine the presence of fractures.

Acute and chronic subdural hematoma

Cerebral angiography is the most reliable diagnostic tool in suspected subdural hematoma.

CAT scan, if available, is as good as cerebral angiography in the diagnosis of subdural hematoma.

Skull x-rays may be helpful in locating fractures or a shift of the pineal body.

CSF examination findings are nonspecific.

EEG and brain scan are not helpful.

Spinal cord injuries

CSF examination reveals elevated protein. A block in the CSF may be elucidated by the Queckenstedt test.

X-ray films of the spinal column should be taken for definitive diagnosis. If cord compression is suspected a myelogram should be done.

Neoplastic diseases

Brain tumor

Skull x-ray films are usually done because they are fairly easy to do, are noninvasive, and very helpful in locating a shift of the calcified pineal gland. They may also help in the diagnosis of increased intracranial pressure, abnormal intracranial calcifications, bone destruction, or change in shape of the sella turcica.

Cerebral angiography is indicated for the definitive diagnosis of intracranial tumors. Serial angiography gives information about the type of tumor.

EEG may show focal abnormalities or may be normal.

CSF examination reveals elevated pressure, protein levels, and some cells. However, findings are too nonspecific for diagnosis.

Brain scan may be helpful in localizing tumors.

CAT scan is very useful in the diagnosis and location of tumors.

Pneumoencephalogram is contraindicated in the majority of tumors.

Spinal cord tumor

CSF examination reveals elevated protein and demonstrates a block by the Queckenstedt test.

Other diagnostic tests include *x-ray of the spine*, *myelogram*, and *elec-*

tromyography (EMG), which may be helpful in localizing the spinal segment involved with tumor.

Infections of the central nervous system

Infections of the CNS are discussed on pp. 228 and 229.

Demyelinating diseases of the central nervous system

[illegible]

inine. Muscle biopsy may be informative if the involved muscles are obtained for biopsy; otherwise, the results of a biopsy may be normal. The EMG is quite specific and will show the typical myopathic pattern. In acute myasthenia gravis the response to neostigmine or edrophonium (Tensilon) aids in the diagnosis.

Seizure disorders

The differential diagnosis of seizures is quite extensive, and a thorough discussion is beyond the scope of this book. Although the seizure disorder is a neurologic manifestation, the cause may be metabolic, cardiovascular, or a primary CNS disorder.

Laboratory investigation will be based on the overall clinical setting. If metabolic disease is suspected, appropriated blood work should include blood glucose, electrolytes, calcium, and phosphorus levels.

If cardiovascular disease is suspected, an ECG and a 24-hour Holter monitor should be done.

If primary neurologic disease is suspected, wakeful EEG, sleeping EEG, or an EEG taken after injection of metrazol will make a diagnosis of seizure disorder and possibly localize the focus.

The CAT scan is often helpful in localizing a lesion.

Headache

The diagnostic approach to headache should depend on the overall clinical picture. An initial period of observation may resolve the diagnosis. However, in persistent headaches, when the decision is made to investigate further, the following are suggested as initial screening tests: skull x-rays, EEG, and radionuclide brain scan (if CAT scan is available, it is preferred). If all of the above are negative, no further work-up may be indicated. However, if the clinical picture suggests a specific neurologic entity, the appropriate tests should be done.

Coma

A comprehensive discussion of coma is beyond the scope of this book. There are numerous conditions, none of them neurologic, which can cause coma and should be looked for.

If a metabolic condition is suspected, blood glucose levels should be determined. Liver function tests, including a serum ammonia level, are done for the diagnosis of hepatic encephalopathy. Serum electrolytes, arterial blood gases, and pH should be obtained.

If a primary neurologic condition is suspected, an x-ray of the skull should be taken.

Before performing a CSF examination, one should weigh the possible diagnostic yield versus the danger of herniation of the brain because of elevated intracranial pressure. If it is deemed necessary to do a lumbar puncture for diagnostic reasons and to implement immediate therapy, then it should be done very carefully, with the smallest possible needle, and with removal of the smallest possible amount of fluid for examination.

11

DIAGNOSTIC TESTS FOR COLLAGEN VASCULAR DISEASES

The systemic rheumatic diseases include rheumatoid arthritis, systemic lupus erythematosus, rheumatic fever, and progressive systemic sclerosis, to name a few. These systemic disorders are also known as connective tissue diseases and were formerly called collagen diseases.

The following laboratory procedures are the ones most commonly used in the diagnosis and management of rheumatic diseases.

LABORATORY TESTS FOR RHEUMATIC DISEASES

Radiologic studies of joints

Although the x-ray film can be of help in the early diagnosis of certain entities, such as sacroiliac involvement in ankylosing spondylitis, seldom can one make a specific diagnosis through radiologic studies.

Usually, in diseases associated with joint involvement one sees erosion of the joint margins, narrowing of joint spaces, and diffuse osteoporosis of the involved joints. A bamboo appearance of spinal joints is characteristic of ankylosing spondylitis, and in certain infectious conditions there will be bony erosion and lytic lesions.

In addition to the initial radiologic evaluation of rheumatic diseases, x-ray films are usually taken to follow the course of the disease.

Synovial analysis

Synovial fluid is contained within articulations having a joint cavity. This viscous dialysate of blood plasma along with hyaluronate from the synovial membrane provides the perfect frictionless film for the bony surfaces. It also nourishes the cartilaginous structures of the joints.

An examination of synovial fluid will give information regarding the underlying synovial tissue reaction.

Routine synovial fluid analysis includes determination of clarity, color, and viscosity; mucin clot formation; cell count; and polarized light microscopy. In special situations synovial fluid complement level, protein, and glucose levels can be measured; rheumatoid factors and the LE cell phenomenon can be looked for. When there is suspicion of septic arthritis, it is essential that a gram stain of the synovial fluid and the appropriate cultures be performed.

The normal synovial fluid is straw-colored, transparent, has normal viscosity, good mucin clot formation, a WBC count of less than 200/cu mm and a neutrophil count of less than 25/cu mm. The glucose content is the same as that of blood.

In disease states clarity is lost and the fluid may be cloudy, milky, grayish, or red, depending on the underlying disorder. Viscosity will be poor in the fluid from chronically inflamed joints.

Polarized light microscopy will aid in the differential diagnosis between gout and pseudogout, since it will distinguish between urate and pyrophosphate crystals. In gout one sees negative birefringence under polarized light, whereas in pseudogout weakly birefringent crystals are seen.

Patient preparation and care for arthrocentesis. The patient should be fasting for 6 to 12 hours; otherwise glucose and lipid evaluations are invalid. The knee joint is most frequently used although any articulation may be aspirated. The area to be aspirated is prepared as for surgery, and rigid aseptic technique is observed to avoid the only complication of this procedure, infection in the joint.

Rheumatoid (RA) factors

Rheumatoid factors are antiglobulin antibodies, which react to immunoglobulins of the IgG class. The principal fractions measured are the IgM rheumatoid factors, although they also exist in the other two major immunoglobulin classes (IgG and IgA), in which case the disease would be milder.

High titers of rheumatoid factors are usually associated with active disease. Low titers are sometimes found in other nonspecific connective tissue diseases, as well as in an estimated 16% to 20% of the elderly population.

Complement

The complement system is a group of nine serum proteins that react with each other to mediate the immunologic response that follows the interaction between antigen and antibody. These serum proteins are inactive in the blood serum. When activated they function as enzymes. Activation occurs when IgG or IgM antibodies are altered following union with their respective antigens. The activated components are designated C1 to C9.

There is also an alternative pathway called the properdin system, which is activated in a wide variety of defense mechanisms.

The C′3 component of the complement correlates very well with the total hemolytic complement. It is diminished in lupus, and is usually associated with kidney involvement.

C′4 component is significantly diminished in lupus nephritis.

The importance of the other components of the complement system, as well as of the alternative pathway, is under intense research.

LE (lupus erythematosus) cell test

This test involves visualization of the LE cell phenomenon, which consists of an autoantibody (LE factor) complexing with leukocyte nucleoprotein as [illegible]

[illegible]

[illegible]

against RNA, DNA, ribosomes, and lysosomes as well as other cytoplasmic constituents.

There are four different types of nuclear fluorescence patterns characteristic of this test:

1. Diffuse or homogeneous. This is the most common pattern and is produced when the antinuclear antibody binds to nucleoprotein. The diffuse pattern is characteristic of systemic lupus erythematosus (SLE), but is seen in other disorders as well.
2. "Shaggy" or peripheral pattern. This pattern is produced by antibody to DNA and is seen almost exclusively in SLE, especially when there is associated lupus nephritis.
3. Speckled pattern. This pattern is produced by an antibody against a nuclear glycoprotein.
4. Nucleolar pattern. This pattern is rare.

Anti-DNA antibodies

Antibodies to DNA (deoxyribonucleic acid) are important in evaluating lupus nephritis. A negative anti-DNA test usually is associated with absence of acute nephritis.

Anti-ENA (extractable nuclear antigens)

The antibodies to extractable nuclear antigens form a speckled pattern with the fluoresent antinuclear antibody test and usually occur in SLE. However, they are also commonly present in the so-called mixed connective tissue diseases.

HLA-B27

This is a tissue transplantation antigen found in human cell C6 chromosome. It is a genetically determined marker that remains unchanged throughout the life of the patient. It has become important in the diagnosis of rheumatology, particularly in the differential diagnosis of seronegative rheumatic variants.

In 90% of patients with ankylosing spondylitis and Reiter's syndrome the findings of this test will be positive and, therefore, it is very useful in distinguishing ankylosing spondylitis from other arthritic conditions, and Reiter's syndrome from gonococcal arthritis.

In some cases of juvenile rheumatoid arthritis, the finding of HLA-B27 antigen indicates the possibility of ankylosing spondylitis.

In patients with psoriatic arthritis or inflammatory bowel disease associated with arthritis, this test will help to predict the development of ankylosing spondylitis.

ASO (antistreptolysin O) titer

The ASO titer is elevated in approximately 80% of those streptococcal pharyngitis patients who develop rheumatic fever or glomerular nephritis. It is elevated in 60% of patients with uncomplicated streptococcal disease, except in streptococcal pyoderma in which only 25% of persons have an elevated ASO titer although acute glomerular nephritis may also be present.

Other streptococcal antibody tests

These include antihyaluronidase (AH), antideoxyribonucleotidase B (anti-DNase B), antistreptokinase (ASK), and antistreptozyme (ASTZ). These tests are most advisable when there is a low or borderline ASO titer. The ASTZ test in particular is a very sensitive indicator of recent streptococcal infection.

Tests performed for muscle disease

The tests performed to determine muscle disease include measurement of the enzymes released when there is muscle destruction. These enzymes (CPK, LDH, SGOT) have been discussed in previous chapters. In addition, aldolase is elevated in certain muscular dystrophies and in polymyositis.

LABORATORY TESTS NOT DIRECTLY RELATED TO RHEUMATIC DISEASES

The following is a brief explanation of some immunologic tests performed by specialized rheumatology diagnostic laboratories; however, these tests have no bearing on strictly rheumatic diseases.

1. *Antimitochondrial antibodies.* These are found in 95% of patients with biliary cirrhosis and also in some patients with chronic active hepatitis.
2. *Antimyocardial antibodies.* Found in 80% to 90% of patients with Dressler's (postmyocardial infarction or postcardiac surgery) syndrome.
3. *Antiparietal cell antibodies.* Found in 84% of pernicious anemia cases.

4. *Antireticulin antibodies.* Found in 60% of children with untreated gluten-sensitive enteropathy and 30% of the adults with gluten-sensitive enteropathy; also in 25% of patients with dermatitis herpetiformis.
5. *Antiskeletal muscle antibody.* Found in patients with myasthenia gravis.
6. *Antismooth muscle antibodies.* Found in patients with chronic active hepatitis.
7. *Antithyroglobulin antibodies.* Found in patients with thyroiditis and [illegible]

[illegible]

[illegible]

In the pathogenesis of rheumatoid arthritis the rheumatoid factors (antiglobulin antibodies) combine with antigen (usually IgG) in the synovial fluid to form immune complexes. Polymorphonuclear leukocytes are thus attracted to the joint space causing a destruction of joint structures.

The *RA factor* is found in significant titer in 75% of patients with rheumatoid arthritis, and in 95% of patients when the disease is associated with subcutaneous nodules. At the beginning of the disease the titers may not be elevated. It will take approximately 6 months for a significant elevation of titer, with a high titer indicating more severe disease. It should be remembered that a positive RA factor test is not diagnostic of rheumatoid arthritis and should be correlated with the total clinical picture.

Antinuclear antibodies will be positive in 20% to 60% of cases; and the *LE cell test* is positive in 10% to 20%. *Serum complement* level is normal or sometimes slightly diminished in vasculitis associated with rheumatoid arthritis.

The *synovial fluid* will have diminished viscosity with poor mucin clot formation. The leukocyte count will be approximately 15,000/cu mm with 75% neutrophils. Glucose levels will be low; the test for RA factor will be positive and complement will be diminished, indicating complement-binding.

In addition to these specific findings the patients also have nonspecific laboratory findings such as anemia, leukocytosis, and elevated sedimentation rate.

Systemic lupus erythematosus (SLE)

SLE is a disease of unknown origin, occurring most frequently in women of childbearing age. It is a disorder of connective tissue with many and varied immunologic abnormalities.

The *LE cell test* is no longer considered the hallmark of SLE, since the LE cells are found in other diseases as well. This test is not helpful in determining prognosis. The test for *antinuclear antibodies* is much more specific, since the titer correlates well with the activity of the disease.

The *anti-DNA antibody test* is highly specific for SLE, since this antibody is not found in any other collagen vascular disease. A positive test result usually indicates associated immune injury to the kidneys.

Serum complement levels, specifically C′3 and C′4, are significantly diminished in lupus nephritis. This actually heralds the exacerbation of renal involvement 1 or 2 months ahead of time.

Rheumatoid factor is found in approximately 20% of patients with lupus.

Synovial fluid examination reveals decreased viscosity, a cell count of around 5,000/cu mm, LE cells, and diminished complement.

X-ray films of the joints are neither characteristic nor of much diagnostic importance.

Nonspecific laboratory findings are leukopenia and elevated sedimentation rate.

Rheumatic fever

Rheumatic fever is an inflammatory disease related to previous infection with group A beta-hemolytic streptococcus, and manifesting with acute migratory polyarthritis. The arthritis, as such, is a self-limiting disease. However, it becomes of clinical importance because of its association with the nonsuppurative complications of streptococcal infection, for example, carditis and glomerular nephritis.

Throat culture is performed for isolation of the beta-hemolytic streptococcus.

ASO titer will be 250 or more Todd units. The other streptococcal antibodies such as antihyaluronidase, antideoxyribonucleotidase B, antistreptokinase, and antistreptozyme can also be measured. Virtually all patients with rheumatic fever have antistreptozyme titers greater than 200 units per milliliter.

ECG findings are important, manifesting a prolonged P-R interval.

C reactive protein is a nonspecific acute phase reaction; *x-ray* studies are unnecessary.

Progressive systemic sclerosis (scleroderma)

This progressive disorder is characterized by alterations in connective tissue leading to fibrosis involving the skin (scleroderma) and internal organs and accompanied by immunologic abnormalities. The diagnosis, however, is strictly clinical.

Immunologic abnormalities include an elevated immunoglobulin G (IgG) level, the RA factor in 20% of cases, and antinuclear antibodies in 40% to 80%. A low titer of extractable nuclear antibodies (ENA) in a "speckled" pattern suggests mixed connective tissue syndrome.

Mixed connective tissue diseases

These patients have clinically overlapping features of scleroderma, SLE, and polyarthritis.

The sera of these patients have high titers of antibody to nuclear ribonucleoprotein. Thus on fluorescent antibody testing a speckled pattern is produced.

Polymyositis and dermatomyositis

[illegible]

Ankylosing spondylitis

This is a chronic inflammatory disease involving spinal articulations, especially the sacroiliac joints. In the past ankylosing spondylitis was classified as a variant of rheumatoid arthritis. However, with the advent of the recently perfected HLA-B27 antigen test, it is recognized as a distinct entity.

Radiologic studies show early sacroiliac joint involvement and typical pathology of the axial skeleton and symphysis pubis. The spine shows a bamboo appearance in later stages.

RA factor is absent and the *HLA-B27* antigen is present in 90% of cases.

Reiter's syndrome

The triad of arthritis, urethritis, and conjunctivitis characterizes this syndrome. The arthritis of Reiter's syndrome has some similarities to ankylosing spondylitis, particularly because of the involvement of the sacroiliac joint.

X-ray films show some soft tissue swelling of the joints along with the sacroiliitis. In longstanding cases there is some bony erosion.

Serologically, RA factor is absent; HLA-B27 antigen is present.

Differential diagnosis. Because of the urethritis differential diagnosis must sometimes be made between gonococcal arthritis and Reiter's syndrome. In gonococcal arthritis the HLA-B27 antigen is absent and usually a positive culture is obtained. However, if there is doubt, the treatment for gonococcal arthritis is indicated. This treatment will not affect Reiter's arthritis.

Psoriatic arthritis

Psoriatic arthritis belongs to the so-called seronegative arthritic diseases, indicating that it is RA factor negative. This disease is associated with hyperuricemia and has characteristic *x-ray features*. There is some destruction of isolated joints, osteolysis, and some ankylosing. *HLA-B27 antigen* is elevated in 40% of cases. This test is also positive in 70% of cases with inflammatory bowel diseases associated with arthritis. This finding may indicate a possible association with ankylosing spondylitis.

Gouty arthritis

Gouty arthritis is an acute clinical manifestation of gout, usually appearing abruptly, with the initial attack involving the great toe in 50% to 75% of cases.

Radiologically, it is impossible to differentiate gouty arthritis from pseudogout. Although in gouty arthritis there is usually an elevation of uric acid, in the final analysis the diagnosis is made by aspiration of synovial fluid. In gouty arthritis there will be negative birefringence of crystals under polarized light. In pseudogout the crystals are those of calcium pyrophosphate, which show weakly positive birefringence under polarized light.

Septic arthritis

Septic arthritis is usually monoarticular and considered a medical emergency.

X-ray films may show soft tissue swelling, bony erosion, and lytic lesions.

Joint aspiration is imperative and usually demonstrates an initially cloudy and later purulent synovial fluid. The leukocyte count is between 50,000 and 100,000/cu mm with 90% or more being neutrophils. Glucose concentration will be decreased. A gram stain and culture should be performed on the synovial fluid right away to establish the definitive diagnosis and treatment.

Degenerative arthritis or osteoarthritis

Degenerative arthritis is found in 85% of persons over the age of 70 and is usually associated with absence of systemic abnormalities. Results of *serologic tests,* including rheumatoid factor, antinuclear antibodies, and sedimentation rate, are usually normal. *Radiologic* changes are quite characteristic. *Synovial fluid* shows decreased viscosity, good mucin clotting ability, and a cell count of less than 200/cu mm. Glucose level is normal.

12

DIAGNOSTIC TESTS FOR INFECTIOUS DISEASES

GRAM STAIN

This staining method permits the classification of bacteria into four basic groups: gram-positive or -negative rods and gram-positive or-negative cocci. After staining with gentian violet and Gram's iodine, the morphology can be visualized. A blue stain is designated gram-positive and a red stain is gram-negative. Such a classification has important clinical implications. For example, identification of a gram-positive chain of cocci immediately narrows down the differential diagnosis of an infectious process, thus guiding therapy 24 to 48 hours before the specific cultural identification and sensitivity testing is completed. The type of groups in which the bacteria arrange themselves can also be seen on gram stain. This is another guide to therapy. For example, the finding of gram-positive diplococci suggests *Pneumococcus* while gram-positive organisms in clumps suggests *Staphylococcus*. Of course, eventually the culture and sensitivity should be performed for definitive diagnosis and adequate treatment, since even after positive gram stain identification it may be very important to have culture identification and sensitivity testing of all isolates.

ACID-FAST BACILLI STAIN (AFB STAIN)

The acid-fast, or Ziehl-Neelsen, stain is mostly used in the diagnosis of tuberculosis, tuberculous infections, and leprosy. These organisms will appear red against a blue background when stained by this method. Since it usually takes 2 to 3 weeks to culture the tubercle bacilli, results of the AFB stain can indicate the need for the immediate initiation of therapy. It is diagnostically most helpful if seen in sputum or the cerebrospinal fluid; the AFB stain is used for follow-up as well.

BACTERIAL CULTURE AND SENSITIVITY

Usually, identification of bacteria and determination of their sensitivity to specific antimicrobial drugs are done after the initial gram stain analysis. Most frequently the identification of a specific organism must be accompanied by a sensitivity study. An exception to this is the beta-hemolytic streptococcus from a throat culture, since the sensitivity of this organism to antibacterial drugs is well known. However, because of the changing patterns of resistance in other bacteria to antibacterial agents, sensitivity studies are essential.

There are two methods of sensitivity testing: (1) the tube-dilution and (2) the agar diffusion methods. The *tube-dilution* method is employed when it is important to know the concentration of the antibiotic that will be effective against the organism. This is a time-consuming and cumbersome method. The *agar diffusion* method is most commonly used clinically. The organism is reported as being either sensitive, intermediate, or resistant to the antibiotic. This is, of course, mainly qualitative and semiquantitative. Sensitivity depends quite a lot on the growth characteristics of the organisms and the diffusion characteristics of the antibiotic.

Blood culture

In fevers of unknown origin, when bacterial infection is suspected, it is usually advisable to take three cultures, aerobically and anaerobically, at 30-minute intervals. This method helps to increase the yield of the organism and confirms the diagnosis when the same organism is obtained in separate blood cultures.

In bacterial endocarditis it is usually easy to identify the organism in culture because of the constant shedding of the bacteria into the bloodstream. In other types of infection, the yield is greatest if cultures are obtained just prior to an expected chill and subsequent rise in temperature. However, since this is difficult to predict, the next best period is during the chill, when the temperature is rising.

Sputum culture

Sputum should be collected after deep cough and production of thick, purulent sputum. It is important that the specimen be truly sputum and not saliva. When accurate bacteriologic diagnosis and sensitivity are of paramount importance, transtracheal aspiration of sputum is done.

Urine culture

Since most urinary tract infections are caused by gram-negative bacilli, identification and sensitivity testing are of primary importance.

A clean-catch mid-stream urine specimen is considered in clinical practice to be an adequate means of obtaining an uncontaminated urine specimen. To obtain such a specimen the urethral meatus is cleansed with an antiseptic solution and the initial one-third of the urine is discarded. The second one-third of urine is then collected for culture and sensitivity studies. The specimen thus obtained correlates well with the catheterized specimen and eliminates the normal bacterial flora of the distal urethra and ureteral meatus from the culture. With this method there is no need to catheterize patients simply for the purpose of obtaining uncontaminated urine. In patients who already have a catheter in place, the specimen is obtained through the catheter. When [illegible]

[illegible]

[illegible] lescent phase of the disease by observing at least a four-fold elevation of titer and then a gradual decrease. Thus in the majority of cases diagnosis will be retroactive and of more epidemiologic use rather than immediate clinical value.

Immunologic methods are employed for detecting antibodies against specific organisms. The choice of tests depends on ease and practicality and has no bearing on the type of infection, organism, or pathogenesis.

The most frequently used serologic tests are discussed below.

Precipitin tests

Precipitates will form when soluble antigens are combined with antiserum containing specific antibody. These tests are used mainly in the identification of bacterial exotoxins and antibodies of certain fungi.

Neutralization tests

An antigen is said to be neutralized when it loses the ability to produce an injurious effect. An antigen-antibody combination causes such an effect. These tests are usually used in viral identification. The incubated known virus and test serum are inoculated into the tissue culture and the effects are noted. Animals may also be used for the test. The test serum is given, and the animal is then challenged with the toxin or microorganism. If the antibody is present in the test serum, the animal is protected against infection.

Agglutination tests

Antibodies are capable of clumping antigen molecules and bacteria together. This process is called *agglutination.* Agglutination reactions can be performed on a slide or in a test tube by mixing the patient's serum with the specific antigen. The presence of agglutination or clumping is then observed.

These tests are used, for example, in the diagnosis of *Brucella* and *Salmonella* infection. The heterophil agglutination tests are used to diagnose infectious mononucleosus.

Complement fixation tests

This test involves a more tedious procedure. Complement is a substance found in normal serum that produces lysis when it is combined with antigen-antibody complexes. The patient's serum is first incubated with the antigen to be tested and a specific amount of complement. If an antigen-antibody reaction takes place, the complement will "fix" to these complexes. Erythrocytes coated with antibodies are then added to the combination and lysis occurs if there is any free complement left in the serum. The failure of lysis to occur implies that all of the complement was used up in the first phase of the test, indicating the presence of the particular antibody for which the test was performed. An example of a complement fixation is the VDRL test.

Fluorescent antibody methods

In this test antibody attachment to an antigen is identified under the fluorescent microscope through the use of a fluorescent dye. A microscope slide is used upon which the clinical material has been fixed and overlaid with a specific preparation of antibody conjugated to dye. An antigen-antibody reaction is noted if fluorescent microorganisms are seen. The FTA-ABS test for the diagnosis of syphilis is an example of a fluorescent antibody method.

An indirect immunofluorescence test uses antibodies to human immunoglobulins, which may be prepared in animals and then conjugated with fluorescein.

Skin tests

A skin test is an intradermal test for delayed hypersensitivity produced by certain infections, such as tuberculosis. This sensitization takes place in the T-lymphocytes.

The antigen is injected intradermally several inches below the elbow in the volar surface of the forearm. Induration of 10 mm or more appearing 48 to 72 hours after injection is diagnostic of delayed sensitivity. In tuberculin testing false negative results (from 5% to 20%) can be caused by depletion of T-lymphocytes because of overwhelming infection, pleural effusions, or an anergic state such as Hodgkin's disease or sarcoidosis.

LABORATORY TESTS IN THE CLINICAL SETTING

Bacterial pneumonias

Chest x-ray is nearly always essential in the diagnosis of bacterial pneumonias. In addition to substantiating the existence of an inflammatory infectious condition, the consolidation pattern may indicate the cause. For example, a lobar distribution usually indicates a *Pneumococcus*, whereas a bronchial distribution will suggest other gram-positive organisms. *Klebsiella* and staphylococci also have some unique radiologic characteristics.

Gram stain of the sputum may be suggestive enough to indicate therapy before culture is available. Occasionally, transtracheal aspiration of sputum will be necessary, especially in anaerobic infections.

An untreated or inadequately treated bacterial pneumonia may resolve into a lung abscess. All of the diagnostic tests helpful in pneumonia are employed in the diagnosis of lung abscess. Occasionally, surgical evacuation is needed for specific bacteriologic diagnosis.

Mycoplasmal pneumonia

This pneumonia has also been called Eaton's agent pneumonia and PPLO. Specific diagnosis is important because the *Mycoplasma pneumoniae* organism does not respond to penicillin. Effective drugs are tetracycline and erythromycin.

Chest x-ray and the clinical picture aid in the diagnosis. *Cold agglutinins* will be positive in up to 90% of severe cases. This test will also be helpful in predicting the possibility of hemolysis associated with the pneumonia.

Serologic tests are available for retrospective diagnosis.

Viral pneumonias

There are at least twelve groups of viruses and 150 different serotypes that can cause pneumonias. In general, viral infections are a common cause of upper respiratory infection that lasts 2 to 3 days and is usually of no clinical consequence. Since there is no specific treatment for viral infections, no specific diagnosis is necessary except for epidemiologic purposes.

Secondary bacterial infection may occur in some patients (particularly in smokers), usually in the form of bronchitis. In such a case there will be purulent sputum and a normal chest x-ray film. The infecting organism is usually *Pneumococcus* or *Hemophilis influenzae*.

Specific serologic diagnosis of viral upper respiratory infections and pneumonias is available for epidemiologic surveys; preventive vaccination is available for specified populations.

Rare types of pneumonias

Tularemia

Tularemia (rabbit fever, deer fly fever, Ohara's disease) is transmitted to humans from animals by direct contact or through an insect host. The causative organism is *Pasteurella (Francisella) tularensis*, a gram-negative bacillus.

The *agglutination test* for this disease uses a suspension of the bacterium *Francisella tularensis*. In patients with tularemia, titers of 1:80 are reached during the second week of infection, rising to 1:640+ in 2 to 3 months and then falling. Since cross-reactions with *Brucella* and *Proteus* OX-19 can occur, both should be tested to make the diagnosis of tularemia.

Cultures from mucocutaneous lesions and sputum should be obtained for definitive diagnosis.

Psittacosis or ornithosis

This disease is transmitted from birds to humans by inhalation and results in a pneumonitis and involvement of the reticuloendothelial system.

Chest x-ray film shows patchy pneumonitis resembling *Mycoplasma* infection.

The diagnosis is made by isolation of the *Chlamydia psittaci* organism from the sputum and by serologic testing (mainly complement fixation of antibodies) in the acute and convalescent stages.

Legionnaires disease

This is a specific bacterial infection that is so named because it caused an outbreak of pneumonia at a convention of American Legionnaires at a Philadelphia hotel. The acute disease is a patchy pulmonary infiltrate and consolidation, which may result in respiratory failure.

After painstaking investigation, a gram-negative bacillus was isolated and documented as the cause. This organism can be isolated directly in vitro on special media. However, this method is difficult. Clinically, the *indirect fluorescent antibody test* of the patient's serum is the most practical method of diagnosis.

Serologic testing has shown that other outbreaks of this disease have occurred and that subclinical infection is not uncommon, but is detectable only by serologic testing.

Viral and bacterial infections of the central nervous system

Meningitis and brain abscesses

In these cases it is extremely important to make an etiologic diagnosis. Common bacterial infections, in order of frequency, are *Meningococcus, Hemophilus influenzae* (especially in children), *Pneumococcus,* and tuberculosis. Less common causitive organisms are *E. coli, Streptococcus,* and

Staphylococcus. Listeria monocytogenes may be found in immunosuppressed and terminally ill patients.

The most important test is the *spinal tap*, discussed on p. 203. The cerebrospinal fluid is analyzed for protein and glucose. Gram stain and acid-fast stain may be diagnostic of the specific bacterial or tuberculous nature of the infection, and india ink stain may be diagnostic of a cryptococcal infection (a fungus). Culture and sensitivity tests are always performed.

[illegible]

[illegible]

[illegible]

In florid bacterial meningitis spinal fluid shows purulent fluid with significant increases in white blood cells (mainly neutrophils) and protein, and a marked decrease in glucose levels.

Tuberculous meningitis

In this condition the WBC count in the CSF is less prominent and consists mainly of monocytes and lymphocytes.

In the differential diagnosis between this and viral meningitis, the glucose level becomes important: It will be decreased in tuberculous meningitis and normal in viral or aseptic meningitis.

Viral meningitis

In the CSF protein is usually elevated, WBC is slightly elevated, mainly with lymphocytes, and the glucose level is always normal.

Brain abscess

CSF pressure is definitely elevated and the white blood cell count is between 50 and 300/μl, mainly lymphocytes. If there is communication of the abscess with the ventricular system the white blood cell count will increase in the CSF with an increase in polymorphonuclear leukocytes and the infecting organism can be cultured. If there is no communication of the abscess, the findings will indicate a space-occupying lesion of the brain (p. 203).

Urinary tract infections

Since this condition is very common in females, the usual practice is to assume that it is a lower urinary tract infection and cystitis with no predisposing factors. It is acceptable practice to treat this condition without elaborate laboratory work-ups. However, in repeated urinary tract infections of females or males, urinalysis should be performed, with gram stain and culture. The necessary tests for possible predisposing factors, such as urinary tract obstruction, should be performed.

In asymptomatic bacteruria a colony count of 100,000/ml or more of gram-negative rods is considered diagnostic of infection. A colony count of only 10,000/ml of enterococci is accepted as diagnostic.

In genitourinary tuberculosis, the most common finding is asymptomatic pyuria and hematuria. In the elderly such a combination should alert the clinician to order the proper cultures to rule out tuberculous involvement of the urinary tract.

Pharyngitis and tonsillitis

The differential diagnosis in acute tonsillitis and pharyngitis is between bacterial infection, mainly beta-hemolytic streptococcus, and viral infection. Unless one is already committed to the use of penicillin, it is essential to identify the organism by throat culture because of the complications of beta-hemolytic streptococcal infection. There is no need for sensitivity testing once the culture identifies the organism. If the culture is negative, a viral infection is usually indicated.

ASO titers will help in diagnosing beta-hemolytic streptococcal infection; however, it takes longer for this titer to be elevated than for the culture results to be obtained.

Diphtheria

Diphtheria is an infection of the mucous membranes of the pharynx with toxin production causing widespread inflammation, trauma, and destruction. If the disease is suspected, antitoxin should be administered immediately, even before attempting any specific diagnosis. However, antibiotics should be withheld until cultures are taken. *Gram stain* will show gram-positive rods.

Testing for *toxigenicity* is done either by animal inoculation or by in vitro testing, the purpose being to demonstrate that the suspected bacteria are capable of producing toxin.

Testing for *immunity* is accomplished through the *Schick test.* Diphtheria toxin is given intradermally. A positive reaction indicates that the patient does not have circulating antibody.

Pertussis

Pertussis, or whooping cough, is an acute infection of the mucous membranes of the respiratory tract.

The organism responsible for this condition *(Bordetella pertussis)* is isolated from the upper respiratory tract and can be cultured only on special media.

Serologic tests are not practical since the antibodies are in low titer and appear only after 2 weeks.

The blood count reveals a leukocytosis from 15,000 to 40,000 cells/cu mm with 90% lymphocytes.

Salmonella infection (typhoidal form)

Salmonella typhi causes typhoid fever. The organisms are ingested, enter [illegible]

Throat cultures will be positive in 10% to 15% the first week, increasing to 75% by the third week.

Serologic tests show an increase in agglutinins against the typhoid bacillus antigens after the first week of illness, rising to a peak by the fifth or sixth week. Such a rise is highly supportive of infection with the typhoid bacillus, but is not specific, since other organisms will also produce such a rise.

The *blood count* reveals leukopenia during the acute febrile phase. A sudden appearance of leukocytosis suggests complication, such as rupture of the bowel.

Salmonella gastroenteritis

Salmonella gastroenteritis usually causes severe nausea, vomiting, and diarrhea. The organism can be isolated from suspected food and from the feces of the patient.

Blood cultures are usually negative.

Shigellosis

The *Shigella* organism will cause acute gastroenteritis with fever, abdominal pain, and diarrhea.

Stool culture will confirm the diagnosis.

The *WBC count* will be from 5,000 to 15,000/cu mm. Usually there will be electrolyte abnormalities, depending on the severity of the nausea, vomiting, and diarrhea.

Venereal diseases

Syphilis

Syphilis is caused by the *Treponema pallidum* organism, is usually transmitted sexually, and is a systemic infection that is initially manifest by a primary chancre.

Microscopic dark field examination is essential in evaluating the moist lesions of primary syphilis. This test must be repeated at least once daily for 3 days before declaring the lesion to be negative.

In the secondary stage, when the lesions are nonpruritic, it is more difficult to obtain the organism from the lesion. However, the diagnosis can be made without the microscopic dark field examination if the lesions are characteristic and results of the serologic tests are positive.

Serologic diagnosis depends on two types of antibodies being produced, the nonspecific reaginic antibody and the specific antitreponemal antibody.

The nonspecific reaginic antibodies are measured by (1) flocculation tests, the most common being the VDRL test (Venereal Disease Research Laboratory); (2) complement fixation tests (Kolmer method); and (3) an agglutination test (Rapid Plasma Reagent test [RPR]). All of these tests are nonspecific with false positives occurring in a significant number of cases.

The specific antitreponemal antibodies are tested by immunofluorescence technique—fluorescent treponemal antibody absorption test (FTA-ABS)—in which only about 1% are false positive reactions.

At present, most institutions and clinics use the VDRL as a screening test. If it is positive the FTA-ABS absorption test is performed. If both are positive then the chances of a false positive become extremely rare.

The treponema immobilization test (TBI) will be diagnostically conclusive, but it is tedious to perform and is not routinely used.

Gonococcal infections

In gonorrhea the organism, *Neisseria gonorrhoeae*, is transmitted by sexual contact, and penetrates the mucous membrane of the urogenital tract. There will be a purulent urethritis in the male, and in the female Bartholin's and Skene's glands and the uterine cervical glands are usually infected.

Gram stain of the urethral or endocervical discharge will reveal intracellular gram-negative diplococci, which is characteristic and nearly diagnostic.

Culture is necessary if one cannot find intracellular gram-negative diplococci on gram stain and the diplococci are extracellular. The culture medium in such a case should have 3% to 10% CO_2 to promote growth. In homosexual patients, cultures must be taken from the throat and anal canal.

Serologic tests (complement fixation or immunofluorescent techniques) are advisable for systemic infections or in patients with gonococcal arthritis when it is difficult to isolate the organism.

Chancroid

This venereal disease is caused by the *Hemophilus ducreyi* organism, which penetrates mucous membranes or broken skin and manifests as a painful ulcer on the genitals.

Diagnosis is made by exclusion of other penile lesions with which it can be confused, such as herpes progenitalis, syphilis, and lymphogranuloma venereum. When all of these have been eliminated, a response to sulfa drugs is diagnostic.

Culture of the *Hemophilus ducreyi* organism is extremely difficult and impractical.

Granuloma inguinale

[illegible]

[illegible]

[illegible] The first manifestation is a genital lesion, with regional lymph nodes being involved weeks to months later.

A *complement fixation* test with rising titers is evidence of active infection, while a negative result rules out lymphogranuloma.

Herpes virus type II progenitalis

In this condition viral isolation techniques are used in the diagnosis. If these are not available, cytologic tests and Pap smear will show multinucleated cells and intranuclear inclusion bodies.

Tuberculosis

Tuberculosis is caused by *Mycobacterium tuberculosis,* which usually infects the lungs but may also involve the kidneys, meninges, spine, and lymph nodes.

Acid-fast stain from sputum and gastric washings is sufficient for a tentative diagnosis and initiation of therapy. However, *culture* of the organism is the only absolute proof of existing infection. For this multiple sputum specimens and gastric washings are needed for sufficient positive yield.

Acid-fast stain of spinal fluid, if positive, is fairly diagnostic and indicates the need for immediate initiation of therapy.

Radiologic methods give valuable information and provide a tentative diagnosis, but never a definitive one. X-ray films are also useful in the follow-up and treatment.

The tuberculin skin test (purified protein derivative; PPD) does not differentiate between present active infection and dormant and subclinical infections, nor does a negative test rule out active tuberculosis, since anergic states such as Hodgkin's disease, sarcoidosis, massive infection, and pleural effusion will cause false negative results.

When routine *urine culture* is negative in the presence of hematuria with pyuria, one should suspect tuberculous infection of the kidney and perform a culture of the urine for the tubercle bacilli.

Biopsy of the liver, bone marrow, or lymph nodes may be diagnostic of miliary tuberculosis.

A pleural biopsy may be very helpful in the presence of pleural effusion, which is usually an exudate. Bacteriologic study and fluid analysis should also be performed.

The pleural needle biopsy usually reveals the typical granuloma of tuberculosis with giant cells showing caseation necrosis. Such findings are sufficiently diagnostic to initiate therapy.

In order to increase the yield, multiple biopsies should be done at one sitting.

Rickettsial diseases

The rickettsias are intracellular parasites maintained by a cycle involving an insect vector and an animal reservoir, with man as an incidental victim. The organism typically invades the endothelial cells of small blood vessels, with perivascular infiltration and thrombosis. Diagnosis is important because the treatment is specific.

Serologic tests are used in the diagnosis because isolation of the organism is difficult, impractical, and hazardous.

The *Weil-Felix test* employs *Proteus* OX-19 and OX-2 and gives positive results in patients with Rocky Mountain spotted fever and murine typhus; and negative results with rickettsialpox and Q fever.

The *complement fixation test* employing group-specific rickettsial antigens will clinically differentiate among the most common infections. A rise of titer in a week or two with a fall in titer later is definitely diagnostic of the specific rickettsia.

Actinomycosis

In the past actinomycosis has been classified under fungi. However, the causative organism, *Actinomyces israelii*, is a gram-positive rod or filament that causes chronic granulomatous infection and is normally present in the mouth. Thus actinomycosis of the face and neck is more common, manifesting a week or more after tooth extraction or mandibular fracture as a painful indurated lesion over the jaw. From there, or from foci in the lung or intestines, actinomycosis may spread to the liver, kidneys, spleen, brain, genitalia, and subcutaneous tissues.

Diagnosis is made by detecting the organism in pus from absesses, by gram stain, anaerobic culture, or by biopsy.

Gram stain is used when clumps of the organism have formed. Such clumps are called "sulfur granules," which are crushed and stained.

Anaerobic culture is utilized when the sulfur granules are not present, and *biopsies* are employed when the culture is negative.

Nocardiosis

Nocardiosis is caused by an aerobic actinomycete found in the soil, which is either inhaled or introduced into the subcutaneous tissue by trauma. Lung abscesses may result and these may spread to the brain.

[illegible]

[illegible]

[illegible]

[illegible] an affinity for the central nervous system, with lesions developing in the meninges at the base of the brain. This is one of the causes of aseptic meningitis.

Diagnosis is made by isolating the organism from the spinal fluid on Sabouraud's agar, and by gram stain and microscopic examination of the spinal fluid.

Blastomycosis

The *Blastomyces dermatitidis* organism, which causes blastomycosis, gains entrance to the body through the lungs to cause systemic infection.

Diagnosis is made by culturing the organism from sputum, pus, or biopsied material on Sabouraud's agar. The value of the skin test is limited. Complement fixation test may also be employed.

Coccidioidomycosis (San Joaquin Valley or desert fever)

This infection is caused by inhalation of the organism *Coccidioides immitis*. After inhalation the organism may be killed or arrested causing an acute respiratory disease; or in some cases it will proliferate and become chronic.

Diagnosis is made by isolating the organism on Sabouraud's agar. Serologic methods include tests for complement-fixing antibodies and precipitin tests.

Histoplasmosis

In this disease the organism, *Histoplasma capsulatum*, after being inhaled from the soil causes pulmonary infection very similar to tuberculosis.

Diagnosis is made by isolating the organism on Sabouraud's agar and by pulmonary radiologic findings. Serologic and skin tests have limited usefulness.

Candidiasis (moniliasis)

Candidiasis is a mild mucocutaneous infection caused by the *Candida albicans* organism. When the mucous membranes are involved, the disease is known as thrush. The disease may enter the bloodstream when it is a complication of other severe debilitating diseases.

The fungus can be isolated from a scraping of the white patches in the mouth. In deep disseminated candidiasis biopsy material from tissues involved will reveal the organism. In *Candida* endocarditis the organism is isolated from blood cultures. Candidiasis is a common form of vaginal infection.

Mucormycosis (phycomycosis)

The Mucorales organism, found in soil, manure, and starchy foodstuffs, may become pathogenic for man in severe underlying disease, particularly diabetic acidosis. The organism enters through the nasal turbinates or paranasal sinus and may eventually spread to the brain or cause pulmonary infection.

Diagnosis is made by demonstration of the organism from biopsied infected tissue.

Viral infections

Most of the viral infections, particularly of the upper respiratory tract, seen clinically are not specifically diagnosed, because of their benign and short duration. By the time the organism could be isolated or serologic test become positive, the infection has subsided. However, for retrospective diagnosis and for epidemiologic purposes isolation and tissue culture techniques of specific viruses, as well as multiple serologic tests, are available.

Another reason for not attempting specific virologic diagnosis is the fact that there is no specific antiviral therapy.

When pericarditis or myocarditis is diagnosed and a viral etiology is suspected, it is helpful clinically to make as specific a diagnosis as possible. This diagnosis is based on serologic testing of sera taken during the acute and convalescent phases. This test could not be used therapeutically, even if specific therapy for viral infections were available.

The main reason for specific diagnosis in such cases is for prognostication and to rule out other possible causes of pericarditis and myocarditis. In this case acute and convalescent sera are usually sent to a reference laboratory with all of the clinical information. In a case of suspected myocarditis or pericarditis, the laboratory is asked to do serologic testing for all possible viruses that could cause these specific conditions. These are: Coxsackie A and B, poliomyelitis, influenza, adenovirus, ECHO, rubeola, and rubella viruses. If the acute and convalescent sera show a four-fold rise in titer of any of the above viruses in a suspected case of myocarditis or pericarditis, a definitive diagnosis is established.

Herpes simplex hominis type I and type II

This virus usually causes mucocutaneous lesions, which may disseminate in the immunosuppressed patient. Type I causes naso-oropharyngeal lesions. Type II causes genitourinary tract lesions and is considered a venereal disease in transmission. This type is associated with carcinoma of the cervix.

A smear from the base of a vesicle shows multinucleated giant cells and [illegible]

[illegible]

[illegible]

[illegible]

[illegible] tuberculin type of reaction.

Mumps

This viral disease results in parotitis, epididymitis, orchitis, and pancreatitis, and is one of the causes of aseptic meningitis.

Diagnosis usually is serologic (complement fixation test). Between the acute and convalescent phases the serum will show a four-fold increase in titer.

Varicella (chickenpox)

The diagnosis of this disease is usually clinical. However, laboratory findings will verify the clinical impression.

A smear from the base of a vesicle demonstrates varicella giant cells with intranuclear bodies.

Serologic tests, mainly immunofluorescent staining, will confirm the diagnosis.

Cytomegalovirus

This virus causes a disease very similar to infectious mononucleosis. It usually occurs in patients who receive large amounts of fresh blood. In the past, patients undergoing open heart surgery would receive large amounts of such blood. The syndrome following open heart surgery was called post-perfusion syndrome. Eventually it was found to be caused by cytomegalovirus.

The diagnosis is made by examining a stained sediment of urine, saliva, or gastric washings, which demonstrate the cytoplasmic inclusion bodies.

Isolation of the virus is possible, and serologic tests include complement fixation and neutralization tests.

Variola (smallpox)

This virus, which gains entrance through the respiratory tract, causes vesicular and pustular eruption, accompanied by fever.

Diagnosis is made by smears taken from the base of the lesions. When stained the typical viral particles are visible. Fluorescent antibody tests, both direct and indirect, may also be used.

Isolation of the virus is possible and serologic tests, mainly complement fixation, hemagglutination, and neutralization tests, show rising titers.

Influenza

Influenza is a generalized, acute, febrile disease sometimes associated with upper respiratory infections. Diagnosis is made mainly clinically in a given epidemiologic setting. However, isolated cases can be definitively diagnosed by isolation of the virus from chick embryos that have been inoculated with sputum or throat washings. Fluorescent antibody staining of nasal epithelial cells will provide a diagnosis in the first days of the disease. Serologic tests require a four-fold increase in antibody titer between the acute and the convalescent sera.

Infectious mononucleosis

This virus has recently been isolated and has been called the Epstein-Barr (EB) virus. It causes sore throat and lymphadenopathy, and may be very mild to severe with hepatomegaly with hepatitis and sometimes meningitis.

The diagnosis is made because of marked lymphocytosis with Downey cells (atypical lymphocytes).

Heterophil antibodies will be present in the serum of 80% to 90% of these patients. These are agglutinins against sheep red blood cells in high titer. This test is called the heterophil antibody test.

Recently, a rapid method of detecting heterophil agglutinins has been developed, which requires a drop of the patient's blood and a reagent. This is called the Spot-Mono test. It is used mainly for screening purposes.

Diagnostic titers of antibodies to the EB virus are 1:80 to 1:160. These are demonstrated by immunofluorescence techniques.

When there is liver involvement and hepatitis, liver function tests are usually abnormal, including elevated SGOT, SGPT, bilirubin and alkaline phosphatase levels.

Parasitic diseases

Malaria

This disease is transmitted by the female *Anopheles* mosquitoe, the causative organism being protozoa of the genus *Plasmodium*. Malaria has a chronic relapsing course with fever, chills, splenomegaly, and anemia.

Blood smear, stained with Wright's, Giemsa's, or Field's stain and taken a few hours after an episode of chills, will usually demonstrate the parasite. There are four species of the *Plasmodium* protozoa, the identification of which requires experience.

Serologic tests, such as the indirect fluorescent antibody test and hemagglutination tests, are available, but not widely used.

Pneumocystis carinii

[illegible]

[illegible]

[illegible]

[illegible]

[illegible] poorly cooked, infected meat. The organism causes lymphadenopathy and myalgia, and can cause central nervous system disease. Transplacental infection causes congenital toxoplasmosis, manifested in the infant by rash, fever, chorioretinitis, and encephalitis.

Diagnosis is made by the indirect fluorescent antibody test. Titers of 1:256 or higher are indicative of recent infection, and titers of 1:1024 or above indicate active disease.

Complement fixation test will become positive in active disease.

Trichinosis

This organism, *Trichinella spiralis,* gains entry to the body by ingestion of undercooked meat, particularly pork.

The most characteristic laboratory finding is that of a marked eosinophilia.

Serologic tests include complement fixation tests, precipitin, and fluorescent antibody test. These tests will become positive about the third week of the disease and are most helpful in the diagnosis if they are initially negative and exhibit a significant change in titer.

Definitive diagnosis is by examination of muscle biopsy. The most frequently involved muscles are those of the extremities, throat, and diaphragm.

Amebiasis

The causative organism of amebiasis is *Entamoeba histolytica,* a protozoon, which causes intestinal disease with diarrhea and colitis, as well as hepatic abscess.

Diagnosis is made by identification of the organism in stools and tissues.

Indirect hemagglutination is usually helpful in diagnosing hepatic abscess. In endemic areas a negative serologic test is important in ruling out the disease.

Trypanosomiasis (sleeping sickness)

This disease is caused by *Trypanosoma brucei,* protozoa that are transmitted by the tsetse fly. In trypanosomiasis the patient has lymphadenopathy followed by encephalitis.

The diagnosis is made by finding the trypanosomes in blood or the aspirate from lymph glands or cerebrospinal fluid.

Serologic tests used mainly are complement fixation and indirect fluorescent antibody test.

Giardiasis

This disease causes "travelers diarrhea" and is the result of infestation of the duodenum and jejunum by the *Giardia lamblia* protozoa. Occasionally malabsorption will result.

Diagnosis is made by finding the trophozoid stage in the duodenal washings.

Trichomonis vaginalis

This protozoon causes vaginal infection with discharge.

Diagnosis is established by examination of the vaginal discharge or seminal fluid by a wet stain or Giemsa-stained preparation.

APPENDICES

APPENDIX A

TABLES OF NORMAL VALUES

Many of the normal values are based on the experience in the Department of Pathology, Mount Sinai Hospital, Chicago, Illinois, and the Division of Clinical Pathology, State University Hospital, State University of New York, Syracuse, New York. Actual values may vary with different techniques or in different laboratories. Although only the more common tests are discussed in the text, others are included here for completeness. Values have been updated according to the current values in use at the Massachusetts General Hospital.

ABBREVIATIONS USED IN TABLES

<	=	less than	mIU	=	milliInternational Unit
>	=	greater than	mOsm	=	milliosmole
dl	=	100 ml	mμ	=	millimicron
gm	=	gram	mU	=	milliunit
IU	=	International Unit	ng	=	nanogram
kg	=	kilogram	pg	=	picogram
L	=	liter	μEq	=	microequivalent
mEq	=	milliequivalent	μg	=	microgram
mg	=	milligram	μIU	=	microInternational Unit
ml	=	milliliter	μl	=	microliter
mM	=	millimole	μU	=	microunit
mm Hg	=	millimeters of mercury	U	=	unit

Adapted with permission from Davidsohn, I. and Henry, J. B. editors: Todd-Sanford Clinical diagnosis by laboratory methods, ed. 15, Philadelphia, 1974. W. B. Saunders Co., and from Scully, R. E., editor: Case records of the Massachusetts General Hospital, N. Engl. J. Med. **298**:34, 1978.

TABLE A-1
Whole blood, serum, and plasma (chemistry)

Test	Material	Normal value	Special instructions
Acetoacetic acid			
Qualitative	Serum	Negative	
Quantitative	Serum	0.2-1.0 mg/dl	
Acetone			
Qualitative	Serum	Negative	
Quantitative	Serum	0.3-2.0 mg/dl	
Adrenocorticotropic hormone (ACTH)	Plasma	15-70 pg/ml	Place specimen on ice and send promptly to lab
Albumin, quantitative	Serum	3.2-4.5 gm/dl (salt fractionation) 3.2-5-6 gm/dl by electrophoresis 3.8-5.0 gm/dl by dye binding	
Alcohol	Serum or whole blood	Negative	
Aldolase	Serum	Adults: 1.3-8.2 U/dl Children: Approximately 2 times adult levels Newborn: Approximately 4 times adult levels	
Alpha-amino acid nitrogen	Plasma	3.0-5.5 mg/100 mg/dl	
δ-Aminolevulinic acid	Serum	0.01-0.03 mg/dl	
Ammonia	Blood	80-110 μg/dl	Collect with sodium heparinate; specimen must be delivered packed in ice and analyzed immediately
Amylase	Serum	4-25 U/ml	
Arginiosuccinic lyase	Serum	0-4 U/dl	
Arsenic	Whole blood	<3 μg/dl	
Ascorbic acid (vitamin C)	Plasma Whole blood	0.6-1.6 mg/dl 0.4-1.5 mg/dl	Analyze immediately
Barbiturates	Serum, plasma, or whole blood	Negative Coma level: phenobarbital, approximately 10 mg/dl; most other drugs, 1-3 mg/dl	
Base excess	Whole blood	Male: −3.3 to + 1.2 Female: −2.4 to + 2.3	
Base, total	Serum	145-160 mEq/L	
Bicarbonate	Plasma	21-28 mM/L	

TABLE A-1

Whole blood, serum, and plasma (chemistry)—cont'd

Test	Material	Normal value	Special instructions
Bile acids	Serum	0.3-3.0 mg/dl	
Bilirubin	Serum	Up to 0.4 mg/dl (direct or conjugated) Total: 0.7 mg/dl [illegible]	
[illegible]		[illegible]	
[illegible] thalein) (5 mg/kg)	[illegible]	[illegible]	
Calcitonin	Plasma	Undetectable in normals. >100 pg/ml in medullary carcinoma	
Calcium	Serum	Ionized: 4.2-5.2 mg/dl 2.1-2.6 mEq/L or 50%-58% of total Total: 9.0-10.6 mg/dl 4.5-5.3 mEq/L Infants: 11-13 mg/dl	
Carbon dioxide (CO_2 content)	Whole blood, arterial	19-24 mM/L	
	Plasma or serum, arterial	24-30 mEq/L 20-26 mEq/L in infants (as HCO_3)	
	Whole blood, venous	22-26 mM/L	
	Plasma or serum, venous	24-30 mM/L	
CO_2 combining power	Plasma or serum, venous	24-30 mM/L	
CO_2 partial pressure (Pco_2)	Whole blood, arterial	35-40 mm Hg	
	Whole blood, venous	40-45 mm Hg	
Carbonic acid	Whole blood, arterial	1.05-1.45 mM/L	
	Whole blood, venous	1.15-1.50 mM/L	
	Plasma, venous	1.02-1.38 mM/L	
Carboxyhemoglobin (carbon monoxide hemoglobin)	Whole blood	Suburban nonsmokers: <1.5% saturation of hemoglobin Smokers: 1.5-5.0% saturation Heavy smokers: 5.0-9.0% saturation	
Carotene, beta	Serum	40-200 μg/dl	

Continued.

TABLE A-1
Whole blood, serum, and plasma (chemistry)—cont'd

Test	Material	Normal value	Special instructions
Cephalin cholesterol flocculation	Serum	Negative to 1+ after 24 hours 2+ or less after 48 hours	
Ceruloplasmin	Serum	23-50 mg/dl	
Chloride	Serum	100-106 mEq/L	
Cholesterol, total	Serum	150-250 mg/dl (varies with diet and age)	
Cholesterol, esters	Serum	65-75% of total cholesterol	
Cholinesterase	Erythrocytes	0.65-1.00 pH units	
Psuedocholinesterase	Plasma	0.5-1.3 pH units 8-18 IU/L at 37° C	
Citric acid	Serum or plasma	1.7-3.0 mg/dl	
Congo red test	Serum or plasma	>60% after 1 hour	Severe reactions may occur if dye is injected twice; check patient's record
Copper	Serum or plasma	100-200 μg/dl	
Cortisol	Plasma	8 A.M.: 5-25 μg/dl 8 P.M.: < 10 μg/dl	
Creatine	Serum or plasma	0.6-1.5 mg/dl	
Creatine phosphokinase (CPK)	Serum	Males: 5-55 mU/ml Females: 5-35 mU/ml	See Chapter 4
Creatinine	Serum or plasma	0.6-1.2 mg/dl	
Creatinine clearance (endogenous)	Serum or plasma and urine	Male: 123 ± 16 ml/min Female: 97 ± 10 ml/min	
Cryoglobulins	Serum	Negative	Keep specimen at 37° C
Doriden (Glutethmide)	Serum	0	
Electrophoresis, protein	Serum	*percent* — *gm/dl* Albumin 52-65 — 3.2-5.6 Alpha 1 2.5-5.0 — 0.1-0.4 Alpha 2 7.0-13.0 — 0.4-1.2 Beta 8.0-14.0 — 0.5-1.1 Gamma 12.0-22.0 — 0.5-1.6	
Ethanol	Blood	0.3-0.4%, marked intoxication 0.4-0.5%, alcoholic stupor 0.5% or over, alcoholic coma	Collect in oxalate and refrigerate
Fats, neutral	Serum or plasma	0-200 mg/dl	

TABLE A-1
Whole blood, serum, and plasma (chemistry)—cont'd

Test	Material	Normal value	Special instructions
Fatty acids			
Total	Serum	9-15 mM/L	
Free	Plasma	300-480 μEq/L	
Fibrinogen	Plasma	200-400 mg/dl	
[illegible]	[illegible]	[illegible]	[illegible]
	Whole blood	60-100 mg/dl	fluoride mixture
Glucose tolerance, oral	Serum or plasma	Fasting: 70-110 mg/dl 30 min: 30-60 mg/dl above fasting 60 min: 20-50 mg/dl above fasting 120 min: 5-15 mg/dl above fasting 180 min: fasting level or below	Collect with heparin-fluoride mixture
Glucose tolerance, IV	Serum or plasma	Fasting: 70-110 mg/dl 5 min: Maximum of 250 mg/dl 60 min: Significant decrease 120 min: Below 120 mg/dl 180 min: Fasting level	Collect with heparin-fluoride mixture
Glucose-6-phosphate dehydrogenase (G-6-PD)	Erythrocytes	250-500 units/10^9 cells 1200-2000 mIU/ml of packed erythrocytes	
γ-Glytamyl transpeptidase	Serum	2-39 U/L	
Glutathione	Whole blood	24-37 mg/dl	
Growth hormone	Serum	<10 ng/ml	
Haptoglobin	Serum	100-200 mg/dl as hemoglobin binding capacity	
Hemoglobin	Serum or plasma	Qualitative: Negative Quantitative: 0.5-5.0 mg/dl	
Hemoglobin	Whole blood	Female: 12.0-16.0 gm/dl Male: 13.5-18.0 gm/dl	
Hemoglobin A_2	Whole blood	1.5-3.5% of total hemoglobin	
α-Hydroxybutyric dehydrogenase	Serum	140-350 U/ml	
17-Hydroxycorticosteroids	Plasma	Male: 7-19 μg/dl Female: 9-21 μg/dl After 25 USP units of ACTH IM: 35-55 μg/dl	Perform test immediately or freeze plasma

Continued.

TABLE A-1
Whole blood, serum, and plasma (chemistry)—cont'd

Test	Material	Normal value	Special instructions
Immunoglobulins	Serum		
IgG		800-1600 mg/dl	
IgA		50-250 mg/dl	
IgM		40-120 mg/dl	
IgD		0.5-3.0 mg/dl	
IgE		0.01-0.04 mg/dl	
Insulin	Plasma	11-240 μIU/ml (bioassay) 4-24 μU/ml (radioimmunoassay)	
Insulin tolerance	Serum	Fasting: Glucose of 70-110 mg/dl 30 min: Fall to 50% of fasting level 90 min: Fasting level	Collect with heparin-fluoride mixture
Iodine			
Butanol extraction (BEI)	Serum	3.5-6.5 μg/dl	Test not reliable if iodine-containing drugs or radiographic contrast media were given prior to test
Protein bound (PBI)	Serum	4.0-8.0 μg/dl	
Iron, total	Serum	50-150 μg/dl	Hemolysis must be avoided
Iron-binding capacity	Serum	250-410 μg/dl	
Iron saturation, percent	Serum	20-55%	
Isocitric dehydrogenase	Serum	50-250 U/ml	
Ketone bodies	Serum	Negative	
17-Ketosteroids	Plasma	25-125 μg/dl	
Lactic acid	Blood	0.6-1.8 mEq/liter	Draw without stasis
Lactic dehydrogenase (LDH)	Serum	80-120 Wacker units 150-450 Wroblewski units 71-207 IU/L	See Chapter 4
Lactic dehydrogenase isoenzymes	Serum	Anode: LDH_1 17-27% LDH_2 27-37% LDH_3 18-25% LDH_4 3-8% Cathode: LDH_5 0-5%	
Lactic dehydrogenase (heat stable)	Serum	60-120 U/ml	
Lactose tolerance	Serum	Serum glucose changes are similar to those seen in a glucose tolerance test	
Lead	Whole blood	0-50 μg/dl	

TABLE A-1
Whole blood, serum, and plasma (chemistry)—cont'd

Test	Material	Normal value	Special instructions
Leucine aminopeptidase (LAP)	Serum	Male: 80-200 Goldbarg-Rutenburg units/ml Female: 75-185 Goldbarg-Rutenburg units/ml	
[illegible]	[illegible]	[illegible]	
phoresis			
Lithium	Serum	Toxic level 2 mEq/L Therapeutic level: 0.5-1.5 mEq/L	
Long-acting thyroid-stimulating hormone (LATS)	Serum	None	
Luteinizing hormone (LH)	Plasma	Male: <11 mIU/ml Female: midcycle peak >3 times base line value Premenopausal: <25 mIU/ml Postmenopausal: >25 mIU/ml	
Macroglobulins, total	Serum	70-430 mg/dl	
Magnesium	Serum	1.5-2.5 mEq/L 3.0 mg/dl	
Methanol	Blood	0	May be fatal as low as 115 mg/100 ml; collect in oxalate
Methemoglobin	Whole blood	0-0.24 gm/dl 0.4-1.5% of total hemoglobin	
Mucoprotein	Serum	80-200 mg/dl	
Nonprotein nitrogen (NPN)	Serum or plasma	20-35 mg/dl	
	Whole blood	25-50 mg/dl	
5′ Nucleotidase	Serum	0.3-3.2 Bodansky units	
Ornithine carbamyl transferase (OCT)	Serum	8-20 mIU/ml	
Osmolality	Serum	280-295 mOsm/L	
Oxygen			
Pressure (Po_2)	Whole blood, arterial	95-100 mm Hg	
Content	Whole blood, arterial	15-23 vol %	

Continued.

TABLE A-1
Whole blood, serum, and plasma (chemistry)—cont'd

Test	Material	Normal value	Special instructions
Oxygen—cont'd			
Saturation	Whole blood, arterial	96-100%	
Parathroid hormone	Plasma	<10 μl equiv/ml	Keep blood on ice, or plasma must be frozen if sent a distance
pH	Whole blood, arterial	7.35-7.45	
	Whole blood, venous	7.36-7.41	
	Serum or plasma, venous	7.35-7.45	
Phenylalanine	Serum	Adults: 0-2.0 mg/dl Newborns (term): 1.2-3.5 mg/dl Male total: 0.13-0.63 sigma U/ml Female total: 0.01-0.56 sigma U/ml Prostatic: 0-0.7 Fishman-Lerner U/dl	
Phosphatase, acid, total	Serum	0-1.1 U/ml (Bodansky) 1-4 U/ml (King-Armstrong) 0.13-0.63 U/ml (Bessey-Lowry) 1.4-5.5 U/ml (Gutman-Gutman) 0-0.56 U/ml (Roy) 0-6.0 U/ml (Shinowara-Jones-Reinhart)	Hemolysis must be avoided; perform test without delay or freeze specimen
Phosphatase, alkaline,	Serum total	Adults: 1.5-4.5 U/dl (Bodansky) 4-13 U/dl (King-Armstrong) 0.8-2.3 U/ml (Bessey-Lowry) 15-35 U/ml (Shinowara-Jones-Reinhart) Children: 5.0-14.0 U/dl (Bodansky) 3.4-9.0 U/dl (Bessey-Lowry) 15-35 U/dl (King-Armstrong)	
Phospholipd phosphorus	Serum	8-11 mg/dl	
Phospholipids	Serum	150-380 mg/dl	

TABLE A-1
Whole blood, serum, and plasma (chemistry)—cont'd

Test	Material	Normal value	Special instructions
Phosphorus, inorganic	Serum	Adults: 1.8-2.6 mEq/L 3.0-4.5 mg/dl Children: 2.3-4.1 mEq/L 4.0-7.0 mg/dl	Separate cells from serum promptly
[illegible]	[illegible]	[illegible]	[illegible]
Renin activity	Plasma	Supine: 1.1 ± 0.8 ng/ml/hr	EDTA tubes on ice Normal diet
		Upright: 1.9 ± 1.7 ng/ml/hr	
		Supine: 2.7± 1.8 ng/ml/hr	Low sodium diet
		Upright: 6.6 ± 2.5 ng/ml/hr	
		Diuretics: 10.0 ± 3.7 ng/nl/hr	Low sodium diet
Salicylates	Serum	Negative Therapeutic level: 20-25 mg/dl	
Sodium	Plasma	136-142 mEq/L	
Sulfate, inorganic	Serum	0.5-1.5 mEq/L 0.9-6.0 mg/dl as SO_4	Hemolysis must be avoided
Sulfhemoglobin	Whole blood	Negative	
Sulfonamides	Serum or whole blood	Negative	
Testosterone	Serum or plasma	Male: 400-1200 ng/dl Female: 30-120 ng/dl	
Thiocyanate	Serum	Negative	
Thymol flocculation	Serum	Up to 1+ in 24 hours	
Thyroid hormone tests	Serum	*Expressed as thyroxine* / *Expressed as iodine*	
T_4 (by column)		5.0-11.0 μg/dl / 3.2-7.2 μg/dl	
T_4 (by competitive binding Murphy-Pattee)		6.0-11.8 μg/dl / 3.9-7.7 μg/dl	
Free T_4		0.9-2.3 ng/dl / 0.6-1.5 ng/dl	
T_3 (resin uptake)		25-38 relative % uptake	
Thyroxine-binding globulin (TBG)		15-25 μg/dl (expressed as T_4 uptake)	
Thyroid-stimulating hormone (TSH)	Serum	0.5-3.5 μU/ml	

Continued.

TABLE A-1
Whole blood, serum, and plasma (chemistry)—cont'd

Test	Material	Normal value	Special instructions
Transaminases			
GOT	Serum	10-40 U/ml	
GPT	Serum	1-36 U/ml	
Triglycerides	Serum	10-190 mg/dl	
Urea nitrogen	Serum	8-25 mg/dl	
Urea clearance	Serum and urine	Maximum clearance: 64-99 ml/min Standard clearance: 41-65 ml/min or more than 75% of normal clearance	
Uric acid	Serum	3.0-7.0 mg/dl	
Vitamin A	Serum	0.15-0.6 μg/ml	
Vitamin A tolerance	Serum	Fasting: 15-60 μg/dl 3 hr or 6 hr after 5000 units vitamin A/kg: 200-600 μg/dl 24 hr fasting values or slightly above	Administer 5000 units vitamin A in oil per kg body weight
Vitamin B_{12}	Serum	Male: 200-800 pg/ml Female: 100-650 pg/ml	
Unsaturated vitamin B_{12} binding capacity	Serum	1000-2000 pg/ml	
Vitamin C	Plasma	0.6-1.6 mg/dl	Collect with oxalate and analyze within 20 minutes
Xylose absorption	Serum	25-40 mg/dl between 1 and 2 hr; in malabsorption, maximun approximately 10 mg/dl Dose Adult: 25 gm D-xylose Children: 0.5 gm/kg D-xylose	For children administer 10 ml of a 5% solution of D-xylose per kg of body weight
Zinc	Serum	50-150 μg/dl	
Zinc sulfate turbidity	Serum	<12 units	

TABLE A-2
Urine

Test	Type of specimen	Normal value	Special instructions
Acetoacetic acid	Random	Negative	
Acetone	Random	Negative	
Addis count	12-hr collection	WBC and epithelial cells: 1,800,000/12 hr [illegible]	Rinse bottle with some [illegible]
[illegible]	[illegible]	[illegible]	[illegible]
[illegible]	[illegible]	[illegible]	
Alpha-amino acid nitrogen	24 hr	100-290 mg/24 hr	
δ-Aminolevulinic acid	Random	Adult: 0.1-0.6 mg/dl Children: <0.5 mg/dl	
	24 hr	1.5-7.5 mg/24 hr	
Ammonia nitrogen	24 hr	20-70 mEq/24 hr 500-1200 mg/24 hr	Keep refrigerated
Amylase	2 hr	35-260 Somogyi units per hour	
Arsenic	24 hr	<50 μg/L	
Ascorbic acid	Random	1-7 mg/dl	
	24 hr	>50 mg/24 hr	
Bence Jones protein	Random	Negative	
Beryllium	24 hr	<0.05 μg/24 hr	
Bilirubin, qualitative	Random	Negative	
Blood, occult	Random	Negative	
Borate	24 hr	<2 mg/L	
Calcium			
Qualitative (Sulkowitch)	Random	1 + turbidity	Compare with standard
Quantitative	24 hr	Average diet: 100-250 mg/24 hr Low calcium diet: <150 mg/24 hr High calcium diet: 250-300 mg/24 hr	
Catecholamines	Random	Epinephrine <20 μg/24 hr	
	24 hr	Norepinephrine <100 μg/24 hr	
Chloride	24 hr	110-250 mEq/24 hr	
Chorionic gonadotropin	First morning voiding	0	Specific gravity should be at least 1.015

Continued.

TABLE A-2
Urine—cont'd

Test	Type of specimen	Normal value	Special instructions
Concentration test (Fishberg)	Random after fluid restriction	Specific gravity: >1.025 Osmolality: >850 mOsm/L	
Copper	24 hr	0-100 μg/24 hr	
Coproporphyrin	Random 24 hr	Adult: 50-250 μg/24 hr Children: 0-80 μg/24 hr	Use fresh specimen and do not expose to direct light; preserve 24-hr urine with 5 gm Na_2CO_3
Creatine	24 hr	Under 100 mg/24 hr or less than 6% of creatinine Pregnancy: up to 12% Children: up to 30% of creatinine	
Creatinine	24 hr	15-25 mg/kg of body weight/24 hr	
Cystine, qualitative	Random	Negative	
Cystine and cysteine	10 ml	0	
Diacetic acid	Random	Negative	
Epinephrine	24 hr	0-20 μg/24 hr	
Estrogens, total	24 hr	Male: 5-18 μg/24 hr Female Ovulation: 28-100 μg/24 hr Luteal peak: 22-105 μg/24 hr At menses: 4-25 μg/24 hr Pregnancy: up to 45,000 μg/24 hr Postmenopausal: 14-20 μg/24 hr	Keep refrigerated
Estrogens Fractionated	24 hr	Nonpregnant, mid-cycle	
Estrone (E1)		2-25 μg/24 hr	
Estradiol (E2)		0-10 μg/24 hr	
Estriol (E3)		2-30 μg/24 hr	
Fat, qualitative	Random	Negative	
FIGLU (N-formiminoglutamic acid)	24 hr	<3 mg/24 hr After 15 gm of L-histidine: 4 mg/8 hr	
Fluoride	24 hr	<1 mg/24 hr	
Follicle-stimulating hormone (FSH)	24 hr	Follicular phase 5-20 IU/24 hr Mid-cycle 15-60 IU/24 hr Luteal phase 5-15 IU/24 hr Menopausal 50-100 IU/24 hr Men 5-25 IU/24 hr	
Fructose	24 hr	30-65 mg/24 hr	

TABLE A-2
Urine—cont'd

Test	Type of specimen	Normal value	Special instructions
Glucose			
Qualitative	Random	Negative	
Quantitative	24 hr	0.5-1.5 gm/24 hr	
Copper-reducing			
[illegible]		[illegible]	
[illegible]	[illegible]	[illegible]	
[illegible]	[illegible]	[illegible]	
17-Hydroxycortico-steroids	24 hr	Male: 5.5-14.5 mg/24 hr Female: 4.9-12.9 mg/24 hr Lower in children After 25 USP units ACTH, IM: a 2- to 4-fold increase	Keep refrigerated
5-Hydroxyindole-acetic acid (5-HIAA)	24 hr	2-9 mg/24 hr (women lower than men)	Some muscle relaxants and tranquilizers interfere with test
5-Hydroxyindolacetic acid, quantitative	24 hr	<9 mg/24 hr	
Indican	24 hr	10-20 mg/24 hr	
Ketone bodies	Random	Negative	Fresh, keep cool
17-Ketosteroids	24 hr	*Age* — *Males* — *Females* 10 — 1-4 mg — 1-4 mg 20 — 6-21 mg — 4-16 mg 30 — 8-26 mg — 4-14 mg 50 — 5-18 mg — 3-9 mg 70 — 2-10 mg — 1-7 mg	Keep refrigerated
Androsterone		Male: 2.0-5.0 mg/24 hr Female: 0.8-3.0 mg/24 hr	
Etiocholanolone		Male: 1.4-5.0 mg/24 hr Female: 0.8-4.0 mg/24 hr	
Dehydroepiandrosterone		Male: 0.2-2.0 mg/24 hr Female: 0.2-1.8 mg/24 hr	
11-Ketoandrosterone		Male: 0.2-1.0 mg/24 hr Female: 0.2-0.8 mg/24 hr	
11-Ketoetiocholanolone		Male: 0.2-1.0 mg/24 hr Female: 0.2-0.8 mg/24 hr	

Continued.

TABLE A-2
Urine—cont'd

Test	Type of specimen	Normal value	Special instructions
17-Ketosteroids—cont'd			
11-Hydroxyandro-sterone		Male: 0.1-0.8 mg/24 hr Female: 0.0-0.5 mg/24 hr	
11-Hydroxyetio-cholanolone		Male: 0.2-0.6 mg/24 hr Female: 0.1-1.1 mg/24 hr	
Lactose	24 hr	12-40 mg/24 hr	
Lead	24 hr	<100 μg/24 hr	
Magnesium	24 hr	6.0-8.5 mEq/24 hr	
Melanin, qualitative	Random	Negative	
3-Methoxy-4-hydroxy-mandelic acid	24 hr	1.5-7.5 mg/24 hr (adults) 83 μg/kg/24 hr (infants)	No coffee or fruit two days prior to test
Mucin	24 hr	100-150 mg/24 hr	
Myoglobin			
Qualitative	Random	Negative	
Quantitative	24 hr	<1.5 mg/L	
Osmolality	Random	500-800 mOsm/L	May be lower or higher, depend-ing on state of hydration
Pentoses	24 hr	2-5 mg/kg/24 hr	
pH	Random	4.6-8.0	
Phenolsulfonphthalein (PSP)	Urine, timed after 6 mg PSP IV		
	15 min	20-50% dye excreted	
	30 min	16-24% dye excreted	
	60 min	9-17% dye excreted	
	120 min	3-10% dye excreted	
Phenylpyruvic acid, qualitative	Random	Negative	
Phosphorus	Random	0.9-1.3 gm/24 hr	Varies with intake
Porphobilinogen			
Qualitative	Random	Negative	
Quantitative	24 hr	0-2.0 mg/24 hr	
Potassium	24 hr	40-80 mEq/24 hr	Varies with diet
Pregnancy tests	Concentrated morning specimen	Positive in normal pregnancies or with tumors producing chorionic gonadotropin	
Pregnanediol	24 hr	Male: 0-1 mg/24 hr Female: 1-8 mg/24 hr Peak: 1 week after ovulation Pregnancy: 60-100 mg/24 hr Children: Negative	Keep re-frigerated

TABLE A-2
Urine—cont'd

Test	Type of specimen	Normal value	Special instructions
Pregnanetriol	24 hr	Male: 1.0-2.0 mg/24 hr Female: 0.5-2.0 mg/24 hr Children: <0.5 mg/24 hr	Keep refrigerated
Protein			
[illegible]	[illegible]	[illegible]	
[illegible]	[illegible]	[illegible]	
[illegible]	[illegible]	[illegible]	
[illegible]	[illegible]	[illegible]	[illegible]
[illegible]	[illegible]	[illegible] gm/24 hr	
Specific gravity	Random	1.016-1.022 (normal fluid intake) 1.001-1.035 (range)	
Sugars (excluding glucose)	Random	Negative	
Titrable acidity	24 hr	20-50 mEq/24 hr	Collect with toluene
Urea nitrogen	24 hr	6-17 gm/24 hr	
Uric acid	24 hr	250-750 mg/24 hr	Varies with diet
Urobilinogen	2 hr 24 hr	0.3-1.0 Ehrlich units 0.05-2.5 mg/24 hr or 0.5-4.0 Ehrlich units/24 hr	
Uropepsin	Random 24 hr	15-45 units/hr 1500-5000 units/24 hr	
Uroporphyrins			
Qualitative	Random	Negative	
Quantitative	24 hr	10-30 μg/24 hr	
Vanillylmandelic acid (VMA)	24 hr	Up to 9 mg/24 hr	
Volume, total	24 hr	600-1600 ml/24 hr	
Zinc	24 hr	0.15-1.2 mg/24 hr	

TABLE A-3
Gastric fluid

Test	Normal value
Fasting residual volume	20-100 ml
pH	<2.0
Basal acid output (BAO)	0-6 mEq/hr
Maximal acid output (MAO) after histamine stimulation	5-40 mEq/hr
BAO/MAO ratio	<0.4

TABLE A-4
Hematology

Test	Normal value		
Blood volume	Male: 69 ml/kg Female: 65 ml/kg		
Coagulation factors			
Factor I (fibrinogen)	0.15-0.35 gm/100 ml		
Factor II (prothrombin)	60-140%		
Factor V (accelerator globulin)	60-140%		
Factor VII-X (proconvertin-Stuart)	70-130%		
Factor X (Stuart factor)	70-130%		
Factor VIII (antihemophlic globulin)	50-200%		
Factor IX (plasma thromboplastic cofactor)	60-140%		
Factor XI (plasma thromboplastic antecedent)	60-140%		
Factor XII (Hageman factor)	60-140%		
Coagulation tests			
Bleeding time (Ivy)	1-6 min		
Bleeding time (Duke)	1-3 min		
Clot retraction	½ the original mass in 2 hr		
Dilute blood clot lysis time	Clot lyses between 6 and 10 hr at 37° C		
Euglobin clot lysis time	Clot lyses between 2 and 6 hr at 37° C		
Partial thromboplastin time (PTT)	60-70 sec		
Kaolin activated	25-37 sec		
Prothombin time	12-14 sec		
Venous clotting time			
3 tubes	5-15 min		
2 tubes	5-8 min		
Whole blood clot lysis time	None in 24 hr		
Complete blood count (CBC)			
Hematocrit	Male: 40-54% Female: 38-47%		
Hemoglobin	Male: 13.5-18.0 gm/dl Female: 12.0-16.0 gm/dl		
Red cell count	Male: 4.6-6.2 $\times$ $10^6/\mu l$ Female: 4.2-5.4 $\times$ $10^6/\mu l$		
White cell count	4500-11,000/μl		
Erythrocyte indices			
Mean corpuscular volume (MCV)	82-98 cu microns (fl)		
Mean corpuscular hemoglobin (MCH)	27-31 pg		
Mean corpuscular hemoglobin concentration (MCHC)	32-36%		
Haptoglobin	100-300 mg/100 ml		
Hemoglobin A_2	1.5-3.5%		
Hemoglobin F	<2%		
Osmotic fragility			
	% Na Cl	*% Lysis (fresh)*	*% Lysis (after 24-hr incubation at 37° C)*
	0.20	97-100	95-100
	0.30	90-99	85-100
	0.35	50-95	75-100
	0.40	5-45	65-100

TABLE A-4
Hematology—cont'd

Test	Normal value		
			% Lysis (after 24-hr incubation at 37° C)
Osmotic fragility—cont'd	*% Na Cl*	*% Lysis (fresh)*	
	0.45	0-6	55-95
	[illegible]	[illegible]	[illegible]
[illegible]	[illegible]		
[illegible]	[illegible]		
Platelet aggregation	Full response to ADP, 1-epinephrine, and collagen		
Platelet factor 3	35-57 sec		
Reticulocyte count	0.5-1.5%		
	25,000-75,000 cells/μl		
Sedimentation rate (ESR) (Westergren)	Men under 50 yr: <15 mm/hr		
	Men over 50 yr: <20 mm/hr		
	Women under 50 yr: <20 mm/hr		
	Women over 50 yr: <30 mm/hr		
Viscosity	1.4-1.8 times water		
White blood cell differential (adult)		*Mean percent*	*Range of absolute counts*
Segmented neutrophils		56%	(1800-7000/μl)
Bands		3%	(0-700/μl)
Eosinophils		2.7%	(0-450/μl)
Basophils		0.3%	(0-200/μl)
Lymphocytes		34%	(1000-4800/μl)
Monocytes		4%	(0-800/μl)

TABLE A-5
Miscellaneous

Test	Specimen	Normal value
Bile, qualitative	Random stool	Negative in adults; positive in children
Carcinoembryonic antigen (CEA)	Plasma	0-2.5 ng/ml, 97% healthy nonsmokers
Chloride	Sweat	4-60 mEq/L
Clearances	Serum and timed urine	
Creatinine, endogenous		115 ± 20 ml/min
Diodrast		600-720 ml/min
Inulin		100-150 ml/min
PAH		600-750 ml/min
Diagnex blue (tubeless gastric analysis)	Urine	Free acid present
Fat	Stool, 72 hr	Total fat: <5 gm/24 hr and 10-25% of dry matter or <4% of measured fat intake in 3 days Neutral fat: 1-5% of dry matter Free fatty acids: 5-13% of dry matter Combined fatty acids: 5-15% of dry matter
Immunologic tests		
Alpha-fetoglobulin	Blood	Abnormal if present
Alpha 1 antitrypsin	Blood	200-400 mg/100 ml
Antinuclear antibodies	Blood	Positive if detected with serum diluted 1:10
Anti-DNA antibodies	Blood	<15 units/ml
Bence-Jones protein	Urine	Abnormal if present
Complement, total hemolytic	Blood	150-250 U/ml
C3	Blood	55-120 mg/100 ml
C4		20-50 mg/100 ml

TABLE A-5

[illegible]

Test	Specimen	Normal value
[illegible]	[illegible]	[illegible]
[illegible]	[illegible]	[illegible]
[illegible]		[illegible]
IgM		[illegible] mg/100 ml Range 39-290
Viscosity		1.4-1.8
Nitrogen, total	Stool, 24 hr	10% of intake or 1-2 gm/24 hr
Sodium	Sweat	10-80 mEq/L
Synovial fluid		
Glucose		Not less than 20 mg/100 ml lower than simultaneously drawn blood sugar
Mucin		Type 1 or 2
Trypsin activity	Random, fresh stool	Positive (2+ to 4+)
Thyroid ^{131}I uptake		7.5-25% in 6 hr
Urobilinogen		
Qualitative	Random stool	Positive
Quantitative	Stool, 24 hr	40-200 mg/24 hr 30-280 Ehrlich units/24 hr

TABLE A-6
Serology

Test	Normal value
Antibovine milk antibodies	Negative
Antideoxyribonuclease (ADNAase)	<1:20
Antinuclear antibodies (ANA)	<1:10
Antistreptococcal hyaluronidase (ASH)	<1:256
Antistreptolysin-O (ASO)	<160 Todd units
Australia antigen	See hepatitis-associated antigen
Brucella agglutinins	<1:80
Coccidioidomycosis antibodies	Negative
Cold agglutinins	<1:32
Complement, C′3	100-170 mg/dl
C-reactive protein (CRP)	0
Fluorescent treponemal antibodies (FTA)	Nonreactive
Hepatitis-associated antigen (HAA or HBAg)	Negative
Heterophile antibodies	<1:56
Histoplasma agglutinins	<1:8
Latex fixation	Negative
Leptospira agglutinins	Negative
Ox cell hemolysin	<1:480
Rheumatoid factor	
Sensitized sheep cell	<1:160
Latex fixation	<1:80
Bentonite particles	<1:32
Streptococcal MG agglutinins	<1:20
Thyroid antibodies	
Antithyroglobulin	<1:32
Antithyroid microsomal	<1:56
Toxoplasma antibodies	<1:4
Trichina agglutinins	0
Tularemia agglutinins	<1:80
Typhoid agglutinins	
O	<1:80
H	<1:80
VDRL	Nonreactive
Weil-Felix (Proteus OX-2, OX-K, and OX-19 agglutinins)	Four-fold rise in titer between acute and convalescent sera

TABLE A-7

[illegible]

[illegible]	[illegible]	[illegible]
[illegible]	[illegible]	
[illegible]	[illegible]	
[illegible]	[illegible]	
[illegible]	[illegible]	
[illegible]	[illegible]	
[illegible]	[illegible]	[illegible]
	[illegible]	[illegible]
[illegible]	[illegible]	
Globulins		
Qualitative (Pandy)	Negative	
Quantitative	6-16 mg/dl	
Glucose	45-75 mg/dl	
Lactic dehydrogenase (LDH)	Approximately 1/10 of serum level	
Protein		
Total CSF	15-45 mg/dl	
Ventricular fluid	8-15 mg/dl	
Protein electrophoresis		
Pre-albumin	4.1 ± 1.2%	
Albumin	62.4 ± 5.6%	
Alpha 1 globulin	5.3 ± 1.2%	
Alpha 2 globulin	8.2 ± 2.0%	
Beta globulin	12.8 ± 2.0%	
Gamma globulin	7.2 ± 1.1%	
Xanthochromia	Negative	

APPENDIX B

NORMAL VALUES FOR ECHOCARDIOGRAPHIC EXAMINATIONS*

The following tables represent normal values for echocardiographic examinations. The adult subjects were examined by Mrs. Sonia Chang between January 1971 and May 1975.

The children whose normal values are listed in Tables B-3 and B-4 were examined by Dr. Lee Konecke between January 1972 and June 1972. All children were examined in the supine position. The values are arranged by both body weight and body surface area. The grouping of the data according to age did not prove to be useful.

The graphs plot echocardiographic measurements against body surface area in a series of children. The data include those measurements in Tables B-3 and B-4 plus a group of patients studied by Goldberg, Allen, and Sahn. These graphs were taken from these authors' book, *Pediatric and Adolescent Echocardiography*. As noted the graphs vary between linear, root, and logarithmic functions.

Notes on Tables: Right ventricular dimension (RVD) is the distance between the echoes of the anterior right ventricular wall and the right side of the interventricular septum at the R wave of the electrocardiogram. The left ventricular internal dimension (LVID) is between the left side of the septum and the posterior endocardium at the R wave of the electrocardiogram. Posterior left ventricular wall thickness is the distance between the posterior left ventricular endocardium and epicardium at the R wave of the electrocardiogram. Posterior left ventricular wall amplitude is the maximum amplitude of the posterior left ventricular endocardial echo. Interventricular septal (IVS) wall thickness is the distance between the left and right septal echoes at the R wave of the electrocardiogram. Mid interventricular septal (IVS)

*Reproduced with permission from Feigenbaum, H.: Echocardiography, ed. 2, Philadelphia, 1976, Lea and Febiger.

amplitude is the systolic amplitude of motion of the left septal echo with the ultrasonic beam traversing the mid portion of the left ventricle. Apical interventricular septal (IVS) amplitude is the systolic amplitude of motion of the left septal echo with the ultrasonic beam directed toward the apex in the vicinity of the papillary muscles. Left atrial dimension is the distance between the posterior surface of the posterior aortic wall echo and the anterior surface of the posterior left atrial wall echo at the level of the aortic valve at end- [illegible]

TABLE B-1

Adult normal values

	Range (cm)	Mean (cm)	Number of subjects
Age (years)	13 -54	26	134
Body surface area (M^2)	1.45- 2.22	1.8	130
RVD-flat	0.7 - 2.3	1.5	84
RVD-left lateral	0.9 - 2.6	1.7	83
LVID-flat	3.7 - 5.6	4.7	82
LVID-left lateral	3.5 - 5.7	4.7	81
Post. LV wall thickness	0.6 - 1.1	0.9	137
Post. LV wall amplitude	0.9 - 1.4	1.2	48
IVS wall thickness	0.6 - 1.1	0.9	137
Mid IVS amplitude	0.3 - 0.8	0.5	10
Apical IVS amplitude	0.5 - 1.2	0.7	38
Left atrial dimension	1.9 - 4.0	2.9	133
Aortic root dimension	2.0 - 3.7	2.7	121
Aortic cusps' separation	1.5 - 2.6	1.9	93
Mean rate of circumferential shortening (Vcf)	1.02- 1.94 circ/sec	1.3 circ/sec	38

TABLE B-2

Adult normal values, corrected for body surface area

	Range (cm)	Mean (cm)	Number of subjects
RVD/M^2—flat	0.4-1.4	0.9	76
RVD/M^2—left lateral	0.4-1.4	0.9	79
LVID/M^2—flat	2.1-3.2	2.6	77
LVID/M^2—left lateral	1.9-3.2	2.6	81
LAD/M^2	1.2-2.2	1.6	127
Aortic root/M^2	1.2-2.2	1.5	115

TABLE B-3
Normal values for children arranged by weight

	Weight (lbs)	Mean (cm)	Range (cm)	Number of subjects
RVD	0- 25	.9	.3-1.5	26
	26- 50	1.0	.4-1.5	26
	51- 75	1.1	.7-1.8	20
	76-100	1.2	.7-1.6	15
	101-125	1.3	.8-1.7	11
	126-200	1.3	1.2-1.7	5
LVID	0- 25	2.4	1.3-3-2	26
	26- 50	3.4	2.4-3.8	26
	51- 75	3.8	3.3-4.5	20
	76-100	4.1	3.5-4.7	15
	101-125	4.3	3.7-4.9	11
	126-200	4.9	4.4-5-2	5
LV and IV septal wall thickness	0- 25	.5	.4- .6	26
	26- 50	.6	.5- .7	26
	51- 75	.7	.6- .7	20
	76-100	.7	.7- .8	15
	101-125	.7	.7- .8	11
	126-200	.8	.7- .8	5
LA dimension	0- 25	1.7	.7-2.3	26
	26- 50	2.2	1.7-2.7	26
	51- 75	2.3	1.9-2.8	20
	76-100	2.4	2.0-3.0	15
	101-125	2.7	2.1-3.0	11
	126-200	2.8	2.1-3.7	5
Aortic root	0- 25	1.3	.7-1.7	26
	26- 50	1.7	1.3-2.2	26
	51- 75	2.0	1.7-2.3	20
	76-100	2.2	1.9-2.7	15
	101-125	2.3	1.7-2.7	11
	126-200	2.4	2.2-2.8	5
Aortic valve opening	0- 25	.9	.5-1.2	26
	26- 50	1.2	.9-1.6	26
	51- 75	1.4	1.2-1.7	20
	76-100	1.6	1.3-1.9	15
	101-125	1.7	1.4-2.0	11
	126-200	1.8	1.6-2.0	5

TABLE B-4

Normal values for children arranged by body surface area

	1.1 to 1.5	[illegible]	[illegible]	29
	over 1.5	4.7	4.2-5.2	11
LV and IV septal wall thickness	.5 or less	.5	.4- .6	24
	.6 to 1.0	.6	.5- .7	39
	1.1 to 1.5	.7	.6- .8	29
	over 1.5	.8	.7- .8	11
LA dimension	.5 or less	1.7	.7-2.4	24
	.6 to 1.0	2.1	1.8-2.8	39
	1.1 to 1.5	2.4	2.0-3.0	29
	over 1.5	2.8	2.1-3.7	11
Aortic root	.5 or less	1.2	.7-1.5	24
	.6 to 1.0	1.8	1.4-2.2	39
	1.1 to 1.5	2.2	1.7-2.7	29
	over 1.5	2.4	2.0-2.8	11
Aortic valve opening	.5 or less	.8	.5-1.0	24
	.6 to 1.0	1.3	.9-1.6	39
	1.1 to 1.5	1.6	1.3-1.9	29
	over 1.5	1.8	1.5-2.0	11

APPENDIX C

NORMAL VALUES FOR CARDIAC CATHETERIZATION

TABLE C-1
Normal values for pressures (at rest) in the cardiac chambers and vessels (mm Hg)

Location	Mean	Range
Right atrium		
Mean	2.8	1-5
a wave	5.6	2.5-7
z point	2.9	1-5.5
c wave	3.8	1.5-6
x' wave	1.7	0-5
v wave	4.6	2-7.5
y wave	2.4	0-6
Right ventricle		
Peak systolic	25	17-32
End-diastolic	4	1-7
Pulmonary artery		
Mean	15	9-19
Peak systolic	25	17-32
End-diastolic	9	4-13
Pulmonary artery wedge		
Mean	9	4-13
Left atrium		
Mean	7.9	2-12
a wave	10.4	4-16
z point	7.6	1-13
v wave	12.8	6-21
Left ventricle		
Peak systolic	130	90-140
End-diastolic	8.7	5-12
Brachial artery		
Mean	85	70-105
Peak systolic	130	90-140
End-diastolic	70	60-90

[illegible]

Measurements	Units	[illegible]
O_2 uptake	143 ml/min/m^2	14.3
Arteriovenous O_2 difference	4.1 vol percent	0.6
Cardiac index	3.5 L/min/m^2	0.7
Stroke index	46 ml/beat/m^2	8.1

TABLE C-3
Oxygen content and saturation

Location	O_2 content (vol %)	O_2 saturation
Superior vena cava (SVC)	14 (±1)	70%
Inferior vena cava (IVC)	16 (±1)	80%
Right atrium (RA)	15 (±1)	75%
Pulmonary artery (PA)	15.2 (±1)	75%
Right ventricle (RV)	15.2 (±1)	75%
Brachial artery (BA)	19.0 (±1)	95%

TABLE C-4

Other measurements obtained during cardiac catheterization

$$\text{Pulmonary arteriolar resistance} = \frac{\text{Mean PA pressure} - \text{Mean PAW pressure (mm Hg)}}{\text{Pulmonary blood flow (L/min)}}$$

where: PA = Pulmonary artery

PAW = Pulmonary artery wedge

Normal values for PAR = Less than 2.0 resistance units (less than 160 dynes sec cm^{-5})

$$\text{Total pulmonary resistance (TPR)} = \frac{\text{Mean PA pressure} - \text{LV mean diastolic pressure (mm Hg)}}{\text{Pulmonary blood flow (L/min)}}$$

where: PA = Pulmonary artery

LV = Left ventricle

Normal values for TPR = Less than 3.5 resistance units (less than 280 dynes see cm^{-5})

$$\text{Mitral valve area, cm}^2 = \frac{\text{Mitral valve flow (ml/sec)}}{31\sqrt{\text{Diastolic gradient across the mitral valve}}}$$

where: $$\text{Mitral valve flow} = \frac{\text{Cardiac output (ml/min)}}{\text{Diastolic filling period (sec/min)}}$$

Diastolic filling period (sec/min) = Diastolic period per beat (sec/beat) × Heart rate (beats/min)

Diastolic gradient across the mitral valve (mm Hg) = Left atrial mean pressure (mm Hg) − Left ventricular mean diastolic pressure (mm Hg)

31 = Empirical constant

$$\text{Aortic valve area, cm}^2 = \frac{\text{Aortic valve flow (ml/sec)}}{44.5\sqrt{\text{Systolic pressure gradient across the aortic valve}}}$$

where: $$\text{Aortic valve flow (ml/sec)} = \frac{\text{Cardiac output (ml/min)}}{\text{Systolic ejection period (sec/min)}}$$

Systolic ejection period (sec/min) = Systolic ejection period per beat (sec/beat) × Heart rate (beats/min)

Systolic pressure gradient across the aortic valve (mm Hg) = Left ventricular mean systolid pressure (mm Hg) − Aortic mean systolic pressure (mm Hg)

44.5 = Gravity acceleration factor

$$\text{Cardiac output (L/min)} = \frac{I}{Ct} \times 60$$

where: I = Amount of indicator injected

C = Mean concentration of indicator for the first circulation (mg/L)

t = Time for the first circulation of indicator (seconds)

$$\text{Cardiac output (ml/min)} = \frac{\text{Oxygen consumption (ml/mm)}}{\underset{\text{(vol \%)}}{\text{Arterial } O_2 \text{ content}} - \underset{\text{(vol \%)}}{\text{Mixed venous } O_2 \text{ content}}} \times 100$$

APPENDIX D

COMMON DRUGS AFFECTING CLINICAL LABORATORY TESTS*

TABLE D-1

Drugs affecting thyroid function tests

Drug	Free thyroxine index	^{131}I uptake	T_3 uptake	T_4 (Murphy-Pattee)
Ampicillin		−		
Aspirin	−†	−	+	−
Barium		−		
Bromides		−		
Cascara		−		
Chlordiazepoxide		−	−	
Corticosteroids	−	−	+	
Coumarin			+	
Dicumarol			+	
Digitalis		−		
Digitoxin		−		
Heparin			+	−
Levodopa				+
Oral contraceptives	+		−	−
Penicillin		−	+	−
Pentobarbital		−		
Phenylbutazone	−	−	+	
Phenytoin sodium	−		+	+
Pregnancy			−	−
Propylthiouracil		−	−	−
Quinidine		−		
Secobarbital		−		
Sulfonamides		−	+	
Thiazides			−	
Thyroid		−	+	

*Sources for the material in these tables are as follows:

Davies, D. M., editor: Textbook of adverse drug reactions, New York, 1977, Oxford University Press.

Wallach, J.: Interpretation of diagnostic tests, ed. 3, Boston, 1978, Little, Brown and Co.

Young, D. S., Pestaner, L. C., and Gibberman, V.: Effects of drugs on clinical laboratory tests, Clin. Chem. **21**(5):240D-399D, 1975.

† +, increased value; −, decreased value; blank, no effect.

DRUGS AFFECTING PROTHROMBIN TIME

Drugs such as salicylates, phenylbutazone, oxyphenbutazone, indomethacin, and some sulfonamides, can displace the anticoagulants from the plasma protein to which they are bound. This will make more anticoagulants available, thus increasing the prothrombin time.

Other drugs, such as barbiturates, griseofulvin, and glutethimide, induce the formation of enzymes by the liver that metabolize coumarin and phenindione derivatives, thus decreasing the prothrombin time. If any of these drugs is withdrawn from a patient who has been stabilized on an anticoagulant plus the drug, a critical fall in prothrombin level may result.

Additionally, vitamin K may be suppressed by broad-spectrum antibiotics and some oral sulfonamides that change the intestinal flora and inhibit the microorganisms responsible for vitamin K production, thus increasing the prothrombin time. By the same token, the patient who is taking vitamin K or daily mineral oil (which enhances vitamin K absorption) may have his prothrombin time decreased.

The commonly used drugs affecting prothrombin time are listed in Table D-2.

TABLE D-2
Most common drugs affecting prothrombin time

Increased time	Comment	Decreased time	Comment
Acenocoumarol		Anabolic steroids	
Acetaminophen		Antacids	May shorten anticoagulant action
Allopurinol	Patients on coumarin	Antihistamines	Anticoagulant metabolism accelerated
Aminosalicylic acid	Suppresses prothrombin formation	Ascorbic acid	Anticoagulant action may shorten
Anabolic steroids		Aspirin	In small doses
Aspirin	In large doses	Barbiturates	Patients on coumarin
Cathartics		Chloral hydrate	Patients on coumarin
Chloral hydrate	Displaces anticoagulants from albumin	Colchicine	Patients on coumarin
Chloramphenicol	May lower prothrombin	Corticosteroids	Anticoagulant metabolism accelerated
Chlorthalidone	Patients on coumarin	Cortisone	Patients on coumarin
Clofibrate		Diuretics	Patients on anticoagulant
Diazoxide	Displaces anticoagulants from albumin	Ethchlorvynol	Patients on coumarin

TABLE D-2
Most common drugs affecting prothrombin time—cont'd

Increased time	Comment	Decreased time	Comment
Dicumarol		Glutethimide	Patients on coumarin
Disulfiram	Patients on coumarin	Griseofulvin	
Diuretics	May prolong action of anticoagulants	Heptabarbital	Anticoagulants metabolized [illegible]
[illegible]		[illegible]	
[illegible]	[illegible]	[illegible]	
[illegible]	[illegible]	[illegible]	[illegible]
[illegible]		[illegible]	[illegible]
[illegible]		[illegible]	
[illegible]	[illegible] proteins		
Mefenamic acid	Displaces coumarin from albumin		
Mercaptopurinne			
Methyldopa			
Methylphenidate	Inhibits metabolism of coumarin		
Monoamine oxidase (MAO) inhibitors			
Nalidixic acid	Displaces coumarin from albumin		
Neomycin			
Oxyphenbutazone	Displaces anticoagulants from albumin		
Phenylbutazone			
Phenyramidol			
Propylthiouracil			
Quinidine			
Quinine			
Streptomycin	May decrease vitamin K synthesis		
Sulfinpyrazone			
Sulfonamides			
Thyroid			
Tolbutamide			

TABLE D-3
Drugs affecting urinalysis

Test	Increased value	Decreased value
Creatine	Caffeine Methyltestosterone PSP	Anabolic steroids Androgens Thiazides
Creatinine	Ascorbic acid* Corticosteroids Levodopa* Methyldopa* Nitrofurans* PSP*	Anabolic steroids Androgens Thiazides
Diagnex blue excretion	Aluminum salts Barium salts Calcium salts Iron salts Kaolin Magnesium salts Methylene blue* Nicotinic acid Quinacrine* Quinidine* Quinine* Riboflavin* Sodium salts* Vitamin B*	Caffeine benzoate
Glucose	Aminosalicylic acid Aspirin Corticosteroids Ephedrine Furosemide Phenytoin sodium	With glucose-oxidase method Ascorbic acid* Aspirin* Levodopa* Mercurial diuretics* Tetracycline*
Hematuria or hemoglobinuria	Acetanilid Acetophenetidin Acetylsalicylic acid Amphotericin B Bacitracin Coumarin Indomethacin Phenylbutazone	
17-Hydroxycorticosteroids	Acetazolamide Chloral hydrate Chlordiazepoxide Chlorpromazine Colchicine Erythromycin Etryptamine Meprobamate Oleandomycin Paraldehyde Quinidine Quinine Spironolactone	Estrogens Oral contraceptives Phenothiazines Reserpine

*Method-affected.

TABLE D-3
Drugs affecting urinalysis—cont'd

Test	Increased value	Decreased value
17-Ketosteroids	Chloramphenicol	Chlordiazepoxide
	Chlorpromazine	Estrogens
	Cloxacillin	Meprobamate
	Dexamethasone	Metyrapone
	[illegible]	[illegible]
	[illegible]	[illegible]
	[illegible]	[illegible]
	[illegible]	
	[illegible]	
	[illegible]	
	[illegible]	
	[illegible]	
	[illegible]	
	[illegible]	
	[illegible]	
	Spironolactone	
pH	Aldosterone	
	Parathyroid extract	
	Prolactin	
	Sodium bicarbonate	
Porphyrins (fluorometric method)	Acriflavine	
	Ethoxazene	
	Phenazopyridine	
	Sulfamethoxazole	
	Tetracycline	
	Antipyretics	
	Barbiturates	
	Phenylhydrazine	
	Sulfonamides	
Pregnancy test (DAP test)	False positive	False negative
	Chlorpromazine (frog, rabbit; immunologic)	Promethazine
	Phenothiazines (frog, rabbit; immunologic)	
	Promethazine (Gravindex)	
Protein	Drugs causing nephrotoxicity such as:	
	Aminosalicylic acid	
	Ampicillin	
	Aspirin	
	Bacitracin	
	Cephaloridine	
	Corticosteroids	
	Insecticides	
	Mercurial diuretics	
	Neomycin	
	Penicillin (large doses)	
	Phenylbutazone	

Continued.

Table D-3
Drugs affecting urinalysis—cont'd

Test	Increased value	Decreased value
Protein—cont'd	Radiographic agents (postaortography)	
	Streptomycin	
	Sulfonamides	
	Turbidimetric procedures* (false positive)	
	Aminosalicylic acid	
	Cephaloridine	
	Chlorpromazine	
	Promazine	
	Penicillin (lg doses)	
	Sulfisoxazole	
	Thymol	
Specific gravity	Dextran*	
	(Diurnal variation)	
	Radiographic agents	
	Sucrose*	
Vanillylmandelic acid (VMA)	Aminosalicylic acid*	Clofibrate*
	Aspirin*	Guanethidine analogs
	Bromsulphaleine (BSP)	Imipramine
	Glyceryl guaiacolate*	Methyldopa
	Mephenesin*	Monoamine oxidase (MAO) inhibitor
	Nalidixic acid*	
	Oxytetracycline*	
	Penicillin*	
	Phenazopyridine*	
	PSP*	
	Sulfa drugs*	

*Method-affected.

TABLE D-4
Drugs affecting blood tests

Test	Increased value	Decreased value
Amylase	Cholinergics	
	Codeine	
	Ethanol	
	Meperidine	
	Methacholine	
	[illegible]	
	[illegible]	
	[illegible]	
	[illegible]	
[illegible]	[illegible]	[illegible]
	[illegible]	[illegible]
	[illegible]	[illegible]
	[illegible]	[illegible]
	[illegible]	[illegible]
	[illegible]	
	Morphine	
	Oral contraceptives	
	Penicillin	
	Phenylbutazone	
	Primaquine	
	Procainamide	
	Quinidine	
	Quinine	
	Radiographic agents	
	Rifampin	
	Streptomycin	
	Sulfa drugs	
	Tetracycline	
	Thiazides	
Calcium	Anabolic steroids	Corticosteroids
	Antacids (Ca containing)	Diuretics (mercurial)
	Calcium gluconate (newborns)	Gastrin
	Estrogens	Insulin
	Hydralazine	Laxatives (excess)
	Oral contraceptives	Mestranol
	Secretin	Oral contraceptives
	Thiazides	Phenytoin sodium (chronic use)
		Sulfates
Chloride	Chlorothiazide (prolonged therapy)	Aldosterone
	Corticosteroids	Bicarbonates
	Guanethidine	Corticosteroids
	Marijuana	Corticotropin
	Phenylbutazone	Cortisone
		Diuretics
		Laxatives (chronic abuse)
		Prednisolone

Continued.

TABLE D-4
Drugs affecting blood tests—cont'd

Test	Increased value	Decreased value
Cholesterol	Anabolic steroids	Allopurinol
	Cinchophen	Azathioprine
	Cortisone	Clofibrate
	Epinephrine	Clomiphene
	Heparin (after cessation)	Corticotropin
	Oral contraceptives	Erythromycin
	Phenytoin sodium	Garlic
	(Pregnancy)	Isoniazid
	Promazine	Kanamycin
	Sulfadiazine	MAO inhibitors
	Sulfonamides	Neomycin
	Thiazides	Tetracycline
	Thiouracil	Thiouracil
CO_2 Content	Aldosterone	Acetazolamide
	Bicarbonates	Dimercaprol
	Ethacrynic acid	Dimethadione
	Hydrocortisone	Methicillin
	Laxatives (chronic abuse)	Nitrofurantoin
	Metolazone	Phenformin
	Prednisone	Tetracycline
	Thiazides	Triamterene
	Tromethamine	
	Viomycin	
Coombs' test	Positive	
	Chlorpromazine	
	Chlorpropamide	
	Dipyrone	
	Ethosuximide	
	Hydralazine	
	Isoniazid	
	Levodopa	
	Mefenamic acid	
	Melphalan	
	Oxyphenisatin	
	Phenylbutazone	
	Phenytoin sodium	
	Procainamide	
	Quinidine	
	Quinine	
	Streptomycin	
	Sulfonamides	
	Tetracycline	
Creatinine	Drugs causing nephrotoxicity such as:	
	Amphotericin B	
	Capreomycin	
	Carbutamide	
	Cephaloridine	
	Chlorthalidone	
	Clofibrate	
	Clonidine	

TABLE D-4
Drugs affecting blood tests—cont'd

Test	Increased value	Decreased value
Creatinine—cont'd	Colistimethate	
	Colistin	
	Doxycycline	
Erythrocyte sedimentation rate	Dextrans	Quinine
	Methyldopa	Salicylates
[illegible]	[illegible]	[illegible]
	[illegible]	
	[illegible]	
	[illegible]	
	[illegible]	
[illegible]	[illegible]	[illegible]
	[illegible]	[illegible]
	[illegible]	[illegible]
	[illegible]	[illegible]
	[illegible]	[illegible]
	Coffee	Sulfaphenazole
	Corticosteroids	Sulfonamides
	Cortisone	Sulfonylureas
	Dopamine	
	Ephedrine	
	Epinephrine	
	Estrogens	
	Ethacrynic acid	
	Furosemide	
	Hydralazine	
	Levodopa	
	Phenylbutazone	
	Phenytoin	
	Prednisolone	
	Reserpine	
	Secretin	
	Thiazides	
	Thyroid	
Lactic dehydrogenase (LDH)	Anesthetic agents	
	Codeine	
	Dicumarol	
	Morphine	
	(Muscular exercise)	
Leucine aminopeptidase	Estrogens	
	Morphine	
	Oral contraceptives	
	(Pregnancy)	
	Thorium dioxide	
Lipase	Cholinergics	Protamine
	Codeine	Saline (at molar concentrations)
	Heparine (10 min post-injection)	
	Meperidine	
	Methacholine	
	Morphine	
	Narcotics	

Continued.

TABLE D-4
Drugs affecting blood tests—cont'd

Test	Increased value	Decreased value
Phosphate	Anabolic steroids Methicillin Phosphates Phospho-Soda	Alkaline antacids Anticonvulsants Calcitonin Epinephrine Insulin (Menstruation) Oral contraceptives Phenobarbital
Potassium	Amphotericin B Epinephrine Heparin Histamine (IV) Marijuana Methicillin Spironolactone Tetracycline	Aldosterone Amphotericin B Aspirin Bicarbonates Corticosteroids Cortisone Diuretics Ethacrynic acid Furosemide Gentamicin Insulin Licorice Polythiazide Sodium bicarbonate Thiazides
Protein	Anabolic steroids Androgens Corticosteroids Corticotropin Digitalis Epinephrine Insulin Oral contraceptives (at 3 months cessation after 3 years administration) Thyroid	Estrogens Oral contraceptives
SGOT/SGPT	Ascorbic acid Cholinergics Codeine Guanethidine Hydralazine Isoniazid Meperidine Morphine Tolbutamide	
Sodium	Anabolic steroids Bicarbonate Clonidine Corticosteroids Cortisone Estrogens	Ammonium chloride Cathartics (excessive) Chlorpropamide Ethacrynic acid Furosemide Mannitol

TABLE D-4
Drugs affecting blood tests—cont'd

Test	Increased value	Decreased value
Sodium—cont'd	Guanethidine	Metolazone
	Marijuana	Spironolactone
	Methoxyflurane	Thiazides
	Oral contraceptives	Triamterene
	Phenvlbutazone	
	[illegible]	
	[illegible]	
[illegible]	[illegible]	[illegible]
	[illegible]	[illegible]
	[illegible]	[illegible]
		[illegible]
		[illegible]
[illegible]	[illegible]	[illegible]
	[illegible]	[illegible]
	[illegible]	[illegible]
	Anabolic steroids	(Pregnancy)
	Androgens	
	Arginine	
	Bacitracin	
	Calcium salts	
	Clonidine	
	Dextran	
	Guanethidine	
	Licorice	
	Marijuana	
	Mephenesin	
	Methoxyflurane	
	Methsuximide	
	Metolazone	
	Minocycline	
Uric acid	Acetazolamide	Allopurinol
	Aspirin	Chlorpromazine
	Ethacrynic acid	Cinchophen
	Furosemide	Clofibrate
	Hydralazine	Corticosteroids
	Propylthiouracil	Corticotropin
	Thiazides	Cortisone
		Coumarin
		Dicumarol
		Phenylbutazone
		Probenecid
		Radiographic agents

REFERENCES

Anthony, C. P., and Thibodeau, G. A.: Textbook of anatomy and physiology, ed. 10, St. Louis, 1979, The C. V. Mosby Co.

Davidsohn, I., and Henry, J. B., editors: Todd-Sanford Clinical diagnosis by laboratory methods, ed. 15, Philadelphia, 1974, W. B. Saunders Co.

Feigenbaum, H.: Echocardiography, ed. 2, Philadelphia, 1976, Lea & Febiger.

Felson, B.: Fundamentals of chest roentgenology, Philadelphia, 1973, W. B. Saunders Co.

Frankel, S., Reitman, S., Sonnenwirth, A. C., editors: Gradwohl's Clinical laboratory methods and diagnosis; a textbook on laboratory procedures and their interpretation, vols. I and II, ed. 7, St. Louis, 1970, The C. V. Mosby Co.

Halsted, J. A., editor: The laboratory in clinical medicine; interpretation and application, Philadelphia, 1976, W. B. Saunders Co.

Harper, H. A.: Review of physiological chemistry, ed. 16, Los Altos, Calif., 1977, Lange Medical Publications.

Hurst, J. W., editor: The heart, ed. 4, New York, 1978, McGraw-Hill Book Co.

Mendel, D.: Practice of cardiac catheterization, ed. 2, Oxford, 1974, Blackwell Scientific Publications.

Ravel, R.: Clinical laboratory medicine: application of laboratory data, ed. 2, Chicago, 1973, Year Book Medical Publishers.

Schottelius, B. A., and Schottelius, D. D.: Textbook of physiology, ed. 18, St. Louis, 1978, The C. V. Mosby Co.

Schwartz, A. R., and Lyons, H.: Acid base and electrolyte balance; normal regulation and clinical disorder, New York, 1977, Grune & Stratton, Inc.

Scully, R. E., editor: Case records of the Massachusetts General Hospital, N. Engl. J. Med. **298**:34, Jan. 5, 1978.

Skydell, B., and Crowder, A. S.: Diagnostic procedures; a reference for health practitioners and a guide for patient counseling, Boston, 1975, Little, Brown and Co.

Slisenger, M. H., and Fordtran, J. S.: Gastrointestinal disease, pathophysiology, diagnosis, management, Philadelphia, 1973, W. B. Saunders Co.

Stollerman, G. H., editor: Advances in internal medicine, vols. 18 and 19, Chicago, 1972, Year Book Medical Publishers.

Tavell, M. E.: Clinical phonocardiography and external pulse recording, ed. 2, Chicago, 1972, Year Book Medical Publishers.

Thorn, G. W., and others, editors: Harrison's Principles of internal medicine, ed. 7, New York, 1977, McGraw-Hill Book Co.

Weisler, A. M.: Noninvasive cardiology, New York, 1974, Grune & Stratton, Inc.

INDEX

C

D

E

H

M

N

O

R

T

U